HEALTH IN AMERICA

A Multicultural Perspective

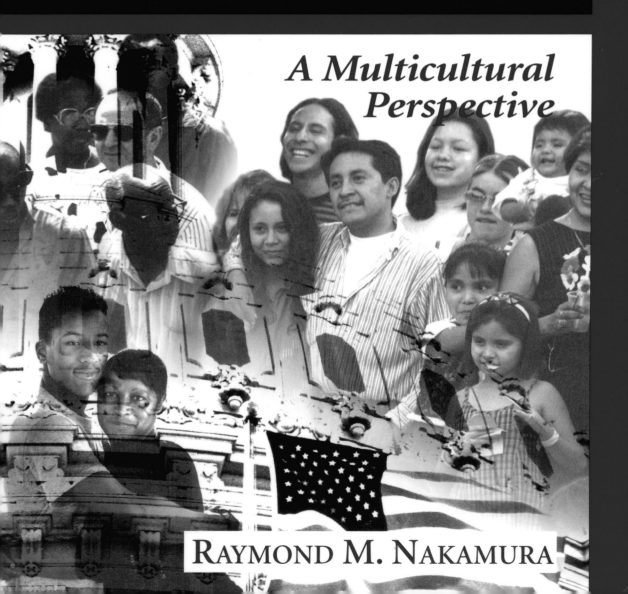

RAYMOND M. NAKAMURA

Health in America

A Multicultural Perspective

Raymond M. Nakamura

California Polytechnic State University

Allyn and Bacon

Boston ■ London ■ Toronto ■ Sydney ■ Tokyo ■ Singapore

Vice President, Editor in Chief: *Paul A. Smith*
Publisher: *Joseph E. Burns*
Editorial Assistant: *Sara Sherlock*
Marketing Manager: *Rick Muhr*
Editorial Production Service: *Chestnut Hill Enterprises*
Manufacturing Buyer: *David Repetto*
Cover Administrator: *Jennifer Hart*

Internet: www.abacon.com

Between the time Website information is gathered and published, some sites may have closed. Also, the transcription of URLs can result in unintended typographical errors. The publisher would appreciated notification where these occur so that they may be corrected in subsequent editions. Thank you.

Library of Congress Cataloging-in-Publication Data

Nakamura, Raymond M.
    Health in America : a multicultural perspective / by Raymond M.
Nakamura.
       p.   cm.
    Includes bibliographical references and index.
    ISBN 0-205-29012-4
    1. Minorities—Health and hygiene—United States.   2. Minorities—
Mental health—United States.   3. Health behavior—United States.
I. Title.
RA448.4.N35   1998
614.4'273'089—dc21   98-26179
                                       CIP

Printed in the United States of America

10 9 8 7 6 5 4 3 2 1   03 02 01 00 99 98

To my wife Connie, who is precious beyond all things—

To my children Kyle and Lindy, who bring me joy—

To my mother Mitsuko, my father Robert,
and my brothers Frank and William, whose consistent love, loyalty,
and support have always been an important part of my life—

Thanks!

I love all of you!

CONTENTS

PREFACE

The purpose of *Health in America: A Multicultural Perspective* is to discuss the health issues and problems that ethnic minority populations face in the United States. Specifically, the health problems of African Americans, Native Americans, Hispanic Americans, and Asian and Pacific Islander Americans are discussed. Ethnic minority Americans make up the fastest growing populations in the United States today. This growth affords all of us the opportunity to make significant personal contributions to the social growth of this nation. It presents challenges as well. One of the most significant challenges ahead is in the delivery of a health care system for all people regardless of age, race, gender, and socioeconomic status.

Ethnic minority Americans, in particular, face a health care system that does not always respond to their needs as individuals or as a community. The plight of certain groups of minority Americans is particularly troubling because they experience a disproportionate burden of poverty, sickness, and early death. These health discrepancies are not only due to unhealthy behaviors but are often a result of social, economic, and political factors. The disproportionate number of health problems faced by minority Americans has often gone unnoticed. In this book I hope to bring into focus (1) the many health problems faced by ethnic minority Americans, (2) an evaluation of what is known and what is not known about the health problems that ethnic minority Americans face, and (3) the need for a reevaluation and reorganization of the health care system to meet the needs of all Americans.

This book is divided into 10 chapters that address the context and health status concerning ethnic minority Americans.

Chapter 1 investigates the dimensions of wellness and, in particular, the cultural differences in rates of morbidity and mortality, differential access to health care, and discussion of the reasons for these differences.

Chapter 2 investigates the traditional healing theories of various cultures and presents a general overview of the lay theories of illness causation. It is important for Western medical practitioners to recognize these traditional practices and understand how they fit into the lives of the believers.

Chapter 3 explores the family and its importance in the health of its members. Particular attention is paid to the family unit, children, traditional gender roles, the care of the elderly, and, finally, death and the grieving process.

Chapter 4 discusses stress and stress factors that are common to ethnic minority Americans, such as discrimination, cultural conflict, immigration, economic oppression, violence, homicide, and gangs. Also included is a section on the mental-health-seeking behavior of ethnic minority Americans and their strategies for coping with stress.

Chapter 5 includes expanded coverage of two personality theories (humanistic and behavioral) and how they apply to the mental health of ethnic minority Americans. Also discussed are the issues of somatization and the expression of depression and suicidal behavior of minority Americans.

Chapter 6 begins with a brief discussion of the Food Guide Pyramid and how the different diets of various cultures also meet the nutritional guidelines of the Food Guide Pyramid. The chapter concludes with a discussion of obesity, anorexia, and bulimia in different minority populations.

Chapter 7 explores the data on the usage patterns of drugs in ethnic minority populations, with special attention to drug-taking behavior in the female population. Special emphasis is placed on tobacco and alcohol. The chapter concludes with recommendations for prevention and treatment of drug abuse in ethnic minority populations.

Chapter 8 explores the data and prevalence of major chronic diseases and disorders, such as heart disease, hypertension, cancer, and diabetes in ethnic minority populations. The chapter concludes with a discussion of some of the hereditary diseases that are unique to minority populations.

Chapter 9 looks at the data and prevalence of the major sexually transmitted infections, tuberculosis, and intestinal infections that are common among ethnic minority populations. The chapter concludes with a discussion of childhood diseases and immunization recommendations.

Chapter 10, the final chapter, explores gender-specific diseases. A special emphasis is placed on women's health problems, both within and outside of the selected ethnic minority populations. Also included is a discussion on fertility control. The chapter concludes with a discussion of men's health problems.

I hope that in the end I have helped you recognize the need for a health care delivery system for all Americans regardless of race, gender, or socioeconomic status.

Acknowledgments

Health in America: A Multicultural Perspective was written and published with the help and assistance of numerous people. I am extremely grateful to be working with the outstanding team at Allyn and Bacon. I wish to acknowledge two senior editors that I had the pleasure to work with. Suzy Spivey who had the vision and confidence in the importance of this book and Joe Burns, whose commitment, high standards of professionalism, and personal attention made it all possible. My personal thanks to both of you. I am grateful to the many people in the production end of this project, in particular, Marjorie Payne and Myrna Breskin for overseeing the development and editing of this book.

I also wish to acknowledge the contributions of the following reviewers whose honest and thoughtful opinions and suggestions are incorporated in every chapter: Richard St. Pierre, Pennsylvania State University; Kathleen Zavela, University of North Carolina; Lee Green, University of Alabama; and Meri Jayne Basti, Cuesta College. A note of special thanks must also be give to Everardo Martinez-Inunza for his generosity in supplying many of the photographs used throughout this book.

A FEW NOTES TO THE READER

A Note on Terminology

It is important that we are sensitive to the names we use for ethnic groups. As the multicultural and intercultural terminology is debated, no single term is deemed acceptable or "politically correct" because it implies that all other terms are disrespectful.

There is much variability in the terminology used in the area of intracultural and intercultural education. The media, professional disciplines, and regions use a variety of terms that influence which ones people use. In addition, there continues to be great discrepancy within and outside of each individual culture. For example, many African Americans still refer to themselves as *blacks* and individuals from various Native American tribes refer to themselves as *Indians*.

Yet, clarification of terminology is important. It is also important that the reader not get stuck on a word or phrase. The terms used in this book are chosen because they are widespread, widely known, and comfortable to the author. The author asks the reader to look beyond the differences in terminology and to view this book in the context of the larger picture. Levels of acceptability with any particular terminology have changed and will change over time. However, feelings of utmost respect for the cultures and people discussed in this book is the primary motivation for writing it.

A Note on Research

Problems of measurement and definition are prominent among the challenges facing researchers who conduct studies on the health problems of the diverse groups in the United States. Presently, the health research on each of the different ethnic groups is limited. There is a relative absence of adequate research. Data are usually drawn from national surveys in which minority groups are underrepresented and often "overlooked" or simply listed as "other." National surveys often ignore the significant differences between and within ethnic and racial groups. As a result, national surveys reflect averages and rates for a category of people, for instance, the death rate for all Asian/Pacific Americans or Hispanic Americans and not, specifically, Japanese Americans or Cuban Americans. It is not enough to say that a person is an Asian or Hispanic American. There are distinct cultural differences that influence health care and prevention. The distinction is critical to the development of appropriate treatment, behavioral change programs, and intervention programs. The failure in the research to make distinctions among specific and cultural groups can lead to faulty conclusions about important health needs among the various ethnic and racial groups. The necessity of examining the health issues of specific groups within groups is imperative in future research.

Because research on both ethnic groups and subgroups within a culture is limited, the information that is available is speculative. It often represents untested theoretical extrapolation from the larger culture. Therefore, the standard "skills" necessary for the development of personal health for some individuals may not always be available, nor can they always be applied. Consequently, thoughtful reflection will be necessary as a substitute for firm data.

1 Health and Wellness: A Multicultural Perspective

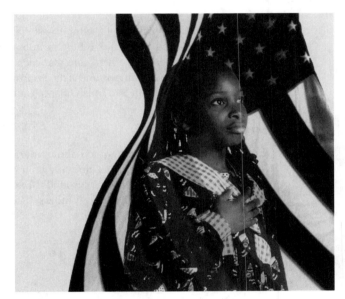

Culture is the first requisite and the final objective of all development.

—Leopold Senghor
and Frantz Fanon

Photo by Chris Cunningham, published in *Cultures* magazine, volume 1, issue 2.

Health and Wellness

The World Health Organization (World Health Organization, 1947) has the most widely recognized definition of *health*. It defines *health* as "a state of complete physical, mental, and social well-being and not merely the absence of disease and infirmity." This definition reveals that health is multifaceted and includes many components beyond just freedom from physical disease and pain. Historically, the definition evolved from a limited perspective that focused on hygiene and sanitation and the prevention of disease to a more contemporary perspective that places greater emphasis on the social, spiritual, emotional, physical, and intellectual actions that lead to good or poor health.

A health-related term that evolved during the 1990s is *wellness*. Wellness is an evolving process in which individuals develop and enhance all aspects of their physical, social, spiritual, emotional, and intellectual well-being. Wellness is viewed as a continuous process in which individuals take control of their own lives by deliberately choosing a lifestyle that leads to a richer, more balanced and satisfying state of being.

Dimensions of Wellness

Each of the five dimensions of wellness—social, emotional, spiritual, physical, and intellectual—are depicted in Figure 1.1. It is important to recognize that each dimension is equally as important as the others, and that each dimension affects and is affected by every other. The following definitions and lists are from the Wellness Project at California Polytechnic State University in San Luis Obispo, California (Wellness Project Committee, n.d.).

Social Wellness

Knowing yourself and feeling good about yourself are fundamental components of social wellness. Social wellness means enjoying your own company and interacting comfortably with people from a variety of backgrounds. Two basic components of social wellness are communication and interaction with others. The university setting contributes to making

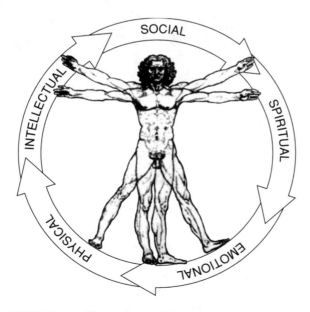

FIGURE 1.1   Dimensions of Wellness

lifelong friends and developing the social dimensions of your life. Provided below are: (1) a personal examination of social wellness, and (2) a social checkup list.

A Personal Examination of Social Wellness.   As you reflect on your social wellness, here are some questions you might wish to ask yourself:

- How do I behave around someone with a disability?
- Have I had lunch with a friend lately?
- Who is the last person to whom I wrote a letter?
- What are the qualities I look for in a friend?
- When was the last time I engaged in a meaningful conversation?
- When was the last time I showed appreciation for someone?
- Do I share ideas, work, play, and possessions?
- Do I share conversations with persons of different cultures, ethnic backgrounds, or religions?

A Social Checkup List.   Being socially healthy means being socially active. Here is a checklist of some questions that may indicate your social wellness:

- Do I know my limits?
- Do I really listen to what others are saying?
- Am I able to laugh at myself and not take myself too seriously?
- Am I comfortable in expressing my opinions with peers, coworkers, administrators, and family members?
- Do I set aside time for myself?
- Do I include people of different lifestyles, ages, and cultural backgrounds within my social circle?

Spiritual Wellness

Spiritual wellness is a dynamic process through which an individual seeks to integrate beliefs and actions. Incorporated into this process is a growing appreciation of aesthetics, nature, the environment, and people of all cultures. A sense of purpose, direction, and awareness contributes to spiritual health, resulting in hope, joy, courage, and gratitude. Provided below are: (1) a personal examination of spiritual wellness, and (2) a spiritual checkup list.

A Personal Examination of Spiritual Wellness.   As you reflect on your spiritual wellness, here are some questions you might wish to ask yourself:

- Have I spent time with someone less fortunate than myself?
- Have I attended a religious service of my choice?
- Have I explored the works of various philosophers, composers, and artists?
- Am I aware of the prejudices I hold, and am I striving to overcome them?
- Do I have a sense of forgiveness toward others and toward myself?
- Have I made an effort to put my convictions into action?

A Spiritual Checkup List.   Being spiritually healthy means being spiritually active. Here is a checklist of some questions that may indicate your spiritual wellness:

- Do I feel my life has meaning and purpose?
- Am I comfortable defining and expressing my spiritual values?
- What are the sources of my inner strength?
- Am I open to people with different ethnic, cultural, and religious backgrounds?
- Is there still a sense of wonder in my life about the world around me?
- Am I satisfied with the direction my life is going?

Emotional Wellness

Learning to cope with the stresses of life is essential to maintaining emotional wellness. Keeping a positive attitude, being sensitive to one's emotional needs, and holding expectations in line with reality all contribute to good emotional health. Emotions influence the way we interact with people, how we perceive our world, and the way we reason. Provided below are: (1) a personal examination of emotional wellness, and (2) an emotional checkup list.

A Personal Examination of Emotional Wellness.   As you reflect on your emotional wellness, here are some questions you might wish to ask yourself:

- Am I comfortable with my sexuality?
- Do I complete projects before the deadline?
- Can I identify how to relieve my tensions?
- Can I share my true feelings with friends?
- Am I comfortable with my intimate relationships?
- Do I find experiences that give me positive strokes?
- Would I consider joining an assertiveness group?

An Emotional Checkup List.   Being emotionally healthy allows identity to develop and feelings to be expressed. Here is a checklist of some questions that may indicate your emotional wellness:

- Do I usually get a good night's sleep?
- Am I able to accept and learn from my mistakes?
- Do I express my anger in a healthy way?
- Do I consider how positive and negative stresses affect my personal growth?
- Is my direction in life clearly identified?
- Am I excited by each day?
- Do I feel pressure to conform?
- Am I working to reduce my fears?
- When I find something is not working, do I try new behavior patterns?
- Do I take on more projects than I can handle?
- Do I have difficulty saying no?

Physical Wellness

A vital component of our daily lives is physical wellness. It is not merely the absence of disease or illness, but a balanced lifestyle focusing on learning about oneself in order to enjoy good health. Being physically well increases resistance to illness and enables one to cope better with stress. Maintaining alertness allows for full participation in learning as well as other situations. Obtaining knowledge and incorporating a healthy lifestyle are essential for assuring physical wellness. Provided below are: (1) a personal examination of physical wellness, and (2) a physical checkup list.

A Personal Examination of Physical Wellness. As you reflect on your physical wellness, here are some questions you might wish to ask yourself:

- Am I familiar with my family's medical history?
- Have I had a wellness physical recently?
- Do I practice relaxation techniques?
- Am I increasing my knowledge of self-health?
- Do I participate in sports or physical activities?
- Does my physical activity contribute to my overall sense of wellness?

A Physical Checkup List. Being physically healthy means being physically active. Here is a checklist of some questions that may indicate your physical wellness:

- Do I contribute to a safe environment?
- Do I exercise regularly?
- Is my sleep sound and restful?
- Do my habits enhance wellness?
- Does feeling good about my body enhance my sexual well-being?
- Do I eat nutritionally balanced meals daily?

Intellectual Wellness

The continuous development of one's knowledge and skills defines intellectual wellness. It is the strong desire to learn from challenges and experiences. By incorporating new ideas into everyday life, the individual follows a pattern of ongoing intellectual growth. Intellectual wellness enables the individual to fully pursue learning about all aspects of life. It creates a broad and open outlook toward all types of learning in all kinds of environments. Provided below are: (1) a personal examination of intellectual wellness, and (2) an intellectual checkup list.

A Personal Examination of Intellectual Wellness. As you reflect on your intellectual wellness, here are some questions you might wish to ask yourself:

- Do I discover new pursuits and challenges?
- Have I joined interest groups?

- Am I becoming well-versed in an area of my choice and interest?
- Do I enjoy exploring the world of art, music, and the classics?
- Do I have confidence in managing my time and planning ahead?
- Do I believe I am achieving my potential?
- Am I able to consider different viewpoints in decision-making?

An Intellectual Checkup List.   Being intellectually healthy means being intellectually active. Here is a checklist of some questions that may indicate your intellectual wellness:

- Am I able to listen to others before making critical judgments?
- Do I exercise my voting privilege and support candidates of my choice?
- Is goal-setting something I do regularly?
- Do I use a sense of humor to put problems into perspective?
- Am I stimulated by new ideas?
- Do I change chores into challenges?
- Do I plan and adhere to a monthly budget?
- Do I seek daily information on current trends and events?

In summary, wellness encompasses one's entire lifestyle. How much we care about ourselves determines whether we eat right, get enough sleep, avoid using tobacco or other psychoactive drugs, wear our seat belts, manage our stresses, and treat others with both dignity and respect. Scientific research continues to reveal new connections between our behaviors and emotions and our level of health. Each of our behaviors becomes a statement of how much we care about living. The way you live today and tomorrow will determine not only the quantity of your life but also its quality.

Health Concerns of the 21st Century

As the year 2000 approaches, the health of our nation is of particular interest to the federal government because its *Healthy People 2000: National Health Promotion and Disease Prevention Objectives* was designed to significantly improve the nation's health in the 21st century. The United States Public Health Service has set many health-related goals for the United States to meet by the year 2000. Some of its goals are to reduce mortality and morbidity rates from various diseases and infections, such as heart disease, cancer, and sexually transmitted infections; to reduce legal and illegal drug use; to reduce homicides, accidents, obesity, and teenage pregnancies; and to improve the personal quality of life for every individual. In general, the purpose was to help Americans live longer and better lives by having better health services and practicing healthier lifestyles. In addition, *Healthy People 2000* specifically points out the inequities in health, especially as they relate to minority groups, and the need to make health services equally available to all Americans.

A major strategy within the report is focused on the concept of prevention. Individuals can prevent illness and promote health and wellness by taking personal responsibility, choosing and living healthier behaviors. Taking personal responsibility can help reduce the number of self-induced illnesses and problems. A second focus is on removing barriers

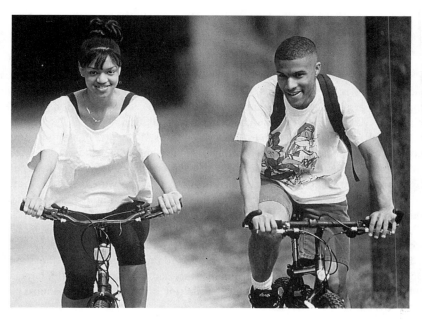

Photo by Tony Nesti.

Health depends on a state of equilibrium among the various factors that govern the operation of the body and the mind; the equilibrium in turn is reached only when man lives in harmony with his external environment.

—Hippocrates

that prevent access to equal education, health care, employment, a reasonable standard of living, and a generally better quality of life.

To develop the needed programs to accomplish the goals of *Healthy People 2000* will not be an easy task because our behavior isn't the only factor involved in our health. Our genetics, access to health care, the environment in which we live, and our economic status are important influences. Each of these factors, acting alone or together, can influence our health and wellness. These factors vary from individual to individual and from group to group. For example, an individual with a genetic predisposition to coronary artery disease is at higher risk of having a heart attack. If this person is not educated about heart disease and lacks adequate health care, he or she is more likely to suffer from more dangerous complications from coronary heart disease and have a lower quality of life.

Diversity in the United States

The United States is one of the most diverse countries in the world. There is no other place in the world where so many different populations live and work together on a daily basis. Trimble (1995) has observed:

America has truly grown into a beautiful complex mosaic of every conceivable skin color from existing populations and descendants of what sometimes appears to be a countless number of countries. To add to the complexity of the mosaic, even the makeup within each diverse group is complex and diverse in its language, norms, mores, and ethnic and cultural traditions.

The four dominant ethnic/racial minority populations (African Americans, Asian and Pacific Islander Americans, Native Americans, and Hispanic Americans) are increasing in size at a rate greater than the dominant Caucasian population. Table 1.1 lists the ethnic/racial demography of the United States population.

Ideally, when it comes to health and wellness, differences among us both as individuals and as members of groups should be insignificant. After all, we all need to eat healthy foods, exercise regularly, manage our daily and long-term stresses, protect ourselves from disease and injuries, and seek adequate health care when we are sick or injured. Realistically, however, there are significant health differences among diverse populations despite our political and cultural ideals.

When viewed from a national perspective health and illness are distributed across populations in predictable ways. The relative proportions of good or poor health among individuals are directly related to those individuals' placement in the social structure. Despite our efforts for justice and equality, there are still very real ethnic/racial disparities in health. Of all the inequalities in the distribution of health, one of the most pronounced is the distribution by race (Reed et al. 1993).

Definition of Terms.   The terms *ethnic, race, culture,* and *minority* to describe groups tend to be used interchangeably and inconsistently by various authors. This suggests the evolving nature of these concepts. Listed below are general definitions for some terms used in this book.

Culture: the collective consciousness of a group of people. A set of invisible patterns that form the normal ways of acting, feeling, perceiving, judging, and organizing the world (Shade, Kelly, and Oberg, 1997).

Ethnic group: Designation of a population subgroup having a common cultural heritage, as distinguished by customs, characteristics, language, common history, and so

TABLE 1.1   Population of the United States (1992)

Population	255,082,000
Men	124,493,000
Women	130,589,000
Whites	188,674,000
Blacks	31,635,000
Hispanic	24,238,000
Asian, Pacific Islander	8,401,000
Native American	2,134,000

Source: Bureau of the Census, Statistical Abstracts of the United States: 1994 (114th ed.) Washington, DC, 1994.

on. Ethnic member: a member of an ethnic group, especially a member of a minority or nationality group that is part of a larger community (*Webster's New World College Dictionary,* 1996).

Minority: A racial, religious, or ethnic group smaller than and differing from the larger, controlling group in a community, nation, and so on. (*Webster's New World College Dictionary,* 1996).

Race: Any of the different varieties of populations of human beings distinguished by a) physical traits such as hair, eyes, skin color, body shape; traditionally, the three primary divisions are Caucasoid, Negroid, and Mongoloid, although many subdivisions of these are also called race; b) blood types; c) genetic code patterns; d) all their inherited characteristics that are unique to their isolated breeding population (*Webster's New World College Dictionary,* 1996).

Anglo refers to non-Hispanic, white U.S. residents of European descent. Although this term carries strong cultural meanings in some contexts, it is most often used neutrally, simply as a shorthand expression to avoid awkward language.

It is important to bear in mind that the labels *Hispanic, African American/blacks, Native Americans/American Indians,* and *Asian Americans and Pacific Islanders* are a designation of convenience, and, while the subgroups to which they are applied show some commonalties, they are culturally, demographically, and linguistically diverse. Because each subgroup differs along so many dimensions, the practice of aggregating data in epidemiological studies of health problems, practices, and prevalence under the above summative labels masks the important differences in at-risk status. National aggregated data for the subgroups listed under these convenient labels is therefore of very limited utility for program planning in regions dominated by a specific cultural subgroup (Watts and Wright, 1989).

Health Status of Minority Americans

Unfortunately, the health status of the ethnic/racial minority populations in the United States has been influenced by the aftermath of past racial restrictions in education, employment, housing, politics, and other institutional systems. Although much progress has been made, continued inequities in the United States can be seen today in the disproportionate numbers of ethnic/racial minority people who are poor, homeless, living in substandard housing, in prisons, unemployed, and/or school dropouts (Ho, 1992). The aftermath of past racism and discrimination has also affected the minorities' help-seeking behaviors and contributes to the underutilization of helping professionals, who are often monolinguistic, middle class, and ethnocentric in problem diagnosis and treatment (Acosta, Yamamoto, and Evans, 1996).

The lingering effects can be measured in terms of mortality and life expectancy. The health status of minorities in the United States is disproportionately lower than the mainstream Anglo population (United States Department of Health and Human Services, 1985). During the 1980s, for example, the gap between the life expectancy of African Americans and Anglos increased. Anglos are living longer, while the average life span of African Americans declined from a high of 69.7 in 1984 to 69.2 in 1988 (Braithwaite and

TABLE 1.2   **Infant Mortality Rates for Selected United States Populations by Gender in 1991**

Year	All Races			White		Black	
	Both	**Male**	**Female**	**Male**	**Female**	**Male**	**Female**
1991	8.9	10.0	7.3	8.3	6.3	19.4	15.7

Source: Adapted from U.S. Dept. of DHHS. PHS, *Healthy People 2000: National Health Promotion and Disease Prevention Objectives,* Full Report. DHHS Pub. No. 91-5212. Washington, DC: USGPO, 1991.

Taylor, 1992). This disparity is reflected in their disproportionately higher mortality rate from many causes, such as cancer, heart disease and stroke, AIDS, cirrhosis, diabetes, unintentional injuries, and homicide.

What is also known in the United States about health and mental health issues is that the health status of African Americans, Native Americans, and Hispanic Americans is disproportionately worse than the mainstream population in almost every area of measurement. Asian and Pacific Islanders have overall measurements equal to white Americans. Infant mortality rate, for example, is a widely accepted indicator of the health status of any group. Although the overall infant mortality rate (both pre- and postneonatal) is declining in the United States, the postneonatal mortality rate, especially among African and Native American infants, is not improving (National Center for Health Statistics, 1993). In fact, the relative discrepancy between African American and white American mortality rates is increasing (National Center for Health Statistics, 1991). Table 1.2 reports the infant mortality rates by race and gender in 1991.

Infant mortality rate is the number of children dying before one year of age per 1,000 live births. This index provides clues about the health care situation, the income level, living conditions, as well as the nutritional status of the mothers in this group. In other words, a consistent high infant mortality rate is a reflection of the health of a particular group. Even though infant mortality rates for all ethnic/racial groups are declining, the gap between African Americans and white Americans is increasing. In other words, the differential ratio between the two groups is wider now than in the past.

A Demographic Profile of the Four Major Ethnic/Racial Minority Groups and Selected Health Concerns

Before profiling each of the four major ethnic/racial minority groups in the United States, Table 1.3 presents the ten leading causes of death and the number of deaths in the United States for all Americans for the year 1994. The table represents the population as a whole and does not distinguish between races. Table 1.3 will allow the reader to make overall comparisons for each of the four major ethnic/racial minority groups discussed in this chapter.

TABLE 1.3   Ten Leading Causes of Death in the United States, 1994

Rank	Cause of Death	Number
1.	Heart disease	734,000
2.	Cancers	536,860
3.	Strokes	154,350
4.	Chronic obstructive lung disease and allied conditions	101,870
5.	Accidents	90,140
6.	Pneumonia and influenza	82,090
7.	Diabetes mellitus	55,390
8.	HIV virus	41,930
9.	Suicide	32,410
10.	Liver Disease and cirrhosis	25,730

The death rate in Table 1.3 is expressed per 100,000 population.—CDC

Source: Centers for Disease Control. (1997) In R. Ballew. *Leading Causes of Death and Suicide.* http://www.sirinet.net/-rballew/deathsum.html

Native Americans/American Indians

The term *Native American* is commonly used to refer to the many peoples of North America whose cultures existed on the continent when Europeans first arrived. It was originally coined as a collective name for the native peoples of the Americas (primarily North America). Yet, as is the case with virtually any collective term suggested, there are problems inherent in the term; for example, literally speaking, anyone of any ethnicity born in the Americas could be considered a "native American."

The late twentieth-century debate over correct terminology is nowhere more evident than in discussions about native peoples. Some authors use the term "American Indians" or "Indians," others discuss "Native Americans," and some authors use them all. All are generalizations that deny the unique, tribal-specific cultural heritage and political legacy of the many original inhabitants of the Americas. The terms *Native Americans* and *American Indians* will be used interchangeably, based on the terminology used in the various studies and quoted authorities.

American Indians from the southwest are quite different from those of the northeast. American Indians from the midwestern plains are quite different from the Indians of Florida. The research on specific American Indian groups is very limited because most national health surveys group them together.

A common but inaccurate perception is that Native Americans are a homogeneous group and that differences between tribes are negligible. Differences between Native American groups are great. There are different languages, customs, and ceremonies, as well as different social, legal, political, and economic concerns. Beyond the cultural diversity among tribes, there is often equal diversity within tribes. For example, there are differences between those individuals who live on reservations as opposed to those who live in urban settings.

The two groups that comprise Native Americans are American Indians and Native Alaskans. Each group, in turn, consists of many subgroups. The 1992 Census registered 2,134,00 Native Americans in the United States. Native Alaskans are Aleuts, Eskimos, and Indians. The Bureau of Indian Affairs recognizes approximately 315 American Indian tribes or bands.

In examining the health circumstances of American Indians and Alaska Natives as a whole, they still lag behind the U.S. general population. Today's Indians are among the poorest, least educated, and most neglected minority groups in America. Unemployment rates are high. Fifty percent are unemployed and a considerable number are underemployed (Olson and Wilson, 1986). When compared to national averages, American Indians have the highest rate of alcoholism (438% greater), tuberculosis (400% greater), diabetes (155% greater), accidents (131% greater), homicide (57% greater), pneumonia and influenza (32% greater), syphilis (300% greater), and suicide (27% greater) (Olson and Wilson, 1986; U.S. Indian Health Service, 1993). Many feel that alcoholism is the number one health problem facing American Indians and contributes to many Indian deaths and illnesses (such as liver disease, suicide, accidents, homicide, diabetes, birth defects, and pneumonia). Table 1.4 lists the leading causes of death for Native American men in 1991. Table 1.5 lists the leading causes of death for Native American women in 1991.

Other data reinforce the fact that Indian women suffer mortality rates higher than all U.S. races from deaths due to accidents, diabetes mellitus, chronic liver disease and cirrhosis, pneumonia and influenza, and tuberculosis (U.S. Indian Health Service, 1993).

Hispanic Americans/Latinos

A controversial issue in the study of Hispanic culture is the question of appropriate language. *Hispanic* is a widely used term, particularly in government statistical reports. How-

TABLE 1.4   The Leading Causes of Death for Native American Men in 1991

Cause of Death	Approximate Number of Deaths in 1991
1. Diseases of the heart	1150
2. Unintentional injuries	875
3. Malignant neoplasms	775
4. Homicide	200
5. Suicide	200
6. Chronic liver disease and cirrhosis	190
7. Pneumonia/influenza	175
8. Cerebrovascular disease	160
9. Chronic obstructive pulmonary disease	150
10. Diabetes mellitus	140

Source: CDC, NCHS: *Vital Statistics of the U.S.,* Vol. 2, PHS, Washington D.C., 1992.

TABLE 1.5   The 10 Leading Causes of Death for Native American Women in 1991

Cause of Death	Approximate Number of Deaths in 1991
1. Diseases of the heart	820
2. Malignant neoplasms	700
3. Unintentional injuries	325
4. Diabetes	225
5. Cerebrovascular disease	225
6. Chronic liver disease and cirrhosis	150
7. Pneumonia/influenza	140
8. Chronic obstructive pulmonary disease	125
9. Certain conditions originating during prenatal period	75
10. Homicide/legal intervention	50

Source: CDC, NCHS: *Vital Statistics of the U.S.,* Vol. 2, PHS, Washington D.C., 1992.

ever, *Latino* is also an accepted term and is commonly used by universities that offer courses in Latino studies. Both terms are used throughout this book to refer to a person of Mexican, Puerto Rican, Cuban, Central or South American, or other Spanish culture or origin, regardless of race. It is further recognized that Latinos prefer not to be categorized as part of such an inclusive group, for example, calling themselves *Americans.* The author has also attempted to use specific designations whenever possible and to avoid generalizations about Latinos as a group that may not be true of particular Latino subgroups or individuals.

The word *American* has been added to the names of immigrant groups, such as Salvadoran Americans, to differentiate people living in the United States from those in the country of origin. Acceptable and preferred group names are constantly in flux, reflecting both changing group identity and social roles. The terms *Hispanic Americans* and *Latinos* will be used interchangeably, based on the terminology used in the various studies and quoted authorities. At other times, specific subgroups, such as Mexican American or Cuban American, will be cited when studies are specific to those groups.

The Hispanic population is the second largest minority population, next to African Americans, in the United States. Hispanics, as an ethnic group, are younger than the United States population, with a median age of 23. One-third of all Hispanics are children under eighteen years who live in poverty (Acosta-Belen and Sjostrom, 1988). This is 2.5 times the rate of poverty among white American children. In addition, 80 percent live in metropolitan areas.

Hispanic is a term that represents a diverse and heterogeneous population including Mexican Americans (Chicanos), who make up 61.1 percent, Puerto Ricans (15 percent), Cubans (6 percent), South and Central Americans (7 percent). The remainder are of "other Spanish" origin. However, what defines the Hispanic American community in national surveys is language and surnames. It is obvious that various Hispanic ethnic groups will differ widely in both intraethnic and regional differences. The 1992 Census registered 24,238,000 Hispanic Americans in the United States. The majority of Hispanics live in the five Southwestern states of Arizona, California, Colorado, New Mexico, and Texas.

The Hispanic population in general has a larger family size, younger median age, families clustered in large U.S. cities, and less favorable socioeconomic status than the majority population. Twenty-two percent of Hispanic-Americans live below the poverty level versus 11 percent of non-Hispanic families. When compared to the majority population, Hispanic Americans have higher infant mortality rates, shorter life expectancies, higher rates of AIDS and other sexually-transmitted diseases, but lower rates of chronic disorders, such as vascular diseases, neoplasms, and heart disease. Table 1.6 lists the leading causes of death for Hispanic Americans in 1990.

Heart disease, all forms of cancer, with the exception of stomach cancer, and cardiopulmonary morbidity and mortality rates are actually lower for Hispanic Americans compared to non-Hispanic Americans, but accidents, diabetes, homicide, chronic liver disease, and AIDS rank higher for Hispanic Americans.

Asian and Pacific Americans

The six major groups that comprise Asian Americans are Chinese, Filipino, Japanese, Asian Indian, Korean, and Vietnamese; there are numerous smaller groups as well. Each of these subgroups is not homogeneous either, but varies internally along a number of dimensions, such as geographical location, country of origin, the period of migration, or, for many Asian Pacific Americans, being native peoples. The 1992 Census listed a total of 8,401,000 Asian Americans in the United States.

Despite limitations, epidemiological researchers and health care policy makers have concluded, on the basis of limited data, that the health status of Asian Pacific Americans as a group is remarkably good (U.S. Office of Disease Prevention and Health Promotion, 1987) and "they are, in aggregate, healthier than all (other) racial/ethnic groups in the

TABLE 1.6   **Leading Causes of Death: Hispanic Americans (1990)**

1. Heart Disease
2. Cancer
3. Accidents
4. Stroke
5. Homicide
6. Diabetes mellitus
7. Pneumonia
8. HIV/AIDS
9. Liver disease

Source: CDC, NCHS: *Vital Statistics of the U.S.,* Vol. 2, PHS, Washington D.C., 1992

United States (U.S. Department of Health and Human Services, 1985). However, more recent health status data of different Asian Pacific Americans has revealed problems with hepatitis B, and that particular Asian Pacific American subgroups suffer equally, and in some cases more, the same problems as the majority population, such as heart disease, cancer, HIV/AIDS, substance use and abuse, domestic violence, suicides, and mental health problems. Two infectious diseases that have seriously affected immigrants of Asian and Pacific subgroups are tuberculosis and hepatitis B. As more immigrants with these infections move to the United States, serious health problems within the Asian communities may arise unless specific health programs that address these issues are developed. Table 1.7 lists the leading causes of death for Asian and Pacific Islanders living in California in the year 1991.

African Americans/Blacks

Controversy over appropriate language also exists in the study of African American culture. In the 1970s, the terms *Afro-American* and *black* were used. The preferred term is *African American.* The term *black,* however, is still a widely used term, particularly in government statistical reports. However, African American studies and black studies are both commonly used terms by universities that offer courses in ethnic studies.

African Americans comprise the largest minority population. The 1992 Census listed a total of 31,635,000 African Americans in the United States. Like the other minority groups, African Americans consist of many subgroups based on geographical location, socioeconomic status, country of origin, and other factors. African Americans come from several specific cultures and differ in language, values, and beliefs. They come from Africa, the Caribbean, and from the Americas, including urban and rural areas.

African Americans are disproportionately concentrated in large cities or Southern states. In 1990, there were 30.8 million African Americans in the United States, with 81 percent living in metropolitan areas. The poverty rate was 28.2 percent compared to the

TABLE 1.7   The Ten Leading Causes of Death for Asian and Pacific Islanders Living in California in the Year 1991

1. Diseases of the heart
2. Malignant neoplasms
3. Cerebrovascular disease
4. Accidents
5. Pneumonia
6. Chronic obstructive lung disease
7. Diabetes mellitus
8. Suicide
9. Homicide
10. HIV (males) and congenital anomalies (Female)

Source: CDC, NCHS: *Vital Statistics of the U.S.,* Vol. 2, PHS, Washington D.C., 1992.

TABLE 1.8   **Leading Causes of Death for African American Men (1991)**

The ten leading causes of death for African American males in 1991 are:

1. Diseases of the heart
2. Malignant neoplasms
3. Homicide/legal intervention
4. Unintentional injuries
5. Cerebrovascular disease
6. HIV infection
7. Pneumonia/influenza
8. Certain conditions originating in perinatal period
9. Chronic obstructive pulmonary diseases
10. Diabetes mellitus

Source: CDC, NCHS: *Vital Statistics of the U.S.,* Vol. 2, PHS, Washington D.C., 1992

United States total of 10.4 percent. When compared to white Americans, they are usually poorer, less likely to graduate from high school or college or to hold professional or white collar positions. Compared to white Americans, African Americans have higher infant mortality rates, lower life expectancies, higher mortality rates at earlier ages, and higher rates of homicide, stroke, cirrhosis, diabetes, and AIDS.

McBarnette (1996) reported that 60 thousand more African Americans than white Americans die each year as a result of cancer, cardiovascular disease, chemical dependency, cirrhosis of the liver, diabetes, homicide, and accidents. African American women are four times more likely to die in childbirth, and their children are three times more likely to die within the first year of life than white children (McCord and Freeman, 1990). Table 1.8 lists the leading causes of death for African American men in 1991; Table 1.9 lists the leading causes of death for African American women in 1991.

TABLE 1.9   **The Ten Leading Causes of Death for African American Women in 1991**

1. Diseases of the heart
2. Malignant neoplasms
3. Cerebrovascular disease
4. Diabetes mellitus
5. Accidents
6. Pneumonia/influenza
7. Certain conditions originating in perinatal period
8. Chronic obstructive pulmonary diseases
9. Homicide
10. Nephritis

Source: CDC, NCHS: *Vital Statistics of the U.S.,* Vol. 2. Washington, DC: PHS, 1992.

Other Ethnic Minorities in the United States

Although the focus of this book is on the four major minorities and their subgroups, there are many other ethnic minority groups about which little or no health research has been done and that are not included in the national health surveys. These groups also face particular health issues that need to be addressed. Listed below are two examples of two growing ethnic groups in the United States whose ancestors came from the Asian continent that are not usually included in U.S. national health surveys.

Iranian Americans and Immigrants

The flow of Iranian citizens into the United States began in 1979, during and after the Islamic Revolution. Thus, most Iranians in the United States are first generation immigrants who share many of the beliefs, values, and characteristics of their compatriots in Iran (Behjati-Sabet, 1990). However, many of the Iranians who came to the United States were educated, from upper- and middle-class families, and familiar with Western culture. Thus, the transition to the United States was somewhat smoother for this group of immigrants than for people from other countries.

Iranians in the United States are very religious. Muslims are very conscious of the different religious subgroups. Even though Iranians are bonded by race, religion and culture tend to keep many of them apart. Because Iranian culture is very class-conscious, members of the upper classes and lower classes do not usually interact socially. However, due to the accessibility of education in the United States, class mobility has become both possible and very common (Behjati-Sabet, 1990). Religion has a strong influence and they strongly believe that their health and life are in the hands of "Allah." Because Western medicine has strong roots in Arabic medicine, Iranians are very familiar with Western medical practices and will seek medical attention when needed. Iranian patients tend to seek Iranian physicians because of their cultural and religious ties.

With the recent military war between the United Nations and, in particular, the United States, Iranian Americans have encountered more open racism. Whether this has had an impact on mental health, psychosomatic disorders, and stress-related depressions has yet to be determined.

South Asians (India, Pakistan, Sri Lanka, Bangladesh, and Nepal)

The whole category of Asian and Pacific Islanders covers a large number of different cultural groups. Often overlooked in this category are the South Asians. Many people tend to visualize Asians only as Eastern Asians (Japan, China, and Korea) or Southeast Asians (Vietnamese, Laotians, Hmongs, and Cambodians). However, this is a limited view. Like the different cultural groups discussed earlier, there is great diversity within the South Asian populations. All South Asians, however, share a common British Colonial heritage, and many migrating South Asians, urban raised and educated, speak English and have a knowledge of Western culture before arriving. However, those who migrate from rural areas are confronted with severe cultural gaps. Most South Asians migrate to the United States for economic and educational improvement rather than for political reasons.

In South Asia, infections and parasitic diseases are prevalent. Typhoid, cholera, tuberculosis, hepatitis, malaria, and amebic dysentery are common. Nutritional deficiency diseases, such as Vitamin A deficiency and rickets, are also common. The incidence of cancer, heart disease, stroke, and diabetes is relatively low. The low rate of chronic diseases may be correlated with their low life expectancy.

Cultural Customs and Behaviors

Culture is the means by which a community communicates, a commonly agreed-on set of meanings in interactions with one another. Each culture has its own history, ideology, traditions, values, lifestyles, and languages that determine how people live and interact together. As a result the cultural group typically feels a sense of unity and has a "will" to survive that is backed up by specific individual and group behaviors (Davidman, 1995).

Culture provides a set of implicit and explicit guidelines that individuals learn as members of a particular group, and that tells them how to view the world and how to behave in it in relation to other people and to the environment. Culture is a lens through which individuals perceive and understand the world they inhabit and learn to live within it.

Individuals become culturally conditioned and this conditioning becomes an integral part of how they interpret and judge the behavior of others. The cultural framework that evolves becomes the "truth" or "belief" by which individuals interpret the world. Therefore, each individual group has its own cultural interpretation of what is "true." Difficulty can arise when individuals encounter a different culture that disregards their cultural truth or when their cultural truth is grossly misinterpreted by others.

The cultural truths or beliefs that constitute "health truths" are often different from the mainstream medical truths of the dominant Western-trained medical profession and society. Cultural factors can be either causal, contributory, or protective in their relation to health and wellness, and they are numerous. Different cultures have different beliefs about such things as family dynamics, gender roles, sexual behavior, diet, personal hygiene, body image alterations (body piercing, cosmetic surgery, tattooing, obesity, slimness), dress, use of drugs (tea, coffee, alcohol, hallucinogens), leisure pursuits, and the use of nontraditional medical practitioners.

Illness is also a sociocultural construct. As a result, each culture provides a culturally relevant diagnosis or cause and a framework for appropriate intervention. Within this framework, different cultures provide explanations for "why" an illness occurred. These cultural beliefs are important in the treatment process of any illness and also in the prevention of illness. In addition, not all cultural beliefs are clearly visible to those outside of the culture. For example, if religion is tightly woven into the culture's view of health, healing may be one of the primary responsibilities of religion. Thus, religious practices may be an integral part of that culture's health care system.

Examples of Cultural Factors That Affect Health

In certain cultures, for example, the male, by virtue of nothing other than his sex, is dominant and, as a consequence, the woman loses control in her sexual relationship. If the man chooses not to use a condom, the woman then loses control of her fertility and her ability to prevent disease.

Many Hispanic, Asian, and African American men come from cultures that reject the use of condoms and believe that extramarital sex with numerous partners enhances their male identity. As a result, the cultural consequence can be seen in an increase in unwanted pregnancies, HIV/AIDS, single mothers, and cervical cancer, all major contributors to morbidity and mortality.

So to argue for the use of condoms without understanding the cultural truth will have little effect. Without knowing the culture, it is impossible to know the people, and to disregard their cultural truths is to disregard *them*. This, in turn, affects how minorities believe they are perceived in mainstream society and, ultimately, affects their self-esteem and sense of self-worth.

Acculturation and Health

Acculturation is loosely defined as the process of becoming adapted to a new or different culture with more or less advanced patterns. In a simple approach, Landrine and Klonoff (1996) viewed acculturation as a continuum from traditional to acculturated (Table 1.10) They defined traditional people as those who remain immersed in many of the beliefs, practices, and values of their own culture. In the middle are bicultural people, who have retained the beliefs and practices of their own culture but also have assimilated the beliefs and practices of the dominant White society and so participate in two different cultural traditions simultaneously. Highly acculturated people have rejected the beliefs and practices of their own culture of origin in favor of those of the dominant white American society. Table 1.10 compares the differences between traditional, bicultural, and acculturated individuals.

Based on this model of acculturation, traditional people will be immersed in their own cultural values, beliefs, and practices, and their health beliefs and practices will differ significantly from the majority society. Minority groups cannot be grouped together to represent a whole. Traditional, bicultural, and acculturated individuals will differ in their health beliefs and practices. The concept of acculturation is important because it not only sheds light on the why of differences between minority Americans and white Americans, but it also highlights and explains differences within a minority group (Landrine and Klonoff, 1996).

The concept of acculturation is also important because it has a direct effect on the health of an individual. Marmot and Syme (1976) did a comparative study of the epidemiological rates of coronary heart disease (CHD) of Japanese men living in Japan (lowest

TABLE 1.10   Traditional, Bicultural, and Acculturated Differences

Traditional	Bicultural	Acculturated
Immersed in culture of origin	Immersed in culture of origin and in dominant culture	Immersed mostly in dominant culture
Usually cannot speak much English	Usually speaks both English (in the world) and native language (at home)	Usually speaks only English and speaks little of or cannot speak native language

rate), Hawaii (intermediate), and California (highest rate). The results of the study showed that, independently of the established coronary risk factors, the incidence of CHD was found to be related most significantly to the degree of adherence to the traditional Japanese culture they were brought up in. The more "Westernized" the Japanese male became, the greater the incidence of CHD. The closer their adherence to traditional Japanese values, the lower was their incidence of CHD. Marmot and Syme concluded that the culture in which a Japanese man is raised affects his likelihood of manifesting coronary heart disease in adult life, and that this relation of culture of upbringing to CHD appears to be independent of the established coronary risk factors.

Landrine and Klonoff (1996) also reported a positive relationship between acculturation and hypertension and smoking. A high level of acculturation in an African American correlated with more smoking and higher blood pressures.

Considering the acculturation continuum and the complex diversity within each minority group, it is possible to make group generalizations only about minority health care in this book.

Factors That Influence Access to Health Care

Equal access to health care in the United States is a noble aspiration. However, implementation of that goal is not without complications. It is not surprising that, because of diversity and related political issues in the United States, particular problems have arisen in implementing this goal. Barriers to achieving it were identified some time ago, yet many still continue to exist today. Some barriers to health care are depicted in Figure 1.2.

Access to health care can be examined in a variety of ways. For the purpose of this chapter, the aspects of access to health care will be discussed by identifying those factors

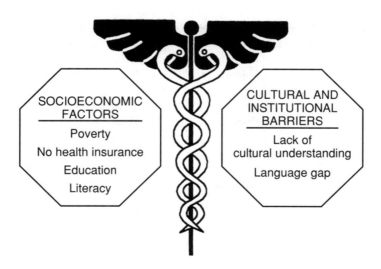

FIGURE 1.2　Factors That Influence Access to Health Care

that influence access to it. Because of the diversity of the various minority populations within the United States, it is difficult to examine the complexity of the health access issues that each minority population faces. Because of the vast differences in such factors as language and culture, the limited data available, and immigration status, only a superficial view of health access issues is possible.

Lack of access to medical care is frequently cited as the single greatest problem that ethnic/racial minority populations face in the health care system. The lack of access results from (1) socioeconomic factors, and (2) cultural and institutional barriers. Each of these factors is discussed below.

Socioeconomic Factors

Poverty.   It is almost impossible to talk about the health and wellness of minority groups without talking about their economic circumstances. Many poor minorities are undereducated, unemployed or work at minimum wage jobs, and are geographically concentrated in large cities and ghetto areas. Substantial evidence suggests that poverty, unemployment, and living in a single-parent home pose significant risks for the development of health problems, particularly in behavioral health areas (Reed et al., 1993). Poverty significantly affects health and wellness, and, in particular, affects the ability to afford preventive and routine health care. Women and children represent 80 percent of the poor people in the United States. The majority of them are people of color. Table 1.11 provides a picture of

TABLE 1.11   Persons and Families Below Poverty Level

Selected Characteristics by Race, Age, and Family	1994	1995*
All persons	%	%
All races	14.5	13.8
White American	11.7	11.2
African American	30.6	29.3
Hispanic American	30.7	30.3
Asian/Pacific Islander	14.6	14.6
Families		
All races	11.6	10.8
White American	9.1	8.5
African American	27.3	26.4
Hispanic American	27.8	27.0
Asian/Pacific Islander	13.1	12.4
Families with female householder, no husband present		
All races	34.6	32.4
White American	29.0	26.6
African American	46.1	45.1
Hispanic American	52.0	49.4

Source: Adapted from U.S. Bureau of the Census: *Poverty in the United States 1996*
www.census.gov/main/www/subjects.html.

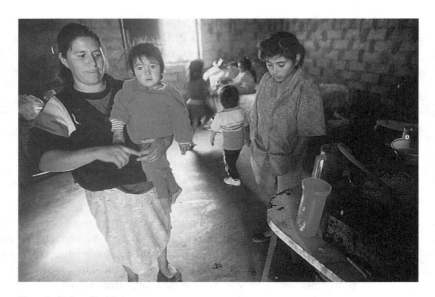

Photo by Robert Harbison.

Poverty is a hellish state to be in. It is no virtue. It is a crime.

—Marcus Garvey

poverty for the years 1994 and 1995. The United States 1994 federal poverty level for one person was $7,500, $9,000 for a couple, and $14,500 for a family of four. The 1995 poverty threshold for a family of four was $15,569.

The 1995 U.S. Bureau of the Census report, *Poverty in the United States,* did not include a separate category for Native Americans. However, according to the 1990 census data, 35 percent of Native Americans live below the federal poverty level, 14 percent live in deep poverty, compared with 9.8 percent of white persons; 21 percent of American Indian and Alaska Native households are headed by women.

Minorities with the worst health status and poorest access to health care live in communities that have inadequate housing, poor nutrition, poor sanitation, and high rates of physical, emotional, and sexual abuse. People living in poverty experience poorer health, which is reflected in a higher incidence of chronic diseases, a higher mortality rate, and poorer survival rates (National Center for Health Statistics, 1991).

Lack of Health Insurance.   "Health insurance is an indispensable key to health care in this country. It opens doors to access, quality, and at least some choice of care. Many Americans, especially members of minority groups, are still locked out of the care they need to live full, healthy lives," said Thomas Chapman, CEO, George Washington University Hospital (Commonwealth Fund Survey, 1994). The lack of insurance is also a primary reason for the failure of many ethnic minorities to seek preventive health care services.

Twenty-nine percent of ethnic/racial minority adults do not have insurance, compared to 12 percent of white American adults (Commonwealth Fund Survey, 1994). Acosta-Belen and Sjostrom (1988) reported that 39 percent of Hispanics under the age of

65 have no health insurance. Brown and colleagues (1991) reported that 20 percent of non-elderly Asian Pacific people and "others" in California, and 21 percent nationally, were uninsured. Although health insurance statistics on African Americans is limited, the Children's Defense Fund (1989) stated that 10 to 12 million African American children are without health coverage and even more are underinsured. They further stated that African American children are 63 percent more likely than white children to be uninsured.

Minority adults are nearly twice as likely to have "very little" or "no choice" in where they obtain their health care, according to the Commonwealth Fund Survey. Many minority groups lack access to a broad array of health services, especially primary care. Many studies have documented that minorities are less likely than any other group to be linked to a regular source of care. The Commonwealth Survey reported minority adults (66 percent) are less likely than white adults (80 percent) to have a regular doctor or other health professional, particularly Asian American (60 percent) and Hispanic adults (59 percent). A regular source of care is an established and identifiable medical source that an individual or a family uses on a routine basis. Having a regular source of care not only improves the continuity and quality of care but also helps facilitate entry into the health care system. Poor and uninsured minorities who turn to public medical facilities for routine care often confront a lack of bilingual and bicultural services, long waiting lines, and distant appointments. These barriers contribute to the advancement of their illnesses and their disproportionate use of costly emergency room services.

Finally, the Commonwealth Survey reported that 46 percent of minority adults are very satisfied with the quality of their health care services, compared with 60 percent of white adults. Fifteen percent of adults in all minority groups—five times the number of whites (3 percent)—believe their medical care would have been better if they were of a different race.

Education and Literacy.   Limited reading skills (in English or native languages) have a negative impact on access. The ability to read and comprehend health-related information and application or registration forms in medical facilities is crucial in a patient's ability to get through the health access process. Even the simple process of reading and comprehending the signs in health facilities can become complicated. Limited education and literacy serve to obstruct the path to health care access.

National standardized tests illustrate continuing gaps in educational attainment measurements between Native Americans, Hispanic Americans, and African Americans, despite improvements by ethnic minorities over the last decade. Disparities occur largely in national achievement test scores in critical areas such as reading, mathematics, and science (U.S. Department of Education, 1992). For many ethnic minorities, schools have become alienating places for them, and the absenteeism, truancy, and dropout rates for these groups is higher compared to white students (Roberts, 1994; Schorr & Schorr, 1988). Roberts (1994) also reported that there is consensus among scholars that, given the proper health care and educational conditions, school performance among black children is comparable with that of their white counterparts, particularly at the elementary level. High school graduation rates are a significant indicator of actual as well as potential socioeconomic status. In 1986, the nonhigh school graduation rate for certain groups of ethnic minorities was still significantly higher than that for whites (United States Department of Health and Human Services, 1990).

A truncated educational experience diminishes prospects for students' success in employment and leads, ultimately, to an increased risk of continued poverty. Deficits in critical cognitive skills restrict opportunities for competitive jobs, improved salaries and, ultimately, social and economic mobility (Turner et al., 1990).

Cultural and Institutional Barriers

Lack of Cultural Understanding.   For many minority groups, Western health care practices conflict sharply with their own cultural health and healing practices. Cultural barriers are built into the very structure of the Western health care model, which emphasizes isolating and treating different ailments through specialized practitioners, rather than a holistic approach. This fragmented health care system is even more formidable for those who possess different conceptions of health care and healing and use different health care-seeking practices. In addition, there is usually a lack of bicultural and culturally competent staff to provide appropriate care. Most health care health professionals are not educated and trained to be culturally sensitive.

Language Gap.   In conjunction with cultural awareness, practitioners face a language gap with some minority groups. The inability of the patient to speak English and the inability of the practitioner to speak the patient's language is one of the most formidable obstacles that immigrants and medical practitioners face. The U.S. Department of Health, Education, and Welfare (1980) stated, "The inability to speak English is a major obstacle for immigrants as most practitioners are not bilingual. As a result, even the simple exchange of information is very difficult without an interpreter. Often, interpreters are not available at crucial times in the delivery of health care. These events further isolate the immigrant, and lead to fragmentation of care."

The Commonwealth Fund survey (1994) reported that language differences are a problem for 24 percent of minority Americans who do not speak English as their primary language. Twenty-six percent of Hispanic adults and 22 percent of Asian American adults need an interpreter when seeking health care services. The survey quoted Grace Wang, the medical director of Chinatown Health Council, as saying, "Talking with your doctor and being understood is basic to getting good care. Many minority Americans do not speak English as a primary language. They are often frightened and confused about their health and problems, and cultural traditions and differences can add to their difficulties in communicating. Patience, empathy, as well as interpreters, can make a real difference in the effectiveness of the treatment that they receive."

Conclusion

The increasing racial and ethnic diversity within our nation has become one of the most significant challenges our teachers, medical practitioners, politicians, and employers face. It is also a challenge that many are ill-prepared to meet.

Every individual should have equal access to quality health care and services, but good personal health is not an entitlement. No individual, regardless of race or sex, can attain good health without a certain amount of personal responsibility and involvement, regardless of the environment and society in which he or she lives. This is not to say that the "victim of poor health is totally responsible" because he or she is the one who chooses to smoke, drink, and eat too much, engage in unprotected sex and violence, and not exercise. This view, of course, is too narrow. Taking control of one's own fate and assuming personal responsibility is one aspect of this effort (Braithwaite and Taylor, 1992). Very few people would argue that economic stratification, politics, and access to health care facilities don't play a major role in one's health. If every citizen is to enjoy an equal opportunity for health, both individual and collective action will be needed to overcome the many obstacles to good health care.

Even though acculturation does take place, structural assimilation or gaining access to U.S. institutions, including medical care systems for prevention, screening, and treatment, continues to be difficult. Sociometric factors, such as lacking health insurance, low income, and lack of a regular health care provider, appear to be the strongest deterrents to gaining entry into the health care system. In addition, the policies and practices in the medical care system have limited flexibility to meet the needs of populations who are poor or may have different illnesses, cultural practices, or languages. Obviously, the needs of all Americans cannot be addressed through a generic approach. The unique characteristics and needs of special populations must be taken into account.

It also appears that, for many minority populations, there are more dimensions to "health" and "wellness" than what traditional Western society considers. Many minority populations practice culturally conditioned health-related behaviors that are different from those of the Western mainstream culture. Therefore, good health must be viewed as a product of cultural considerations, such as behavior and customs, human ecological systems, education, exercise, proper diet, healthy self-esteem, social supports, healthy lifestyles, and acceptable health care services. Policies must support strategies that will increase cultural, linguistic, and geographic access to care while attempts are being made to remove financial obstacles that deprive tens of millions of people of excellent health care.

Finally, quality health care should be accessible to everyone and should not vary depending on the language, culture, race, and financial status of the patient. Providing equal access to ethnic/racial minority populations must be seen in the context of improving health care access for all Americans.

REFERENCES

Acosta, F., Yamamoto, J., and Evans, L. Effective psychotherapy for low-income and minority patients. In Ho, M. *Minority children and adolescents in therapy.* Newbury Park, CA: Sage, 1996, p. 26.

Acosta-Belen, E., and Sjostrom, B. *The Hispanic experience in the United States.* New York: Praeger, 1988.

Behjati-Sabet, A. The Iranians. In N. Waxler-Morrison, J. Anderson and E. Richardson (Eds.) *Cross cultural caring: A handbook for health professionals.* Vancouver, BC: UBC Press, 1990, pp. 91–115.

Braithwaite, R., and Taylor, S. (Eds.). *Health issues in the black community.* San Francisco, CA: Jossey-Bass, 1992.

Brown, E., Valdez, R., Morgenstern, H., Wang, C., and Mann, J. *Health insurance coverage of Californians in 1989.* Berkeley: University of California, California Policy Seminar, 1991.

Bureau of the Census. *Poverty in the United States 1996. Current population reports.* P-60, No. 185. Washington, DC: U.S. Government Printing Office, 1993.

Bureau of the Census. *Statistical abstracts of the United States: 1994.* Washington, DC: U.S. Government Printing Office, 1994.

Centers for Disease Control. *Vital statistics of the United States.* Vol. 2, Public Health Services. National Center for Health Statistics. Washington, DC: U.S. Government Printing Office, 1992.

Centers for Disease Control. In R. Ballew. (Ed.), *Leading causes of death and suicide,* 1997. http://www.sirnet.net/-rballew/deathsum.html

Children's Defense Fund. *Lack of health insurance makes a difference.* Washington, DC: Author, 1989.

Commonwealth Fund Survey. *A comparative survey of minority health.* New York: The Commonwealth Fund, 1994. http://www.cmwf.org:80/minhlth.html

Davidman, L. "Culture, Education, and Learning," unpublished paper. San Luis Obispo: California Polytechnic University Center for Teacher Education, 1995.

Ho, M. *Minority children and adolescents in therapy.* Newbury Park, CA: Sage, 1992.

Landrine, H., and Klonoff, E. *African American acculturation.* Thousand Oaks, CA: SAGE, 1996.

Marmont, M. Culture and illness: Epidemiological evidence. In Christine, M. and Mellett, G. (Eds.), *Foundations of psychosomatics.* New York: Wiley, 1981, pp. 323–340.

Marmot, M., and Syme S. Acculturation and coronary heart disease in Japanese Americans. *American Journal of Epidemiology,* 104 (1976), 225–247.

McBarnette, L. African American women. In Bayne-Smith, M. (Ed) *Race, gender, and health.* Thousand Oaks, CA: Sage, 1996. (pp. 43–67)

McCord, C., and Freeman, H. Excess mortality in Harlem, *New England Journal of Medicine,* 322 (1990), 173–177.

National Center for Health Statistics. *Health, United States,* 68. DHHS publication; PHS 91-1232, Hyattsville, MD: 1991.

National Commonwealth Fund. *A comparative survey of minority health,* New York: The Commonwealth Fund, 1994 http://www.cmwf.org:80/minhlth.html

Olson, J., and Wilson, R. *Native Americans in the twentieth century.* Chicago: University of Illinois Press, 1986.

Reed, W., Darity, W., Sr., and Robertson, N. *Health and medical care of African Americans.* Westport, CT: Auburn House, 1993.

Roberts, V. A. Emeritus scientists, mathematics and engineers program: Evaluation report. In D. Jones and V. Roberts (Eds.), "Black Children: Growth, Development, and Health. In I. L. Livingston (Ed.) *Handbook of Black American health.* Westport, CT: Greenwood Press, 1994, pp. 331–343.

Schorr, L., and Schorr, D. *Within our reach: Breaking the cycle of disadvantage.* New York: Anchor Press Doubleday, 1988.

Shade, B., Kelly, C., and Oberg, M. *Creating culturally responsive classrooms.* Washington, DC: American Psychological Association, 1997.

Trimble, J. Ethnic Minorities. In R. Coombs and D. Ziedonis (Eds.), *Handbook on drug abuse prevention,* Boston, MA: Allyn and Bacon, 1995. pp. 379–409

Turner, R., Grindstaff, C., and Phillips, N. Social support and outcome in teenage pregnancy. *Journal of Health and Social Behavior,* 31 (1990), 43–57.

U.S. Department of Education. *Digest of education statistics, 1992* (NCES Publication No. NCES 92-097). Washington, DC: Government Printing Office, 1992.

U.S. Department of Health and Human Services. *Report of the secretary's task force on black and minority health,* Vol. 1. *Executive summary* (Publication No. 491-313/44706). Washington, DC: Government Printing Office, 1985.

U.S. Department of Health, Education, and Welfare. *Special report to Congress on the primary health needs of immigrants.* Washington, DC: Government Printing Office, 1980.

U.S. Indian Health Service. *Trends in Indian health.* Washington, DC: U.S. Department of Health and Human Services, 1993.

U.S. Office of Disease Prevention and Health Promotion. *ODPHP's prevention fact book: Life expectancy in the United States.* Washington, DC: Government Printing Office, 1987.

Watts, T., and Wright, R. *Alcoholism in minority populations.* Springfield, IL: Charles C. Thomas, 1989.

Wellness Project Committee, Dean of Students Office. *Wellness.* San Luis Obispo, CA: California Polytechnic State University, n.d.

World Health Organization: Constitution of the World Health Organization, *Chronicle of the World Health Organization,* 1:29–43, 1947.

CHAPTER

2   Healing and Culture

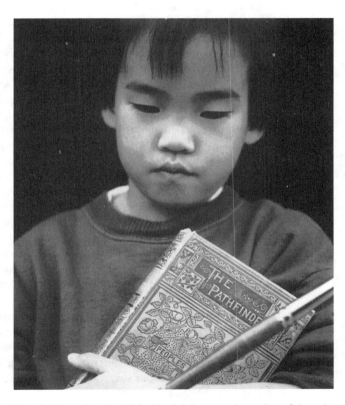

Destroy the culture and you
Destroy the people.
—Frantz Fanon, *Wretched of the Earth,* 1963

Photo by Marcy Israel, published in *Cultures* magazine, volume 2, issue 1

Why do we become sick? Who or what can make us well? The answers to these questions differ significantly depending on who asks them and when and where.

In a Mexican American barrio, a man with terrible stomach pains seeks a *curandero* (folk healer) to heal his illness. The curandero listens to the man's complaint, then massages the man's body with a mixture of daisies, violets, poppies, and blessed rosemary, all

27

soaked in alcohol. After the massage, she pours the blood of a black hen into a dish mixed with pineapple. The patient must take the mixture to the church in hopes that the blessed virgin at the church will cure the illness. The hen is then cooked until it is so black that it would drive out the evil spirits. Almost miraculously, the man's symptom's disappear.

On an American Indian reservation, a woman believes she is ill because she is possessed by an evil spirit and she seeks a shaman for help. The shaman brings the woman, her family, and many of her acquaintances to the sweat lodge to heal her. Slipping into a trance, the shaman communicates with the spirits of another world to gain healing experience and to gain an ally to rid the woman of the evil spirit. Drumming, chanting, rattles, and dancing are used to help direct the shaman's travels. The sweat ceremony purifies the body of evil or malignant influences. Dramatically, the shaman, with song and prayer, helps to release the evil spirits from her body.

Some people, of course, think that the above two examples are irrational and even silly. How can evil spirits create sickness and how can trances be used to diagnose illness? After all, in our logical and rational Western society, an illness is diagnosed through X rays, laboratory tests, and physical examinations, and treated with medications and surgery. If you go in for a severe inflammation, the rational approach is to use an anti-inflammatory drug. A benign growth can easily be surgically removed.

Those who have grown up with Western medicine tend to make assumptions about Western versus non-Western approaches to disease and treatment. They judge one to be modern and the other primitive; one scientific and the other based on superstition. But patients being treated by practitioners of either approach get better for reasons that have little to do with the objective cause of the discomfort (Institute of Noetic Sciences, 1993).

Regardless of the culture, each patient believed in the powers of the healer. The treatments may be different, but each patient has faith in both the practitioner and the process. Western society believes in the supremacy of medical technology in the same way that traditional Native Americans or Hispanic Americans believe in the rituals and incantations of the shaman or curandero. In either case, much of the relief hinges on beliefs or on healing practices that are not completely understood.

As we approach the year 2000, Western medicine views the body essentially as a machine, an exceedingly complex mechanism that can be understood and, as appropriate, modified and repaired. Specificity is Western medicine's greatest asset: Our physicians work best when they can identify and eliminate a known cause of disease that comes from outside the body, and our surgeons are unsurpassed in dealing with acute trauma (Smolan, Moffitt, and Naythons, 1990).

The issues that lie at the very heart of non-Western traditional medicine are concerned with the spirit and the soul and a person's interaction between the environment and the cosmos, issues that are dismissed by modern Western medicine because they do not fit into the scientific model. Non-Western traditional medicines also have commonalities shared with Western medicine: the importance of belief in healing, the healing power of the unconscious, health as an adjusting balance between a multitude of physical, psychological, and spiritual variables (Institute of Noetic Sciences, 1993).

Western scientific medicine has much to teach and contribute to the world. At the same time, there is much to learn from other cultures, especially from other types of healers who, lacking the technical ability of modern medicine, choose to embrace the human being as a whole, an embrace that has existed for thousands of years.

Two Theoretical Explanations for Ritual Healing Success

1. Neurobiological. A growing number of scientists, biochemists, pharmacologists, psychiatrists, and anthropologists have speculated that another key to the lay healer's success may be found in the biochemistry of endorphins, endogenous morphinelike substances that act on the nervous system and are generated by the human brain in response to pain, stress, or certain kinds of peak experiences (Laderman & Roseman, 1996). Given the proper cues, through psychological means, the brain may also generate other endogenous chemicals as effective as Librium and Valium in their tranquilizing effect. Endorphins are one such class of identified neurochemicals that are produced by the brain. Endorphins resemble opium in effects. A full understanding of the role of the endorphins in pain perception has not yet been fully developed, but they seem to be one of the brain's mechanisms for producing pain relief.

2. Psychological. The placebo effect refers to those effects caused by people's beliefs or expectations. A person's expectancy can trigger effects independently of any effect of the treatment or medicine itself. The placebo effect is capable of helping the body's ability to heal itself. Western physicians have used placebos for relieving anxiety, headache, fever, and warts. The placebo effect is not necessarily limited to the administration of substances, but may also include words and actions, such as occur in a shamanistic seance or a Western physician's diagnosis. The healer, in engaging the mind and affecting the emotions of his or her patient, might also initiate physiological repair (Laderman & Roseman, 1996).

The field of psychoneuroimmunology (PNI) studies the relationship between psychosocial processes and nervous, endocrine, and immune system functioning. Research (Ader and Cohen, 1985; Buck, 1988) has recently demonstrated that the immune system does not operate independently of the central nervous system. Rather, there are centers in the brain that are critical to the regulation of hormones and neurotransmitters that affect immune responses. The immune system is subject to modulation by the brain (DiMatteo, 1991). Because of this effect, mood states can influence an individual's susceptibility to disease and the progression of disease once it has developed.

Traditional Medicines

It is important to remember that no cultural group is homogeneous, and that every ethnic group contains diversity (Randall-David, 1989). It is not possible to provide a complete review of all traditional practices or to give a comprehensive review of each individual traditional practice, because each is so complex. In addition, this book does not wish to stereotype or imply that all members of a group hold certain beliefs or follow certain practices.

Chinese Medicine

One of the earliest civilizations to practice holistic medicine was the Chinese. More than 5,000 years ago traditional Chinese medicine did not distinguish between the mind and the body but viewed illness as manifestations of both within the individual's environment. The traditional Chinese concepts of health and disease are intimately tied to the constructs of classical Chinese thought. A human being is a reflection of the universe, a microcosm in the macrocosm, and both are subject to the same universe, the divine law, the law of Tao (pronounced "dow"). To live according to Tao is to follow the "order of nature" and live in harmony with the "ultimate principle." If one does not live according to Tao, the resulting disharmony may be manifested as physical or psychological disease. Therapy must then be directed toward the reestablishment of balance and harmony if it is to have long-term effectiveness (Hastings, Fadiman, and Gordon, 1980).

In daily usage, Tao means "way," "path," or "discourse." But on a more spiritual level it symbolizes the absolute Way of nature, the primeval law that regulates all heavenly and earthly matters. "You may rest with the Tao, but you cannot define it," said the philosopher Chuang-tzu. The Tao is the foundation of Chinese medicine (Palos, 1971). Where Western medicine is concerned with identifying and conquering specific causes of disease, in Chinese medicine health is seen not as an absence of disease but as a way of life.

The ancient Chinese healing arts were not founded on a knowledge of human anatomy. The Chinese revered their ancestors, so gross dissection of a corpse was not only unacceptable but unthinkable. Instead the concept of an energy system within and outside of the body evolved. They believed that matter and energy were just two different manifestations of the same thing. Rather than focus on the anatomical aspects, they focused on the vital life energy that creates and moves the physical body.

Taoist philosophy describes health as the manifestation of the harmony of heaven, attained by the proper balance of internal and external forces. Taoists find unity in the diversity of natural phenomena by inferring a basic universal energy (called the Chi) underlying all of them. Chi (pronounced "chee" or "key") flows into and throughout all parts of the human body (Wallnofer and von Rottauscher, 1965). Good health requires that the Chi be in balance. If body parts have too much or too little Chi, the balance will be disrupted and a malfunction (disease) of the body will occur. Each morning in many Chinese American communities, people gather in the parks and squares to practice ancient exercises known as Tai Chi. The purpose is to promote the flow of Chi.

In essence, diagnosis in Chinese medicine is concerned with identifying the location and nature of energy imbalances in the body and, in particular, specific organs. Treatment involves restoring the energy balance between body parts by bringing more Chi to deficient organs and drawing energy away from organs with too much Chi. It is difficult for Westerners to think about Chi, because there is no comparable concept.

The universe is conceived of as a vast indivisible entity in which each single being has its definite function. However, no one thing can exist without the others, and to each thing, in turn, is linked a chain of concepts that correspond to each other in harmonious balance. To violate this harmony is to bring chaos, wars, catastrophes, and sickness on humanity and individuals.

The Chinese believed in the Five Evolutive Phases or the "five elements" (*wu-hsing*), stretches of time and divine conventionally and unequivocally energetic qualities that succeed one another in cyclical order (Porket, 1979). Individuals must therefore strive to adjust themselves wholly within the world of those correspondences, in which the five elements—wood, fire, earth, metal, and water—constitute the guiding principles. These are said to create one another, but also destroy each other, depending on the sequence of enumeration.

All substances and objects are referable to these five elements alone or in combination. The Chinese rigorously classify foods, drugs, and organs of the body according to this scheme. The bladder and the kidney are assigned to the realm of water, and the gall bladder and liver are assigned to the realm of wood. Because each bodily organ is assigned one of these elements, the functional relationships among organs can be shown in a schematic chart.

The Chinese term for organ is *tsang*. Its meaning, however, is clearly different than Western conceptions. It means something like "sphere of function" and does not equate specifically with an anatomical identification and function. The Chi within the tsang of the liver refers to a sphere of bodily function that may not correlate with Western ideas of liver function. In fact, of the twelve organs that the Chinese have identified, two have no anatomical correspondence at all (Weil, 1983). They are called "triple-heater" and "circulation-sex." The circulation-sex (also called the "heart constrictor" or "pericardium") probably relates to the endocrine system, while the "triple-heater" relates to the "heat" of respiration, digestion, and reproduction.

The liver (wood) controls the spleen (earth) and is controlled by the lung (metal); it also generates the activity of the heart (fire), and its own activity is generated by the kidney (water). The gall bladder (wood) controls the stomach (earth) and is controlled by the large intestines (metal); it also generates the activity of the small intestines (fire), and its own activity is generated by the bladder (water). These relationships indicate the direction of the flow of Chi energy from one organ to another.

FIGURE 2.1

Creation:

Wood creates Fire	Two pieces of wood rubbed together create sparks
Fire creates Earth	Fire transforms burning matter into ashes
Earth creates Metal	Within the earth, ore is "born"
Metal creates Water	Melting metal becomes liquid
Water creates Wood	Through being watered the tree grows

Destruction:

Wood destroys Earth	The tree sucks strength from the earth
Earth destroys Water	Earth can halt the flow of water
Water destroys Fire	Water extinguishes the flame
Fire destroys Metal	Fire causes metal to melt
Metal destroys wood	The ax fells the trees

Taoist philosophy also identifies two opposite and complementary qualities to all aspects of being, called the Yin and Yang. If Yin and Yang are not in harmony, it is as though there were no autumn opposite the spring, no winter opposite the summer. When Yin and Yang part from each other, the strength of life wilts and the breath of life is extinguished. If the balance between Yin and Yang are disturbed, illness will set in.

The concept of Yin and Yang is fundamental to an understanding of Chinese medicine. They are preexistent twin polarities that regulate things within the Universe. Nature is seen in terms of balance and that nature appears to group into pairs of mutually dependent opposites. Each opposite in nature gives meaning to the other. Thus, for example, the concept of night has no meaning without the concept of day, smallness has no meaning without the concept of bigness, and the concept of up has no meaning without the concept of down. The concept of cold has no meaning without the concept of warm and the concept of masculine has no meaning without the concept of feminine. The concept of Yin literally means "the dark side of the mountain" and represents such qualities as negative, darkness, cold, small, and empty. The character for Yang means the "bright side of the mountain" and represents such qualities as positive, light, warm, big, and fullness. Accordingly, everything has existence because everything manifests both Yin and Yang qualitites. Yin and Yang may vary but both aspects are always present in and throughout nature.

It is important to note that Yin is feminine and Yang is masculine but this philosophy is not androcentric. The terms are used in the same sense that modern physics describes an electron as "negative" and a proton as "positive." Neither is superior to the other. In the same manner, Yin and Yang refer to the opposing polarities, forces, or tendencies contained in all living things (Wallnofer and von Rottauscher, 1965).

Yin and Yang only exist in relation to each other. Yin is perceived as flowing into Yang even as Yang approaches its zenith, while Yang begins to flow in, even as Yin is approaching its zenith. Yin cannot be without Yang, nor Yang without Yin. Within each Yang there exists Yin and within each Yin there must be a Yang (Wallnofer and von Rottauscher, 1965). For example, no one is completely male or female; rather, masculinity and femininity are both present in each individual in varying degrees.

All substances, objects, times, places, and other aspects of creation are mixtures of these Yin and Yang qualities. Proper classification of them allows the Chinese physician to combine them in ways that promote general balance. For example, hollow organs are Yang and solid ones are Yin. All foods and medicinal herbs are so classified, along with all other

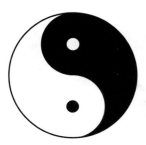

FIGURE 2.2   Symbol for Yin and Yang

FIGURE 2.3   Yin and Yang and the Human Body

Yin	Yang
the body's surface	inside the human body
back part of the body	front part of the body
liver	gall bladder
heart	stomach
spleen	large intestines
lungs	small intestines
kidneys	bladder
circulation-sex	triple-heater
diseases of winter and spring	diseases of summer and autumn

variables relevant to health and treatment. For example, an overly Yang Person should eat more Yin food. A brief discussion of Chinese food in relationship to the concept of Yin and Yang is found in Chapter 6. A discussion of herbs is discussed later in this chapter.

As Yin and Yang ebb and flow, the undulating nature affects not only individual health but all the events in the universe. This pulsation, for example, can be found in the contraction and dilation of the heart (systole and diastole) and in the inhalation and expiration of the lungs.

The theory of Chinese medicine is primarily concerned with the flow of Chi from organ to organ and ways to influence it. These pathways are deduced from the theory of Yin and Yang polarity and that of the five elements. Figure 2.4 depicts the interconnections between Yin and Yang and the five elements. Methods to correct the problems commonly include massage, herbal drugs, and dietary regimens, with selection of foods and herbs based on Yin and Yang and the five elements. A patient who appears deficient in wood may be given a wood herb; if the problem is in a particular wood organ like the liver, selection of a wood herb believed to have special affinities with the liver will be given.

Acupuncture.   An important theoretical concept of Chinese medicine is that the flows of energy in the interior of the body are mirrored in the flows on the surface. This is crucial because the deep flows are inaccessible to direct medical intervention, but the superficial flows can be changed by the unique Chinese medicine called *acupuncture.* Changing the superficial flows will indirectly affect the energy of ailing organs (Davis, 1975). Acupuncture involves the stimulation of specific points on the body, usually by the insertion of thin needles, often no thicker than a human hair. According to Chinese medical theory, Chi circulates through the body along the acupuncture meridians. Chi controls the blood, nerves, and all organs and must flow freely for good health to be maintained. It is the insertion of special needles into specific points of the body in order to draw energy to or from internal organs by changing the related flows on the surface. These points relate to the twelve organs (tsang) and are connected in lines called *meridians* (Bresler and Kroening, 1976).

Each of the twelve organs has a superficial meridian with many numbered points. The meridians end and begin at the fingers and toes, where the polarity of Chi is said to

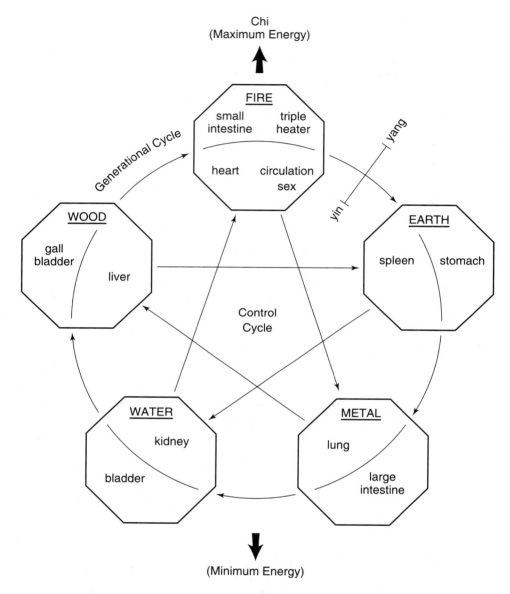

FIGURE 2.4   The Interconnection of Yin and Yang and the Five Elements

change (Mann, 1964). Most needling is done below the elbows and knees because energy circulation is most easily influenced near the origins and termination of the meridians. Accuracy of insertion is paramount. Even slight errors in needle placement will result in ineffective treatment. Needles are usually left in place for several minutes and, frequently, the acupuncturist will move or twirl them to increase the stimulation (Weil, 1983).

The needles are made up of solid stainless steel with a rounded point that pushes the tissue aside without cutting it. Needles must be sterile and disposable for the prevention of transmission of the AIDS virus, hepatitis, and any other transferrable blood-borne pathogens. Some patients have reported a slight pricking sensation on insertion and a characteristic tingling or feeling of heaviness that occurs once the needle is properly placed. After 20 to 30 minutes, the needles are removed without discomfort. Patients have reported experiencing light-headedness or euphoria, but most describe a feeling of contentment or relaxation after treatment. The number of treatments will vary according to the individual and the problem he or she is having. For acute ailments, only a few treatments—sometimes just one—are necessary. Chronic problems usually require more treatments.

Acupuncture is gaining acceptance by many contemporary U.S. medicinal practitioners. Acupuncture is routinely used to treat a wide variety of medical problems throughout the Far East, in Great Britain, Europe, Russia, and Asia. As a medical system, acupuncture has withstood the test of time, and it is likely that more individuals have been treated by acupuncture in the course of human history than by all other known systems of medicine combined (Weil, 1983).

Herbal Cures.   All Chinese medicinal herbs have specific properties and flavors that are important signs of their actions. There are hundreds of different herbs used in Chinese medicine. Knowing their properties and flavors helps to guide medical practice. There are many books available that provide a comprehensive list of Chinese herbs and their usage. Three available comprehensive books are listed below:

1. *The essential book of traditional Chinese medicine* by Liu Yanchi. Published by Columbia University Press, 1988.
2. *The chemical constituents of oriental herbs* by Yu-Pan Chen and Mei-na Hung. Published by Oriental Healing Arts Institute, 1985.
3. *Chinese herbs, their botany, chemistry, and pharmacodynamics* by John D. Keys. Published by C. E. Tuttle, 1976.

Because Chinese medicine has used herbs for centuries, many have survived the test of time and have even become popular in the United States. Four of the most popular Chinese herbs used in the United States are Ginseng (*Panax ginseng*), Dong Quai (*Angelica sinensis*), Ginger (*Zingiver officinale*), and Ma Huang (*Ephedra*).

> *Ginseng* is used to increase energy, relieve stress, resist illness, enhance sexual behavior, reduce cholesterol, regulate blood sugar, and protect the heart and liver. Overuse of this herb may cause nervousness, insomnia, breast pain, and diarrhea.
>
> *Dong Quai* taken as a tea is used to treat cramps, PMS, irregular periods, hot flashes, and fatigue.
>
> *Ginger* is used to relieve motion sickness, indigestion, and nausea. Ginger works best before vomiting begins.
>
> *Ma Huang* is used to treat respiratory conditions such as bronchial asthma and congestion. It is also used as an herbal weight loss remedy. This herb was the forerunner

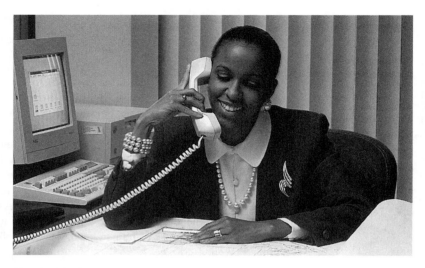

Photo by John Coletti.

He who has health has hope, and he who has hope has everything.

—Arabian Proverb

to pseudoephedrine, the active ingredient in over-the-counter decongestants such as Sudafed. This herb should be taken with caution, especially in individuals with heart problems or high blood pressure.

Caution! Deadly Herbs. Even though herbs have been used by all cultures and for thousands of years, they still can be dangerous to your health. Herbs, like prescription and over-the-counter drugs, need to be taken with caution. According to Varro Tyler (1994), the following herbs may be dangerous to your health:

Comfrey root: Used to treat stomach ulcers and as a blood purifier. Evidence indicates it can cause liver cancer.

Sassafras: Promoted as a blood purifier and anti-infective, it is carcinogenic in rats and mice.

Chaparral is used to treat cancer, colds, arthritis, sexually-transmitted diseases, and cramps. It can cause severe liver damage.

Germander is used for weight loss but is linked to hepatitis.

Pokeroot is used for arthritis, cancer, swollen breasts, and other ailments. It is highly toxic and has been associated with illness and death among children.

Other Asian Healing Practices

The traditional healer in the Cambodian immigrant community is the "loke kruu." These practitioners, like practitioners in other cultures, are greatly revered and trusted. Many common ailments are treated in some interesting ways that most Western practitioners don't understand. Cambodians and Laotians use mentholated balms to treat a variety of conditions, including bruises, upset stomachs, the flu, colds, and insect bites. Ginseng is also used as a preventative and cure-all tonic. One of the most interesting treatments is known as "coin rubbing": A coin or spoon is used to rub over a preselected body part, depending on the symptom or problem. The mentholated balms or other ointments are used to massage the area first before the skin becomes red from the rubbing. For example, the skin between the eyes is rubbed or pinched until it becomes red for the treatment of headaches.

Ayurveda: Traditional Indian Medicine

Ayurveda has its roots in India and dates back to 1500 B.C. Loosely translated, it means " "the science of life." It is important to make the distinction between treatment of disease and living life completely. Ayurveda focuses on living a true and naturally balanced life and Ayurveda treatment of disease is based on bringing life back into balance. Ayurveda unifies the knowledge, nature, and divinity within us. Health is defined as soundness of body (*shira*), mind (*manas*), and self (*atman*). Each of these must be nurtured if the individual is to create health (CyberIndia, 1996). Ayurveda offers a holistic approach based on the understanding that no single agent by itself causes disease or brings health.

Ayurveda views the person as a composite of three forces or humors (called *doshas*). These terms are difficult to translate into English because they can be understood, experienced, or felt only from their qualities, behavior, and actions in the body (Chauhan, 1996). No two individuals are alike because each is a unique combination of the three forces. Therefore, an individual with a predominantly *pitta* constitution will experience symptoms that are quite different than those for *vata* and *kapha*.

1. *Vata* is the force compared to air;
2. *Pitta* is the force compared to fire;
3. *Kapha* is force compared to mucus and water.

The quality and the relative balance of these forces determines health and disease. When the equilibrium of the doshas is upset, disease or disorder of the body occurs. When these forces act harmoniously, the functions of digestion, absorption, and elimination (physically and mentally) create health. As these three forces are responsible for specific areas of body/mind function, the symptoms of imbalance indicate which of these forces is deficient or excessive (CyberIndia, 1996). For example, excess vata causes arthritis and excess pitta causes acidity, ulcers, and liver disorders (Chauhan, 1996). The disruption of the doshas can be caused by a variety of factors, such as eating too much of certain foods, problems with relationships, environmental factors, such as noise or too much television, or having too much sex. Remember, Ayurveda is about putting balance in all the things that you do in life. Too much or too little of any one thing leads to a disruption of balance in the body, mind, or self.

Eating too much of raw foods, watching excessive TV, being surrounded by loud noises, having too much sex, participating in too much sports, and taking too much medicine are some factors that are responsible for increasing vata, resulting in some of the following conditions: weakened nervous system, constipation, vertigo, insomnia, and dry skin.

Drinking too many caffeinated drinks or excessive smoking can increase pitta of the body, which will cause such disorders as fever, ulcers, and liver disorders. Eating too many fatty foods or not being physically active can increase kapha in the body. Some of the symptoms of this condition include congestion in the chest and obesity.

Once a person recognizes what increases or decreases each of the doshas and understands the symptoms associated with each, he or she can apply Ayurveda treatments to restore balance. Treatment is based on removing the cause of the disruption of the doshas. Treatments may also include natural medicines comprised of powders, tablets, medicated oils, herbs, plants, and minerals. Yoga and meditation are also used to help individuals deepen the knowledge of who and what they are within nature.

American Indians and the Concept of Harmony and Health

American Indians consist of many different tribes that share both similar and different beliefs, languages, traditions. The following discussion is based on common beliefs about traditional medicine and provides generalizations about traditional medicine among American Indians that can be used as a guideline in understanding tribal beliefs about illness and health.

For centuries, American Indian cultures understood health to mean simply the balance or beauty of all things physical, spiritual, emotional, and social. Sickness was seen as something out of balance, the absence of harmony. The concept that all things are connected, just as the blood that unites one family, is common, despite the heterogeneity of culture, language, and values of the many Indian tribes. The notion that an individual is merely a part of the web of life means that what each person does to others, he or she does to himself or herself. Thus, he or she not only becomes one with the ultimate harmony, but is the harmony.

This belief can best be summarized by the words of Gladys Reichard (1959), a lifelong student of Navaho religion:

> The Navaho religion must be considered a design in harmony, a striving for rapport between man and every phase of nature, the earth and the waters under the earth, and the sky and the land beyond the sky, and of course the earth and everything on it. (p. 6)

This interrelatedness between people and the environment and the inclusion of a greater spirit is a common thread in the concept of wellness and well-being for many American Indians and Alaskan Natives. Many healing ceremonies and ritualistic dances seek to reaffirm oneness with the universe and restore harmony and balance as a part of treating illnesses and misfortune. Most importantly, most traditional Indian beliefs focus on prevention and wellness, not illness.

Many American and Alaska Native groups believe that there is a reason for every illness. Every illness is the consequence of a past, present, or future act. Reasons for illness can range from violating cultural taboos to supernatural interventions by sorcery. For example, the visible congenital anomalies of a child may be attributed to the child's parent who failed to obey tribal taboos concerning tribal prenatal customs.

Native Americans believe that illness is caused by either natural or unnatural causes. Natural causes of disease or misfortune are easily explainable. They occur as a result of natural consequences. If a person eats something disagreeable, it may cause diarrhea. If a person accidentally hits his or her finger with a hammer, it will hurt and possibly bleed. Natural diseases are easily treatable with folk remedies. However, "why" the accident happened may require the assistance of a special healer.

Unnatural causes of disease or misfortune are thought to be a result of evil forces, angry gods, or ancestors as a form of punishment for violating certain rituals or customs. Witchcraft, demons, and malevolent supernatural forces are the major causes of disease. Demons and evil spirits may enter the human body and bring ill health with them or sorcerers and hostile *shamans* may entice souls from the bodies. *Shamans* are special healers who are called on to remove the unnatural causes. For example, it might be necessary to call for rituals of exorcism to remove seizure disorders or other violent outbursts that have been caused by a supernatural force.

The special healers within most tribes go by different names, *medicine man, medicine woman, shaman,* and *Native practitioner.* However, they are not all the same. Each has special responsibilities, A medicine man or woman is not a true shaman. Shamans have the ability to journey in a meditative state to another world that is filled with objects, individuals, and various kinds of spirits. While visiting this other world, the shaman communicates with the spirits and gains both experience for healing as well as an ally who can intercede on the community's behalf. Shamans often use hallucinogenic plants as a tool to help change their consciousness. Drumming, chanting, rattles, and dancing are used to direct the travels. Medicine men and women do not ascend or descend into other worlds or talk to supernaturals. They need no special trance, ecstatic vision, or mystic vocation to enter their role as healers. Medicine men and women do, however, use the vast amount of symbolic material and rituals associated with Native American beliefs (Sander, 1979). Historically, tribal medicine men and women practice some aspects of shamanism for various reasons: physical, psychic, or spiritual healing; divining new hunting grounds; and ridding their communities of evil spirits. This symbolic healing complex could be called "symbolic shamanism" (Sander, 1979).

In modern Native American communities, the term *shaman* is usually used for healers whose primary practice is treating illnesses associated with malevolent spirits. Medicine men and women, on the other hand, are religious leaders as much as doctors, treating spiritual and physical ailments at the same time. They tend to treat illnesses caused by both natural and supernatural causes. Herbalists and diagnosticians are specialists within the healing community who practice a specific form of intervention.

Shamans have been an integral part of many cultures through eons of human life and throughout the world. More amazing is that the techniques used are similar and these techniques have existed from the very beginnings of history to modern day shamans. The approaches may be different and yet they are amazingly alike. Most ceremonies are similar in that they include dancing, drumming, singing of songs, the telling of great mythologies that explain the cosmos, and healing of individuals. Even healing techniques by shamans around the world are similar. They suck bad spirits out of the bodies of the sick with their mouths, use rattles and drums around the body of the sick, use herbal remedies from local plants, and sing songs of power in order to dominate the spirits that have entered the body of the sick person. Of course, each society has its own particular methods known only to them, but, for the most part, many of these things are shared by people who have never had any contact.

The sweat lodge ceremony, which is still practiced today, is an important part of healing for Native Americans. A sweat ceremony is a communal affair in which many persons who know the patient will expect the patient to benefit from it. The sweat ceremony is one of physical and spiritual purification practiced by Native Americans to overcome illness and other problems. The sweat lodge ceremony is performed in a tentlike structure with a round pit dug in the center of the floor. Rocks are heated in a fire outside the structure then brought into the sweat lodge by a fire keeper. The medicine man or woman throws water and cedar and other herbs on the hot rocks. There are specific prayers, sand paintings, and drumming, and songs are sung and specific rituals are performed. The sweat ceremony purifies the body of evil or malignant influences. The songs, paintings, and religious pieces are used for evocation. Through specific ceremonial practices the patient is brought into psychic union with the powers that have been called forth by the medicine man. Then the transformation (freedom from disease and disharmony) is described through song and prayer. The final stage is one of release, in which the power built up in the patient must be released back into nature. The patient must observe some special restrictions for several days after the ceremony before he or she is finally released. The use of drugs or alcohol, for example, may be restricted for at least 24 hours.

The most recognized contribution by Native Americans to modern medicine has been in the area of herbal medicines. Before colonialism in American, many Native American tribes had their own remedies for different ailments, using plants and herbs. Some of the most well-known drugs include digitalis, quinine, belladonna, cocaine, curare, and ipecac. Unfortunately, as time passed, forced tribal relocations resulted in the loss of knowledge of plants and herbal remedies. However a few remedies are still practiced in many Native American homes today and are being passed on to the next generation. For example, sage tea is still used for colds, sore throats, and decongestion. Peppermint tea is still used for diarrhea, upset stomachs, and colic for babies.

FIGURE 2.5 A Partial List of Traditional Indian Medicines Still Used in Canada

Plant	Symptom	Preparation	How Used
Black Spruce	Cough	Soft inner bark	Chewed
Sage	Colds	Boiled	Inhaled
Soapberry	Diarrhea	None	Eaten
Spruce needles	Eye infection	Needles boiled	Eye wash
Strawberry leaf	Safe pregnancy	Dried and boiled	Drunk
Tamarack bark	Stomach trouble	Beaten, tea added	Drunk
Wild rhubarb	Arthritis	Boiled as tea	Drunk
Willow leaves	Insect stings	Chewed and applied	As poultice

Source: Duane Champagne, ed., *The Native North American Almanac.* Detroit: Gale Research, 1994.

Hispanic Americans/Latinos

Giachello (1994) reported that good health, according to some Hispanic cultures, means that a person is behaving to his or her conscience, God's mandate, and the norms and customs of his or her group-church, family, and local community. Illness, then, according to Giachello has been perceived as the result of the following causes: (a) psychological states, such as embarrassment, envy, anger, fear, fright, excessive worry, turmoil in the family, improper behavior, and violations of moral codes; (b) environmental or natural conditions, such as bad air, germs, dust, excess cold or heat, bad food, or poverty; and (c) supernatural causes, such as malevolent spirits, bad luck, witchcraft, and living enemies (believed to cause harm out of vengeance or envy).

Although there may be similarities in traditional Latino medical systems, there are important differences among subgroups. The Mexican American system is called *curanderismo*. According to modern Western medicine, germs cause illness. Many Mexican American patients believe they may be a victim of malevolent forces or suffer from soul loss. Several unique illnesses are reported by Mexican Americans. *Susto* is sometimes called *magical fright* or *soul loss* and occurs when an apparition or a frightening event causes the soul to leave the body. Symptoms include sleepiness, anorexia, insomnia, loss of appetite, palpitations, and depression. Susto is the most-studied psychosomatic illness.

> *Bilis* is the result of excessive bile in one's system. A person can become ill with bilis if he or she becomes angry or frightened.
>
> *Empacho* is an illness caused by food that sticks to the stomach lining. This occurs most frequently when a person consumes a "hot" food instead of a "cold" food or vice versa. Symptoms include stomach aches, diarrhea, vomiting, and fever.
>
> *Envidia* (envy) is set off when a person is envious of another. Harm can occur to the object or person admired. Touching the object or person after admiring it is thought to remove the harmful force.
>
> *Mal aire* (bad air) is caused by an evil wind or by the air being at a different temperature from the individual, such as a cool breeze or draft passing over a warm or hot person. Symptoms can range from a common cold or flu to pains in a joint or in the eyes and ears.

Puerto Ricans have a medical religious system called *espiritismo,* which is a belief in an eternal good God, that emphasizes the spiritual over the material and considers "do unto others as you would have them do unto you" as its highest ethical rule. Espiritismo believes in the spirit world of help and protection and harm and danger. Everyone is believed to have a guardian spirit. Through spiritual *espirista* mediums who are usually women, individuals help patients with emotional, interpersonal, and social problems, as well as physical problems such as fatigue, aches, pains, and rashes. Mediums can exorcise evil spirits or call them forward in revengeful sorcery as well as connect with good spirits.

Many Cuban Americans believe in Santeria, a belief system similar to espiritismo except that they go to a priest (*santeros*) instead of a medium. The priest will, hopefully, change life's events in their favor by connecting with the *orishas* (the evil spirits that are causing problems). Cuban Americans believe the Santeros can undo evil spells (*bilongo*) as well as perform an *ebbo* (protective spell). Spirit diseases are also believed to be caused by magic (a person can harm another by using a picture or object), soul loss (a person's soul can be taken by a witch), spirit intrusion (the spirits of the dead are angry with the living), and the evil eye.

Not all Latinos, of course, believe in traditional medical systems. Research has shown that Latinos are more likely to believe in the traditional folk medicine system if they have lived in the United States for only a short time, have little formal education, or come from lower socioeconomic or rural backgrounds. Researchers also report that Hispanics in the United States who prefer to speak Spanish tend to be fatalists. That is, they attribute illness to luck, supernatural powers (such as spirits), and God, rather than their own actions and activities.

Mexican Americans do not typically go directly to a physician when they are ill. There is a hierarchy of lay healers who are sought out first. The first contact is usually a neighbor or relative. If the family or friends cannot treat the condition, the patient is referred to an herbalist (*yerbero*), massage therapist (*sobador*), or midwife (*patera*). If these specialists cannot handle the problem, the patient is referred to a special lay healer called a *curandero* (Chavira & Trotter, 1981). These special folk healers have the ability to treat not only natural diseases, with such treatments as herbs and massage, but unnatural diseases caused by evil spirits.

Two different but related concepts about diseases have evolved in Hispanic culture. The first concept, that disease is caused naturally by an imbalance of hot and cold principles, evolved from the ancient Greek concept of an imbalance of the four humors. The second concept is that disease is caused by supernatural factors such as evil spirits, the evil

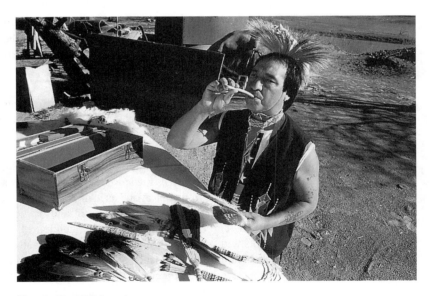

Photo by David Weintraub.

It is part of the cure to wish to be cured.

—Seneca (3 B.C.–A.D. 65)

eye, or black magic. The latter cause of illness must be cared for magically. Regardless of the cause, many Hispanic cultures have used folk medicine as part of the healing process.

Diseases are classified as either "hot" or "cold." A "cold" disease is characterized by vasoconstriction and a low metabolic rate while a "hot" disease is characterized by vasodilation and a high metabolic rate. Examples of "hot" diseases are hypertension, diabetes, and acid indigestion. Some "cold" examples are menstrual cramps, pneumonia, and colic. The goal of treatment is to restore balance. Thus, "hot" diseases are treated with "cold" remedies and "cold" diseases are treated with "hot." It is also important for individuals to avoid being exposed to extreme temperatures.

Curing illness with herbs is still common practice among many Hispanic cultures. The medicinal practice of using herbs has its foundation in early Spanish medical practice. Eighteenth century Spanish explorers tapped the knowledge of the Indians' native herbal remedies. The Meso-American Indians, for example, had established a pharmacy of over 5,000 well studied herbal medications well before the colonials settled in the America. Herbs are used to balance "hot" and "cold" diseases. Hypertension, for example, is defined as a "hot" illness. Cool remedies such as bananas and lemon juice are popular as well as passion flowers. Menstrual difficulties are "cold" problems and can be countered with "hot" remedies such as oregano.

Curanderos.   Folk healers called *curanderos* are special individuals in the community who are called on to use their gift of healing to tell whether an illness is caused by nature or an evil *brujo* (witch or sorcerer). Among very traditional Mexican American families and, often, low-income families, witchcraft, hexes, the evil eye, and fright are common sources of disease and disorder. Curanderos are the clearly acknowledged experts in diagnosing and treating these illnesses in the *barrio* (Chavira & Trotter, 1981). The curandero has the special ability to determine whether the illness is natural or supernatural. If it is a natural disease, the curandero may use herbal remedies, make referrals to a medical doctor, or, on occasion, use supernatural intervention. If the disease is determined to be supernatural, it is the curandero's job to rid the cursed patient's body of the *brujo*.

The curanderos use methods of healing such as massaging the body with specially blended plants and oils, bleeding, sweating, prayers and offerings to pagan gods, good and evil spirits, and Christian saints. Curanderos will also use magic, herbs, and minerals, and other objects to perform their healing (Chavira & Trotter, 1981). However, curanderos

FIGURE 2.6   Examples of Folk Remedies

Herb	Use
Garlic	Cough
Chamomile	Nausea, flatus, colic
Passion flower	Anxiety
Peppermint	Dyspepsia, flatus
Aloe vera	External cuts, burns
Mullein	Asthma

know what they can handle and what they cannot and will refer severe health problems to a medical professional.

Curanderismo has its roots in the Spanish ideology concerning the power of the devil to do harm and Spanish Catholicism and its concept of "divine healing," which is the ability of a human, with the grace of God, to heal. Curanderos with the power to heal claim God gave them that power. They cite the following passage in the Bible to justify their activities:

> *(1 Corinthians 12: 7–11)* In each of us the Spirit is manifested in a particular way, for some useful purpose. One man, through the Spirit, has the gift of wise speech, while another, by the power of the same Spirit, can put the deepest knowledge into words. Another by the same Spirit, is granted faith; another, by the one Spirit, gifts of healing, and another miraculous powers; another has the gift of prophecy, and another ability to distinguish true spirits from false; yet another has the gift of ecstatic utterance of different kinds, and another the ability to interpret it. But all these gifts are the works of one and the same Spirit, distributing them separately to each individual at will. (Chavira & Trotter, 1981) (p. 27)

Many Mexican Americans are Catholic. This means that the Catholic church and its many beliefs and rituals (mass, baptism, communion, confirmation, and confession) are strongly integrated into the lives of many families. Prayer and the celebration of the many sacraments of the Catholic church are part of the health process.

Central America.   Immigrants from Central America classify illnesses based on hot and cold qualities. Certain sicknesses or conditions are considered "hot" and others "cold." Food and medicines also fall into these categories. Like Chinese medicine, treatment is based on balancing the temperature equilibrium between foods and medicines. But the most important disturbance is from foods one chooses to eat. Some foods are hot, others cold, so careful choice is required to retain, or regain, equilibrium. Herbs are an important part of the treatments. Childbirth and the postpartum period are seen as very cold times, and sometimes new mothers in the hospital are shocked to be served ham, a notoriously cold food (Gleave & Manes, 1990). Lay healers also exist within immigrant communities and are often the main source of medical care, especially for the poor and uneducated.

African American Medicine

Traditional African American health beliefs and practices stem from the West African cultures of the slaves and persisted through slavery to the present (Mbiti, 1975). West African cultures maintain a holistic belief and see no real separation between the mind, body, and spirit (Jacques, 1976). Health is attained when one can achieve a state of harmony with nature and oneself. Illness occurs when this harmony is disrupted. They see themselves as children of mother nature. The medicine of African natives claims to be based on the highest conception of life and the universe (Sakurazawa, 1966).

Folk health among African Americans has survived for centuries, and folk healers continue to exist in many Southern African American communities, many of them older African American women. This role began in the days of slavery when older women, called *slave doctors,* used herbs and roots to maintain the health of the other slaves (Bailey, 1991). These female indigenous healers continue to use prayer and teas in their treatment. Minor illnesses are believed to have natural causes and cures, whereas major illnesses have supernatural causes and cures (Landrine et al., 1992).

Religion is an integral part of the African American community. Belief in Jesus is a prerequisite for acquiring the power; one cannot heal without faith in God. As a result, prayer is a common method of healing illness in the rural South. It is not uncommon for members of church congregations to gather to pray for the recovery of a fellow parishioner. Often these group prayers, accompanied by singing, are highly emotional. Through the spirituality provided by religion, African Americans also recognize and worship powers beyond themselves. The preacher is a positive life force in the health of community members (Harrison, 1992).

African Americans in Southern Rural Communities.   Folk medicine has persisted in some rural Southern African American communities in spite of the rise of modern medicine. Folk practitioners still provide services that meet an important human need. Within some rural southern communities, three types of healers exist: (1) those who have learned the ability from others; these are the individuals considered to have the least amount of power, (2) older persons who received the gift of healing from God during a religious experience in later life; these have medium power, and (3) those who are born with the gift of healing, the most powerful (Snow, 1984).

Root and herb doctors are included among those who learned to heal from others, and are believed to have the least healing power (Snow, 1974). Faith or spiritual healers, practitioners with the greatest power, are believed to have received the gift of healing from a God (Mitchell, 1978/1984). The laying on of hands and frequent use of prayer are methods most used to treat illness. Most individuals who acquire the power through learning or apprenticeship are able to treat natural and/or occult illnesses, but the person who is born with the power or who receives the gift from a god can cure all illnesses, natural, occult, and spiritual (Watson, 1984).

Elderly African Americans, in particular, who were exposed to the historical traditions of early folk healers use a variety of herbs and over-the-counter preparations that appear to be unique to their ethnic group. Some of their basic drugs includes such ingredients as spirits of turpentine, camphor, flowers of sulfur, oil of cloves, and assafetida (Watson, 1984). Watson listed the following home remedies used by folk practitioners:

- Honey and lemon and whiskey tea, used to handle a cold
- Warm salt water, for a fever
- Garlic cloves, for blood pressure
- Eucalyptus oil and honey, for colds
- Fat meat or potatoes, for boils
- raw egg, for boils
- Penny and chewed tobacco, for a rusty nail wound
- Strings tied on the leg, for cramps
- Coins, keys, for a bleeding nose
- Beer, for prevention of worms

- Turpentine and sugar, to promote healing of open wounds
- Kerosene and sugar, for colds
- Silver dollar and belly band, for protruding navel
- Mustard seed, for asthma
- Dirt and clay rocks, for headaches
- Standing on head, for headaches

In spite of the fact that medical doctors are available in southern rural communities, this has not significantly diminished the presence and/or use of these folk remedies. Physicians who work with patients from these rural areas generally have a better understanding of the importance of folk medicine because they realize that it is based on a system of cultural knowledge and an integral feature of the social life and health care in small, poor, and ethnically homogeneous communities.

Voodoo.   Although the religion of Voodoo is not a major force in the lives of most West Indians, Voodoo does have African roots. Because it still has some influence in some communities, a brief history and description is necessary. Voodoo developed in the United States around 1700, when African slaves from the African kingdom of Dahomey (now the Republic of Benin) were transported from the French West Indies to the Louisiana territory. Louisiana, especially New Orleans, is most associated with Voodoo. Vodu (now known as voodoo) was the religion of the Dahomean slaves. Vodu religion included gods, cults, rituals, sorcery, black magic, and the belief that illness or bad luck is caused when one person places a hex or spell on another. Voodoo ceremonies are often exotic and include fires, boiling cauldrons, chanting, Congo drums, and whirling dances. The python, a primary god in voodoo, is an integral part of ceremonies. Coffins, bones, torches, and animal blood add to the mystique and fear.

Voodoo leaders called *queens* and *kings* have the power to cast spells and remove hexes through the use of their powerful *gris-gris* (charms, potions, and powders). It is believed that these special kings and queens can literally "voodoo" someone to death. Individuals have actually laid down to die because they believed that sorcery had been worked on them. They died that day for reasons science cannot fully explain. Scientists sometimes call such deaths "voodoo deaths," a reference to the magical religion of voodoo. Voodoo deaths do not result from heart attacks or other understood diseases. Some voodoo deaths are sudden, others result from a nervous collapse before overwhelming fright. As in so many mind/body mysteries, belief seems to be the key.

Voodoo flourished in the 1800s in the New Orleans area but is no longer the force that it once was. However, Voodoo still persists in some African American communities.

Muslims.   Many African Americans have embraced Islamic practices and the teachings attributed to Allah. It is estimated that there are over 900 Muslims in the world, including about 8 million in North America. The holy book of the Quran teaches that all must live in accordance with the laws enacted by Allah. When there is any disturbance or deviation from the inherent discipline of Tasbeeh, then there is disease. *Tasbeeh* refers to the glorifying and praising of Allah. In humans, such a disease can be moral (psychological), pathological, or a combination of both. If a patient is suffering from a moral disease, he or she must turn to the Quran because it is a guide and healing to those who believe.

When a practicing Muslim becomes sick, he or she goes to a qualified medical doctor (preferably a practicing Muslim). Islamic medicine and Western medicine have many similarities because they have the same historical roots. Therefore, Muslim doctors are not lay healers. They are medically trained in the same manner as Western physicians are trained. According to Islamic teachings, all diseases have a cure because Allah would not inflict a disease without prescribing a cure for it. The cure is known to whoever knows it, and known to whoever does not know it. By accepting this concept, every Muslim patient maintains hope of recovery, which is essential to the healing process.

Muslim doctors believe they are the agents of God and that the act of healing is not entirely in their hands. They may prescribe the treatment but the will of Allah is the ultimate healer. This spiritual conviction certainly improves the psychological state of the patient and will increase hope of recovery, and thus help him or her overcome weakness or sickness.

General Overview of the Lay Theories of Illness Causation

In general, lay theories of illness have a four-layer etiology. The four layers are: (1) the patient, (2) the natural world, (3) the social world, and (4) the supernatural world. Illness can be caused by one of these factors or illness can be a combination of all four factors. The social and supernatural etiologies are usually found in non-Western societies, while natural and patient-centered explanations are in the Western world. The four layers are briefly discussed below.

1. *The patient.* The cause of the illness is mainly (though not completely) the patient's responsibility. The patient has created much of his or her own illness through poor diet and negative health behaviors, such as smoking, drinking, carelessness, and poor hygiene. The patient is generally reminded of his or her unhealthy behavior and is often made to feel guilty.
2. *The natural world.* This includes the natural aspects of one's environment. Common conditions, such as excess heat, cold, wind, rain, and snow, are related to certain illnesses (e.g., excess exposure to the sun can cause sunstroke). Natural etiologies also include illnesses caused by outside organisms (e.g., germs, viruses, parasites, worms, animals, pollens, poisons, fumes, and smoke).
3. *The social world.* In non-Western worlds, the most common causes of illness are witchcraft, sorcery, voodoo, and the evil eye. The social etiology may also include physical injuries, such as poisoning or war wounds, caused by other people. In Western society, stress conflicts between family, friends, children, or other people may be included in the social world.
4. *The supernatural world.* Supernatural entities, such as Gods and malevolent spirits, are the causes of illness. The invasion of these supernatural entities has been brought on by some type of moral or social misbehavior by the patient. Repentance, prayer, and exorcism are needed to remove these supernatural entities.

In most lay theories of illness, the cause is multifaceted. This means that several causes are acting together, and that the patient, the natural world, the social world, and the supernatural world are not mutually exclusive, but usually linked together in a particular case.

Conclusion

As the immigrant population increases in various cities and hospitals, doctors are regularly faced with individuals who also seek treatment from curanderos, voodoo doctors, shamans, faith healers, and herbalists. As a result, some doctors have begun to recognize how important these lay practitioners are in the lives of their patients and have consulted with and invited lay practitioners to the hospital. Although most Western physicians do not believe in the methods of these healers, they find that cooperating is healthier for the patient. Patients have a tendency to comply with the medications or treatments when the lay healer sanctifies them. The medical profession is beginning to recognize that these lay healers may provide patients with psychological and emotional counseling. With the aid of the lay healers, the healing focuses on the individual as a spiritual whole and not as a dysfunctional body part.

REFERENCES

Ader, R., and Cohen, N. (1985). CNS-immune system interactions: Conditioning phenomena. *Behavioral and Brain Sciences,* 8, 379–395.

Baca Zinn, M. *Problems of inequality: Race and ethnicity.* In D. Stanley & M. Baca Zinn (eds.), *Social problems* (4th ed.). Boston, MA: Allyn & Bacon, 1989.

Bailey, E. J. *Urban African-American health care.* New York: University Press of America, 1991.

Bresler, D., and Kroening, R. Three essential factors in effective acupuncture therapy. *American Journal of Chinese Medicine,* 4(1), 81–86, 1976.

Buck, R. *Human motivation and emotion.* New York: Wiley, 1988.

Champagne, D. (Ed.) *The Native North American almanac.* Detroit: Gale Research, 1994.

Chauhan, P. *Home menu: Ayurvedic medicine.* 1996. http://www.ayurvedic.org/

Chavira, J., and Trotter, R. *Curanderismo.* Athens, GA: University of Georgia Press, 1981.

CyberIndia. *Ayurveda.* 1996. http://www.cyberindia.ne...ia/healthsc/ayurveda.htm

Davis, D. The history and sociology of the scientific study of acupuncture. *American Journal of Chinese Medicine* 3: 5–26, 1975.

DiMatteo, M. *The psychology of health, illness, and medical care.* Pacific Grove, CA: Brooks/Cole, 1991.

Giachello, A. Hispanics' access to health care: Issues for the 1990s. In C. Molina and M. Aguirre-Molina (Eds.), *Latino health: America's growing challenge for the 21st century* pp. 83–114. Washington, DC: American Public Health Association, 1994.

Gleave, D., and Manes, A. The Central Americans. In N. Waxler-Morrison, J. Anderson, and E. Richardson, (Eds.), *Cross-cultural caring: A handbook for health professionals.* Vancouver: UCB Press, 1990.

Harrison, I. Community AIDS education: Trials and tribulations in raising consciousness for prevention. In H. Baer and Y. Hones (Eds.), *African-Americans in the south: Issues of race, class and gender.* 72–93. Athens, GA: The University of Georgia Press, 1992.

Hastings, A., Fadiman, J., and Gordon, J. *Health for the whole person.* Boulder, CO: Westview Press, 1980.

Institute of Noetic Sciences, with William Poole. *The heart of healing.* Atlanta, GA: Turner Publishing, 1993.

Jacques, G. Cultural health traditions: A black perspective. In M. Branch and P. Paxton (Eds.), *Providing safe nursing care for ethnic people of color.* New York: Appleton-Century-Crofts, 1976.

Laderman, C., and Roseman, M. The performance of healing. New York: Routledge, 1996.

Landrine, H., Klonoff, E., and Brown-Collins, A. Cultural diversity and methodology in feminist psychology, *Psychology of Women Quarterly,* 16, 145–163, 1992.

Mann, F. *The meridians of acupuncture.* London: William Heinemann Medical Books, 1964.

Mibti, J. S. *African religions and philosophies.* Garden City, NY: Anchor, 1975.

Mitchell, F. Hoodoo medicine: Sea Islands herbal remedies. Berkeley, CA: AND/OR Press, 1978. In W. Watson (Ed.), *Black folk medicine.* New Brunswick, NJ: Transaction, 1984.

Palos, S. *The Chinese art of healing.* New York: McGraw-Hill, 1971.

Porket, M. Chinese medicine: A traditional healing science. In D. Sobel (Ed.), *Ways of health.* New York: Harcourt Brace Jovanovich, 1979.

Randall-David, E. *Strategies for working with culturally diverse communities and clients.* Association for the Care of Children's Health, Bureau of Maternal and Child Health and Resources Development, Publication No. MCH11373. Washington, DC: U.S. Department of Health and Human Services, 1989.

Reichards, G. A. *Navaho medicine man.* New York: J. J. Augustine, 1959.

Sakurazawa, Yukikazu. *The book of judgment.* Los Angeles, CA: Ignoramus Press, 1966.

Sander, D. *Navaho Indian medicine and medicine men.* In D. Sobel (Ed.), *Ways of health.* New York: Harcourt Brace Jovanovich, 1979.

Smolam, R., Moffitt, P., and Naythons, M. *The power to heal: Ancient arts & modern medicine.* New York: Prentice-Hall, 1990.

Snow, L. Folk medical beliefs and their implications for care of patients: A review based on studies among black Americans. *Annals of Internal Medicine 81,* (1974): 82–96. In W. Watson (Ed.), *Black folk medicine.* New Brunswick, NJ: Transaction, 1984.

Tyler, V. Caution! deadly herbs. In T. R. Rand, (Ed.), *The healing power of herbs. Redbook* (November 1994), p. 102.

Wallnofer, H., and von Rottauscher, A. *Chinese folk medicine.* New York: Bell, 1965.

Watson, W. (Ed.) Black folk medicine. New Brunswick, NJ: Transaction, 1984.

Weil, A. *Health and healing: Understanding conventional and alternative medicine.* Boston: Houghton Mifflin, 1983.

3 Ethnic Minority American Families

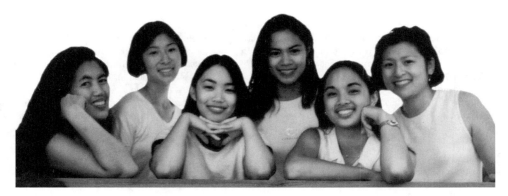

When a child has no sense of how he should fit into society around him, he is culturally deprived.
—Ralph Ellison

Photo by Courtesy of Alpha Kappa Delta Phi, published in *Cultures* magazine, volume 2, issue 1.

As we move into the 21st century, the concept of family has changed considerably. The traditional view of the ideal American family embraces the image of a lifelong monogamous marriage and the nuclear family pattern of husband and wife living together with their children in the same home. Research has shown that white American families have undergone dramatic changes in the last 30 years. There has been a shift from traditional, nuclear families to families consisting of single people, single older people, and unmarried couples (Sweet & Bumpass 1987). Divorce, remarriages, single-parent families, especially many headed by women, and various configurations of the blended family have changed this traditional image.

Minority American families have also experienced these same dramatic changes, which have implications for their economic status and security. Coupled with deteriorating economic conditions, there has been a deterioration in the well-being of minority families (Ortiz, 1995), but, the extent varies considerably by national origin, regional concentration, and other factors. Minority families, in particular, value the extended family, which has a long tradition and includes grandparents, cousins, uncles, aunts, and others.

The traditional view of families is no longer applicable as we move into the 21st century. The diversity of values, characteristics, and lifestyles that arises from such elements as geographic origin, level of acculturation, socioeconomic status, education, religious background, and age level reveals such traditional categorization to be inaccurate and ultimately unproductive (Boyd-Franklin, 1989).

Family structure also has a tremendous influence on the physical and mental health of its members. There are many myths about certain minority families that have painted a negative portrait of their functioning and the health problems that they encounter. In addition, many ethnic minority families are being referred to health clinics, hospitals, and mental health centers. It is important that practitioners and policy makers understand the family structure (both its strengths and weaknesses) of minority families. This understanding can serve as a foundation for preventive and therapeutic work.

Cultural Diversity within Minority Families

It is important to recognize that there is tremendous cultural diversity within and between each minority community in the United States. There is a tendency to categorize racial and cultural groups along stereotypical lines. Given the heterogeneity of cultural variables that are present in each minority American family, it should be clear that there is no such entity as a single kind of minority (Asian, African, Native, Hispanic) American family.

Although it is virtually impossible to write about a single minority family structure, it is possible to acknowledge a certain level of cultural similarity within each minority (Asian American, African American, Hispanic American, Native American) group without reducing the group in question to a simple singular configuration. Each family unit described in the following section will include the basic family unit and children, traditional sex roles, the elderly, and death and grief.

The Family Unit and Children

The family unit is more difficult to define than we think, because people have found so many different ways to organize "familylike" groups. The nuclear family consists of a single married couple and their children. The extended family can consist of relatives, friends, and members of the community who often assist with childcare responsibilities, finances, care of the elderly, and emotional support.

It is almost impossible for minority families in America to maintain a traditional family structure. This is true, in particular, with children. As children become more acculturated to mainstream society through school and peers, conflict often arises between them and their family when traditional customs, behaviors, and values differ from the dominant culture. Vega (1995) cited numerous studies that indicated that acculturation and the associated changes in household structure are linked with family dysfunction, low family pride, and higher levels of personal disorganization, especially adolescent pregnancy, deviant behavior, and drug use.

Conflicts in interpersonal relationships often occur for minority children because many traditional behaviors and values are unconsciously modeled and learned and become a natural part of their emotions and may conflict with the dominant culture. It can be as simple as an African American not looking another person in the eye as a recognition of that person's authority, which white Americans interpret as shiftiness and unreliability. The differences can be extreme and volatile, such as when traditional cultural expectations of men and women clash with the egalitarian view of Western society.

Ethnic minority families and, in particular, children must also make psychological sense out of the dominant culture's sometimes disparaging view of them, deflect negative messages about themselves, and negotiate racial barriers under all kinds of conditions (Greene, 1992). Ethnic minority children must face particular challenges in the course of their development that are not encountered by their white counterparts.

Traditional Sex Roles

Many anthropologists agree that, historically, within the family structure, males held formal authority over females in almost every society. Although the degree of masculine authority may vary from one group to the next, males always have more power. In most societies females are subordinate. Male dominance is so widespread that it is virtually a human universal. However, in many countries, including the United States, women are no longer devoting most of their productive years to childbearing, and childrearing; they are beginning to demand a change in the social relationships of the sexes. As women gain access to positions that control the exchange of resources, male dominance may become archaic, and industrial societies may one day become egalitarian. Many traditional minority families are facing this revolution, as minority females are now commonplace in the workforce. The traditional minority female role is now changing as they become co-wage earners in the financial survival of the family. Many are rightfully demanding that the male now share in many of the household chores and responsibilities.

The Elderly

Historically, the elderly have played a prominent role in families. In many cultures, the elderly are to be respected and revered as their age increases. They play important roles in decision-making in all matters. However, as many minority Americans have become acculturated, the feelings and responsibility to care for the elderly have diminished. In addition, older minority Americans face a higher rate of poverty, chronic illness, and disability. Many are unable to afford adequate health care and services.

Death and Grief

Although the experience of loss is universal, the expression of loss is culturally defined. Each culture uniquely frames the social group process, the prescribed roles of those affected by the loss, and the desired scenario and location in which this final transition occurs (Kawaga-Singer, 1994). Every culture has developed rituals to guide its members, both the dying and the bereaved. Across cultures, people differ in what they believe and understand about life and death, what they feel, what elicits those feelings, the appropriateness of certain feelings, and the techniques for dealing with feelings that cannot be directly expressed (Irish et al., 1993). However, when a member dies, across all cultures, death rituals reestablish emotional synchrony and a sense of equilibrium for the dying and the bereaved, and ensure group welfare and continuity (Kagawa-Singer, 1994). Grief is expressed so differently from culture to culture that one must be sensitive to making judgments about how people from another culture respond to the loss of a loved one.

The trends of minority families described in this chapter will demonstrate the unique social, economic, familial, and health characteristics that have shaped, and will continue to shape, the development of these families in the United States. The profiles of the following minority families will provide a context for understanding and interpreting the dynamic evolution of individual minority families over time.

The Hispanic American/Latino Family

The family is considered the single most important institution in the social organization of Latinos. It is through the family and its activities that all individuals relate to significant others and the community. The family is the central thread that connects all of its members to each other and the culture with all of its values. But this broad statement hides the specific and rich cultural diversity and the complex cultural adaptations of Mexicans, Cubans, Dominicans, Puerto Ricans, and Central and South Americans to the United States. Even though Latinos have broad similarities, each culture within the Latino population has its own broadly identifiable "Latino family" that is different from the others.

Each group has its own particular history and, in particular, a different socialization process within the United States. Mexican Americans, for example, originated in an area that is directly connected to the United States, while Puerto Ricans, Cubans, Dominicans, and Central and South Americans immigrated to the United States. Puerto Ricans are U.S. citizens and move freely between the island of Puerto Rico and the mainland. These factors have played an important role and affected the socialization process of each group. Puerto Ricans, for example, migrated to urban barrios (Spanish Harlem) in New York and were affected by high unemployment, poverty, and a lack of housing. Many Mexican families moved to rural settings. Cubans, on the other hand, settled in Miami and set up thriving businesses in "Little Havana." Each "Latino family" is different and expresses itself in different ways because of the variety of adaptations that each has to make to the environmental and economic conditions in which they live. The following section is a broad description of a common theme that runs through Hispanic culture.

The Family

The concept of *la familia* (the greater family) is the most important institution in life and it is the means of cultural and social existence for Latinos. *La familia* includes the extended family of parents, grandparents, brothers and sisters, cousins, and other blood relatives. The foundation of *la familia* is pancultural in Latino families, although the structure may vary, depending on the subculture. This broad concept has important consequences for actual social and cultural behavior. The extended family provides a network of social relations within which mutual support and reciprocity occur. Although the nuclear family and household is preferred to the extended family household by most Latino families, the ideology of *la familia* plays an important role in the lives of Latinos living in the United States.

As a result of *la familia*, Latinos place a great deal of value and pride on membership in the family. The importance of family membership and belonging cuts across caste lines and socioeconomic conditions (Keefe & Padilla, 1987). Individuals' relationships to other family members influence their self-confidence, sense of self-worth, security, and ethnic identity. The well-being of the Hispanic family comes before the needs of the individual.

The connecting threads of *la familia* in Mexican Americans includes: (1) the extended family of blood kin (*parientes*), (2) *parentesco* or the concept of familism, (3) *compadrazo* (godparents), (4) *confianza* (trust), and (5) family ideology. A very important characteristic of *la familia* is the *compradazo* or the institution of *compadres* (companion parents or godparents). Although the nuclear family is the basic and most significant familial unit, and normally constitutes the household (Ho, 1992), relatives sometimes interact as a social group and are often relied on for assistance in times of need. Important friends outside of the family become part of the family through a binding kinship (Keefe & Padilla, 1987). Often a godfather or godmother of a child shares in the raising of the child through economic assistance and emotional support. To become a godparent is an honor and a creates a deep sense of obligation to the family. Mexican Americans place much value on familism and interact with many relatives, see them often, and rely on them for mutual aid.

Parentesco is similar to *la familia* except that it is a kinship sentiment that is extended to nonrelatives, who become part of the family network. The institution of marriage also plays an important role in *la familia* because it strengthens extended family ties and incorporates individuals and their kin into network alliances under parentesco. *Confianza* (trust) is the underlying factor that builds relationships and forms the basis of trust in the institutions of *parentesco* and *compadrazo*. *Confianza* with someone goes beyond ordinary trust, it signifies a special relationship of sentiment and importance involving respect, dignity, and intimacy.

Family ideology among Latinos defines the ideals, roles, and behaviors of family members by providing a model of how people should act. It holds all individuals together and tells them that they should put family before their own concerns. Family ideology also defines the ideal roles and behaviors of family members. Traditional views on the ideal family revolve around a strong male figure who is responsible for the well-being of all family members who live in his household.

Children

Because children are such an important part of *la familia*, Latinos, and, in particular, Mexican Americans, tend to have large families. Mexican American families average almost five people per family, which is the largest family size for all Americans. White Americans average 2.6 people per family. Latino populations are growing, and some estimates predict that Latinos will be the largest minority in the United States by the year 2000.

The basic family theme that Mexican American children are expected to accept includes a focus on the strength of the family, a respect for the family hierarchy, the development of an interconnected extended family, and most importantly, a belief in an authoritarian, just God (Ramirez & Casteneda, 1974). The age-old dictum, "children are to be seen but not heard," summarizes the role of children in the Mexican American family. Children are to be subservient and respectful (*respecto*) to all elders.

Children are cherished and revered in the usually large families. They are taught to share and work together, and sibling rivalry is minimal. The father disciplines and controls while the mother supports and nurtures both the children and the husband. Often the father is very playful and loving to the children when they are small, but is more stern and strict with older children, especially daughters (Fitzpatrick, 1981). Grandparents play an important role in the raising of the children and it is not uncommon for extended family members to be welcomed into the home. Caribbean Islanders, such as Puerto Rican and Cuban American families, have family values similar to those of Chicano families. New immigrants are most likely to settle where their relatives have become established.

One of the new roles that children have inherited in Latino culture is to be the social brokers or go-betweens for their parents and the outside world. Because the children are educated in the American school system, they often speak better English and are more comfortable with and knowledgeable about American culture.

The development of a child's sexuality is also greatly influenced by Latino culture and values. Respect and dignity are important components of sexuality, and physical modesty

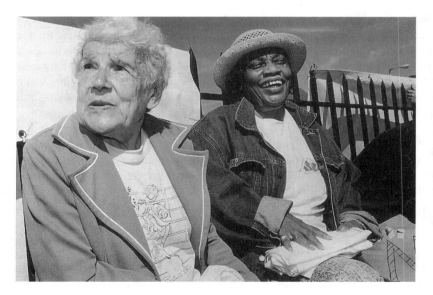

Photo by Robert Harbison.

As minorities, we must be concerned with the preservation of our culture, traditions, and identity, but we must also learn how to understand and get along with members of other groups if we are to swim successfully in the mainstream.

—Clarence Page

is an important part of one's physical presence, especially for the female. Nudity is inappropriate, except for young children. Few parents talk with their children about sex and reproduction. Females are placed under great scrutiny and control because evidence of inappropriate sexual behavior on a girl's part brings dishonor and disrespect to the family. Females are given less freedom than their brothers. Girls begin to play the role of mother and homemaker by caring for younger brothers and sisters and by helping with the housework. A boy is encouraged to join with others of his age to help socialize him into becoming an adult male (Ho, 1992).

One of the growing concerns for Latino children is the increased rate of teenage pregnancies. While the growing rate of teenage pregnancy confronts all adolescent populations in the United States, the fertility rates among Mexican American adolescents reflects the national trend. The Hispanic teen birth rate rose slightly in 1994 and matched the African American teen birth rate of 108 per 1,000 females, ages 15–19 (Child Trends, 1996). This, of course, has a direct effect on the Latino family. Latino families tend to be younger and have more children.

Traditional Sex Roles

In traditional culture the Mexican American father is the head of the household and the primary decision-maker. He is *machismo*. Machismo is a quality of personal magnetism that impresses and influences others. It is a style of personal daring by which one faces challenge, danger, and threats with calmness and self-possession (Ho, 1992). Machismo ideally encompasses a strong sense of personal honor, family, loyalty, and care for children, and is expressed as exaggerated masculinity, virility, and aggressiveness (Trankina, 1983).

The traditional hierarchical role of Mexican American males and female submission rooted in Spanish customs defines the husband–wife relationship. The man is to be the provider and protector of the family and the wife is the homemaker and the caretaker. It is his responsibility to ensure that the family has enough to eat, has clothing, and that the children get a good education. A woman is expected to be in the home looking after the family, the house, doing the sweeping, cooking, and taking care of the children.

In real life, however, this is rarely realized. Although the wife appears to be submissive to the husband in the family structure, she often assumes power behind the scenes and makes major family decisions. She often is the internal authority figure in the family. The concept of machismo is disappearing from many Mexican American families. Many Mexican American males feel that machismo is no longer necessary and that it is a thing of the past. Mexican American women also see machismo as something that is more prevalent in Mexico than in the United States (Vega, 1995).

Acculturation to white American values and society has been a major force in challenging machismo. Latinas have been forced to enter the labor force out of economic necessity because their husbands often hold disadvantaged positions in the labor market. The fact that increasing numbers of Latino families are headed by females may increase egalitarian gender participation in families, posing a direct challenge to the male dominance that once was the preferred mode (Vega, 1995). As a result, traditional sex roles in the home and the workplace are in transition.

The Elderly

Older Latinos are highly respected within their own community and often act as the "family historians" who pass on the history of the family and community to younger children and adults. There is often great pride and courage in the stories that relate the struggles and obstacles that Latinos have faced in the past and present. It is not uncommon for the elderly to be a significant part of family and community affairs. In addition, the ideology and practice of *la familia* and religious beliefs offer strong social and emotional support for the elderly.

Unfortunately, many older Mexican Americans live in poverty without Social Security and access to adequate health care. They also suffer from high rates of chronic illness and disability, such as cardiovascular disease and diabetes.

Death and Grief

Finally, because *la familia* is the basis for life, when death occurs, great effort is put into the rituals that honor the passing of a soul. In Mexican American culture, for example, everything possible is done to bring a priest to the bedside of the dying person in order to administer the last rites. Family members, the extended family, and friends are usually expressive and demonstrative about their loss and crying and grief are often animated as opposed to a "stoic" posture. Death and bereavement in Mexico and among Mexican Americans, whether in rural or urban settings, generally follow the patterns of the orthodox Catholic service. Demographic projections predict that 50 percent of American Catholics will be Hispanic by the year 2000 (Weyer, 1988).

The Catholic church does not recommend cremation. Funeral directors who are sensitive to the culture allow the family and other close friends to stay as the casket is lowered into the ground. Relatives will throw a handful of dirt on the casket before the cemetery men come to fill the grave (Younoszai, 1993). Family members also tend to stay at the gravesite for longer periods of time to look at other graves and to reminisce, recalling who died and when and from what cause (Younoszai, 1993). Novenas are said during the nine-day period following the death, and people take candles to church to light the altar.

In many Latino cultures, *Dios de Los Muertos,* or Day of the Dead, is celebrated on the first and second day of November. Community members form a procession to the graveyard where families decorate the graves of their loved ones. In addition, the Day of the Dead is celebrated with festive feasts and decorations placed on artifacts representing death. This celebration also reinforces the belief that death is a part of daily life.

The African American Family

The Family

There is a great deal of diversity among African American—families derived from geographic origins, religious values, level of acculturation, intermarriage, and socioeconomic status. This section focuses primarily on African Americans whose ancestors were brought here as slaves and who have their roots in the South. African Americans from the South represent the largest group. In addition, while disproportionate segments of African American families are poor, many younger African Americans have become affluent, college-educated, and have nuclear families. These upper income African American families have been less researched, even though they are a growing segment of the nation's consumer population. The focus of this section will be on families from the lower economic strata.

In the mid-1960s, Moynihan (1965) published a report for the U.S. Department of Labor in which he painted a dismal picture of African American families as highly unstable disorganized, deprived, and approaching breakdown, and described the continual expansion of welfare programs as a measure of the "steady disintegration of the Negro family structure over the past generation." Moynihan labeled the black family as a "tangle of pathology" because he viewed it as a matriarchal culture that ran counter to the "normal" family structure of the dominant culture. Moynihan blamed African Americans for their own social conditions while others argue that the effects of racism, segregation, and economic inequities are the major contributors to the plight of African American families.

White (1972) challenged the characterization of African American families as "matriarchal" by pointing out that many African American families are viewed from a middle-class frame of reference, which makes the assumption that a "psychologically healthy" family must consist of two parents. It is true that many African American families are headed by single mothers, but Lindblad-Goldberg and Dukes (1985) have reported that a healthy single parent and a sufficient extended family and/or community support system can lead to healthy family functioning. Jaynes and Williams (1989) believe that current differences in African American family structure are also due to poor economic conditions in many black communities and to residential segregation.

A strength of African American families is that of strong kinship bonds and extended family relationships. Extended families include other relatives, such as grandparents, uncles, aunts, nieces, nephews, cousins, or other relatives. African American families have historically taken in other children and the elderly, and "doubling up" has been a common practice among these families (Boyd-Franklin, 1989). Boyd-Franklin also states,

> as a result of these strong kinship bonds, many Black families have become extended families in which relatives of a variety of blood ties have been absorbed into a coherent network of mutual emotional and economic support.

Kennedy (1980) described the African American family as a complex pattern of relationships among a wide range of people who may or may not be related by birth or marriage. The major adaptive strengths of the African American family are strong kinship bonds and flexibility of family roles. African American couples are usually more egalitarian with respect to family roles than other couples in mainstream America (Staples, 1988). Family life for African American families is still greatly affected by discrimination and oppression and the family and extended family provide protection from the effects of racism and support.

Hill (1977) reported that economic necessities forced African American families to be more versatile in assuming and fulfilling family roles. For example, older children stand in as parents and caretakers; mothers fill the shoes of both parents or trade traditional roles with fathers, and so on. Hill believes that "such role flexibility helps to stabilize the family." Hill further stressed the importance of viewing this adaptation from a positive perspective and not a pathological one.

Another important strength of the African American family is religion and spirituality. African Americans have used Christianity and spirituality as a survival mechanism for generations. Knox (1985) stated,

> The organized church is by far the most profound instrument available to Blacks when it comes to coping with the multiplicity of problems that beset their lives. Church members as well as non-members accept their spirituality embodied in the church and use the church to confront their own helplessness and depressive attitudes and oppressive practices toward them by others. (pp. 34–35)

The African American family has evolved into the following types of families over the years (Billingsley, 1987): nuclear, extended, and augmented. The nuclear family consists of related family members only. The extended family has other relatives living with the family. The augmented family has nonrelated friends living with a family. A fourth type of family has also been evolving in the last few decades, the single-parent family.

The extended family, a trait that has been maintained since tribal times, is an integral part of African American life. During slavery, many nuclear families were disrupted and extended families provided support for dislocated parents and children. Many African Americans live in an extended family situation in which other in-laws share the same household with the nuclear family. The extended family includes grandparents, aunts, uncles, sisters, brothers, religious leaders, and friends. The extended family, as in the past, continues to protect young African American children from the problems of a discriminatory society. This structure forms a cooperative interface and provides strength, vitality, resilience, and continuity within the African American family. However, children in extended families can be exposed to extended family conflicts over discipline and autonomy because of the many different adult caretakers. This can create conflict, stress, and anger in the family. African American parents also tend to be strict and direct with discipline. In disciplining the children, African American parents may use physical measures, but this is done with love and care (Ho, 1992).

Martin and Martin (1978) interviewed members of 30 extended families and noted the following characteristics:

- Members depend on each other for emotional, social, and material support.
- The typical household consists of at least four generations.
- A dominant family figure keeps the family together, and all members look to this person for leadership.
- Family members do not have to live in the base household to be active participants in family activities.
- The subextended family may resemble the nuclear family in that members are obligated to assist in family crises.
- Adult children are expected to perform duties for their parents as reciprocal acts.

Today, the majority of African American families are headed by women. A high rate of unemployment, separation and divorce, unmarried parenthood, and early deaths of African American men have contributed to this dramatic increase in single-parent families (Billingsley, 1987). Single-parent families are becoming the fastest growing structure among African American families (Moore, 1986). However, a fatherless child does not significantly suffer from the absence of the father, in part, because of male models that are among the male kinsmen in the extended family network (Rubin, 1974). Many African American single parents raise their children to become capable and well-adjusted adults.

More than half of all African American children are born to single mothers and nearly half of those to teenage girls. Teenage females in single families may be required to become surrogate parents with detrimental effects on their educational and occupational outcomes.

The 1994 birth rate for African American teenagers was 108 per 1,000, ages 15–19, down from 111 in 1993, 116 in 1992, and 118 in 1991. The birth rate for white American teenagers in 1993 and 1994 was 40 per 1,000, ages 15–19, down from 42 in 1992, and 43 in 1991 (Child Trends, 1996). Although birth rates to African American teenage females actually have dropped since 1960, they are still nearly five times as likely as white American females to have a child out of wedlock (Children's Defense Fund, 1988). Having a child at such an early age has been found to interfere with sexuality, income, and educational and occupational opportunities for a more productive, satisfying life for young African American mothers (Furstenberg and Gellas, 1987). For many low-income African American teenagers, early parenthood is seen as a rite of passage to adulthood. An African American teenager, therefore, may not experience the same degree of anxiety, shame, and social stigma normally experienced by middle-class white American adolescents (Franklin, 1982). However, Staples (1988) reported that the birth rate of college-educated black women is lower than that of their white counterparts.

In addition, Cummings (1983) reported that 26 percent of black women had abortions as compared to 41 percent of white women. Cummings concluded that African American women in the South have tended to seek abortions less often than women in the North and less often than white women in general. Wattleton (1992) thought that because of inadequate contraceptive usage, African American women are also twice as likely as white women to experience unplanned pregnancies.

Children

African American children, in particular, face a difficult task. They must learn to grow up within their own culture and, at the same time, learn to imitate the dominant culture, whether they accept its values or not. This is complicated by the dominant culture's history of devaluating people of color. In addition, many African American children are raised in poverty, which produces feelings of intense alienation from mainstream society. Children living in poverty do not have a protected childhood in which they can grow up in a safe and healthy environment. Many children of poverty have poor educational experiences that lead to high dropout rates. Children raised in poverty will often lose hope because they see their parents and others fail at combating many of the problematic situations generated by poverty and discrimination. In this atmosphere, it may require exceptional performance to succeed.

Some African American children may more easily resign themselves to frustration, hostility, and self-destructive behavior. Edelman (1985) reported that African American children have a 75 percent higher occupancy rate in state and county psychiatric and health care facilities compared to their white counterparts. Edelman also suggested that 10 to 25 percent of African Americans are at significant risk for developing clinical depression.

Racial issues require the African American child to interpret the world differently than the majority white American child, because they make it more difficult for the African American child to determine who he or she is and what his or her respective place in the world can be. African American families must help their children identify racial discrimination and distinguish it from other life problems. Once distinguished, effective strategies and role models must be provided to show children how to cope with discriminatory practices.

Traditional Sex Roles

The role of African American males as fathers and husbands has been much misunderstood. There is, of course, a wide variety of fatherhood behaviors, as there is in all ethnic groups. There is so much variability in how African American males adjust to fatherhood that it is impossible to generalize. The African American male, however, has often been assumed to be someone who is peripheral to the family as both a father and husband. The literature does not support this assumption.

The identity of the African American male is tied to his ability to provide for his family. Because of economic circumstances for many African American families, the male expends a great deal of time and energy trying to provide the basic survival necessities for his family. This investment of time and energy contributes to his absence in family activities. This, however, should not imply that he is not family-oriented or uncaring (Hines and Boyd-Franklin, 1982). There is clear evidence that many African American men are involved in an egalitarian manner in childrearing, particularly in decision-making patterns (Gary, 1981). There are, of course, many African American males who are disinterested in childrearing, which is common in all ethnic groups, but it is a serious error to assume that most African American fathers are not involved with their children.

The Elderly

The elderly in the African American community are respected and valued. They are seen as wise individuals who have kept the African American tradition alive through years of struggle and survival against poverty, discrimination, oppression, and racism. They are seen as assets to the community because they can pass on their knowledge and experiences, especially to the young, that have withstood the test of time. They are important members of the extended family and their wisdom is cherished. Hill (1977) found that the African American elderly are more likely than Caucasian elderly to describe themselves as "happy," with few problems adjusting to aging. Perhaps one of the reasons is that they often continue to play an important role in the extended family for advice and child care.

Although statistics show that whites live longer than blacks, African American elderly, men and women, who live to be 70 to 75 years or older, have longer life expectancies than their white counterparts (Watson, 1990). The health status of older African Americans, unfortunately, is poor. Chronic diseases are not only more prevalent within this population, but the onset of them usually occurs much earlier when compared to the majority population. The African American elderly, generally, don't fear death. They have seen it in their communities throughout their life time and are not terrified by the eventuality of their own death. In essence, they have seen much of it and they're ready for it.

Death and Grief

Death in the African American community is perceived as a celebration of life. Those who serve as witnesses in the presence of death—extended family, friends, and church members—to affirm the essences of the person's existence are ready to testify to the fact that the deceased has fought the battle, borne the burden, and finished the course; they are ready to understand and say, "Well done" (White and Parham, 1990). Funerals are followed by the gathering of mourners to eat, drink, and talk joyously about their happy times with the deceased.

For Muslims, the first morning prayer begins with the contemplation of one's own death. Muslims believe that Allah determines when death will occur, and one must always be in the right frame of mind to accept His decision. Grief, however, is expressed in loud keening and wailing to indicate how much pain the loss has caused the bereaved.

African Caribbeans generally fear death, especially if it occurs prematurely. If a person dies from natural causes, such as old age, he or she is feared less than someone who dies early from an accident or violence. It is believed that the soul or spirit of those who die early wanders the earth and has the ability to take the living to the next world or to lead them astray (Glaskow and Adaskin, 1990). Therefore, being near a deceased person is approached with great caution. Many West Indians are also superstitious about death. If, for example, a shooting star appears to fall on someone's house or a dog howls, these are interpreted as signs of impending death. If one dies from a painful illness, it may be seen as divine retribution for sins committed while living (Glaskow and Adaskin, 1990).

African Caribbean families will gather the night of the death to provide moral support for the grieving family and to affirm the life of the group, even though a member is dead. This may go on for days and nights until the body is buried or cremated. During this gathering, the family and friends may eat special foods, drink, talk, pray, gamble, and celebrate life in a happy manner. As a result, the outward grieving process is less noticeable (Glaskow and Adaskin, 1990). Postmortem procedures are usually not requested because the family is usually not interested in knowing the cause of the death.

The Native American Family

The Family

The last part of the 20th century has brought about great diversity in the Native family structure because of education, economics, government control, and urbanization. Each of the many Native societies have had to make adjustments to the changes imposed on them. Native families can be patrilineal, matrilineal, or bilateral. However, the family still represents the cornerstone for the social and emotional well-being of every family member and the community. This concept is pancultural to the many Native American cultures. A primary social unit of Native Americans is the clan, which is still found in many tribes. The Navajo, for example, the largest culturally intact nation numerically, have maintained a functional clan system. Many Native Americans identify themselves by their clan affiliation. The clan is a functional extension of the nuclear family and influences education, socialization, marriage, and ritual structures.

The clan is similar to the extended family concept, characteristically including several households. It is important that each person be a good relative. Every other consideration is secondary—property, personal ambition, glory, good times, and life itself (Champagne, 1994). The caring and sharing aspects that are basic to the nuclear family and clan structure have allowed many Native American families and tribes to function under extreme conditions of poverty.

The multiple family structure provides family members with a strong sense of belonging. The extended family network fosters intense personal interactions between many individuals and this can have lasting effects on a child's life and behavior. This structure allows the biological parents to engage their children in a different manner because the disciplining of the children is shared among relatives of the extended family network.

All blood kin of all generations are considered equal and there is no differentiation between close and distant relatives. Aunts and uncles are considered like second parents and cousins are treated as brothers or sisters. There is no such thing as an in-law because families are blended, not joined. Through marriage, one becomes a sister or brother. Even unrelated individuals can become a family member by being a namesake for a child. This individual then assumes family obligations and responsibilities just as other family members do. In many Native American societies, an individual without relatives is considered poor (Sutton and Broken Nose, 1996).

American Indians also believe that each individual is unique and an integral part of nature and the universe. Each person serves a purpose and therefore should not be controlled. No person, therefore, should have another person's power imposed on him or her. Parents do not impose power or control over their children or relations. Children are given the freedom to make their own decisions and solve their own problems in life. Children, therefore, are taught not to feel guilt (Attneave, 1982).

Getting along with others and working together are highly valued traits. The family and group are more important than the individual. This concept of collaboration reflects the integrated view of the universe in which all people, animals, plants, and objects in nature have their place in creating a harmonious whole (Ho, 1992).

Sharing is also an important part of many Native American tribes. There is great respect for those who give the most to others and families. Sharing holds greater esteem than the white American ethic of saving. Because one's worth is measured by one's willingness and ability to share, the accumulation of material goods for social status is alien to the American Indian. Sharing, therefore, is neither a superimposed nor an artificial value, but a genuine and routine way of life (Ho, 1992). Native Americans do not place value on time in terms of minutes or hours. Therefore, if an American Indian is on his or her way to an appointment and meets a friend, the conversation takes priority over the appointment. The relationship and the sharing of one's self are more important than punctuality.

The Children

Many Native American cultures are accustomed to observational or imitative learning in their home cultures. It is a process of doing. Children, for example, in most Native American families participate in most family and community affairs. In fact, children are revered and welcome to such occasions. It is not uncommon, then, for children to accompany their parents to community meetings, bingo nights, or even their place of employment. In sharp contrast, a mainstream white American teenager would "rather die" than have to bring a younger sibling to a teenage gathering, but this would be acceptable to Native American teenagers, who do not generally exclude younger children. As a result of this constant and close proximity, the child has the opportunity to observe, evaluate, and then practice skills in a multitude of situations with a minimum of verbal preparation or interchange.

This observational and imitative style of learning, of course, contrasts sharply with the learning styles often fostered in most mainstream American schools. Even though this style of learning is universal to all people, according to Scribner and Cole (1973), "observation is a very limited technique in the overwhelmingly linguistic environment of the school."

The expectations of Native American children are often in direct contrast to what is expected in schools. For example, many Native American children enter school expecting freedom of movement, but encounter restricted movement; they expect visual–spatial kinesthetic learning but encounter verbal learning; they expect to "learn by doing" but receive indirect and vicarious learning. Pepper (1986) also reported that Native Americans learn faster when the teaching style is based on the concrete approach and moves to the abstract—from practice to theory—but most schools follow the Western European American model and move from theory to practice.

In addition, many Native Americans do not traditionally converse by asking each other questions in their day-to-day speech. This may stem from their cultural value of not interfering with or intruding into another person's affairs. As a result, Native American students do not like being involved in strategies that involve questioning. However, question-asking is one of the dominant verbal strategies employed in most schools. As a result of cultural differences, Native American children may not ask questions in class.

Thus, many Native Americans find it difficult to transform their knowledge from one performance style to another. As a result, the format of written tests or activities may be more of a problem for them than the content and substance of the learning task. Incorporating collaborative/cooperative learning, group projects, lessons that incorporate manipulative devices, experiments, practical, as opposed to theoretical, lessons, experiential activities, and informal settings that allow movement are conducive to a Native American learning style.

Native American children have great difficulty adapting to the mainstream school system and, consequently, have a dropout rate that is substantially higher than the general population. The dropout rate among Indian students ranges from 15 percent to 60 percent (U.S. Commission on Civil Rights, 1978). Whitaker (1989) also reported that Indian children are more likely than Anglo students to perceive public schools as a hostile environment infested with alcohol, drugs, property destruction, violent acts, and theft.

Traditional Sex Roles

Sex role variations within Native American cultures are highly diverse. No clear demarcation of sex-role behavior can be generalized. In some families sex roles may be ambiguous or interchangeable, while in others they are clearly defined, with the male being the dominant force. Some tribes treat females as inferior (Hippler, 1974) and, in some instances, the female plays a submissive, supportive role for the male (Hanson, 1980/1992). The historical roots of many North American tribes are founded in a matriarchal society in which women owned the property and home and men married into the clan and lived in the home and cleared the land of trees and readied the fields for planting, which was done by the women, who cultivated the crops. In modern Navajo tribes, the patriarchal model is evident, but women hold the decision-making power in the clan or matrilineally oriented kin group. Open displays of affection between men and women are limited. This, however, does not mean that relations are not close, affectionate, and satisfying.

In some Native Alaskan communities, women are treated almost exclusively as objects to be used, abused, and traded by men. After puberty, Native Alaskan girls are fair game for any interested male. A man shows his intention by grabbing the belt of a woman, and, if she protests, he cuts off her trousers and forces himself on her. These encounters are considered unimportant by the rest of the group. Men offer their wives' sexual services to establish alliances with trading partners and members of hunting and whaling parties (Friedl, 1997).

The Elderly

Elders are shown great respect, and children are highly valued by both the family and community. Grandparents, for example, do much of the training and disciplining of the children. It is also important to recognize that American Indians may be considered as elders by their communities at 45 or younger, if warranted by impaired health and functional abilities (Kramer, 1991). Although the elderly tend to live apart from their children, but within the same reservation or community, they often live in poverty and substandard living conditions. Older Native Americans generally have a lower life expectancy than white Americans and have a higher rate of chronic disease and disability.

Death and Grief

Death in Native American communities is understood to be a natural and cyclical part of human existence. Native Americans believe in the afterlife as a natural part of a person's lifecycle, something that need not be earned. For the living, the focus is on how to live here and now, not on a reward in the afterlife (Brokenleg and Middleton, 1993).

Because observation is a primary way of learning, from an early age children observe the rituals and ceremonies that surround death. They learn how to behave in such situations. Mourning is considered natural, and unrestrained expression is appropriate and regarded as a good thing for both sexes. Women will typically wail loudly; men will often sing emotional, mournful songs. Cutting the hair, cutting or scratching the forearms and face, tearing clothing, and wearing black are common and appropriate outward displays of grief. This, like everything else, is done in the presence of the whole community (Brokenleg and Middleton, 1993).

A person's death is sacred and family and friends go to whatever lengths are necessary to be at the wake and funeral. The community gathers to support the grieving. It is not unusual to see hundreds of people attending the services. It is important that all members behave appropriately at such ceremonies; misbehavior brings great shame to the individual. Alcohol or other drugs are also forbidden to the mourners from the moment of death until after the burial (Brokenleg and Middleton, 1993).

The human body is considered sacred; therefore, cremation and postmortem procedures are avoided whenever possible. It is a major concern that mourning and burial take place on the home reservation because no one should be buried alone. At the wake and funeral site, significant objects (jewelry, locks of the mourners' hair, etc.) are placed in the casket or near it to be later buried with the deceased. However, most personal possessions of the deceased are distributed to others because, in Native American cultures, possessions are accorded little importance and are understood to be communally shared. What the community has given the person in life is returned through the life of the person and that person's involvement in the community. The material possessions also are returned at death so that the cycle is complete (Brokenleg and Middleton, 1993).

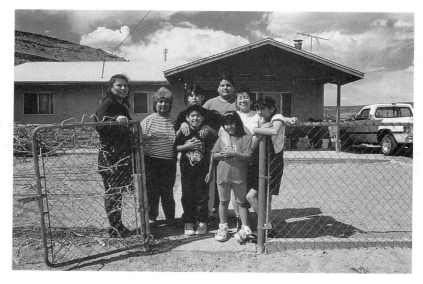

Photo by Will Hart.

One of the greatest strengths of American Indian cultures is the extended family. It is not uncommon to find grandparents, aunts, uncles, cousins, or even friends of the family rearing the Indian child.

—Jeanne Bearcrane (Crow Indian)

The Asian American Family

The Family

Filial piety is a cornerstone in traditional Asian cultures. Filial piety refers to the dutiful or obligatory responsibilities of the family members to each other. It means loyalty and devotion to parents, family, and others. It means, in particular, reciprocity and a sense of obligation that children feel toward their parents. In the traditional filial piety model, it is the responsibility of the son to carry on the family name, and women are expected to be submissive to their husbands. Children are to behave in ways that are not shameful to the family. Asian culture puts the family's needs above individual needs. Traditionally, the Asian family unit is the pillar of strength and stability for all its members and plays a critical role in the ongoing development and support of the child, even into adulthood. These concepts of filial piety have shaped many of the Asian cultures. In addition, many Asian families have been influenced by the teachings of Buddhism, which stresses moderation in behavior, self-discipline, modesty, selflessness, and balance in nature and living.

Traditional Asian American families have a hierarchical structure in which the male is dominant and parental ties are extremely important (Strom, Park, and Daniels, 1987). The father is the head of the family. He makes the decisions, and his authority generally is unquestioned (Ho, 1992). He is usually the disciplinarian and the mother is the nurturer and caretaker of both her husband and children. The rigidity of the hierarchical structure does not provide for expression of feelings on many issues, and conflict resolution is difficult, leaving the wife and children often vulnerable, angry, and unhappy.

Children

Children are taught to be obedient to elders and to put their family's needs above individual needs. Concepts of working hard, responsibility, and collaboration are a part of the child–parent relationship. Children are taught not to fight or cry, and showing emotion is discouraged. When children are small, they are pampered and cared for without hesitation. However, as they grow older, the children are expected to be more responsible and "grown up" and less affection is shown toward them (Okabe, Takahashi, and Richardson, 1990). Tidiness and good manners are encouraged, as well as being considerate to others. Teenagers are expected to be diligent in their school work and generally do not have many responsibilities. There is a strong emphasis on achievement, and schoolwork takes priority over peer relationships.

Asian American youths who experience a gap between what is expected of them and what they have actually achieved may suffer from high levels of emotional stress, specifically a fear of failure. Because Asian parents are very strict, and children are taught not to dishonor the family, conflict often arises as Asian children become acculturated to American society. The process of immigration and cultural transition has created a great deal of turmoil in the structure of many Asian American families.

There generally seems to be more emphasis on education among Asian Americans than among some other ethnic groups in the United States. Many Asian parents hope for fulfillment in their own lives through the success of their children. Japanese, Korean, and Chinese parents instill in their children very early the idea that parental acceptance is contingent on their educational performance. Low performance by the child will elicit not only parental disapproval and criticism, but also disappointment and sometimes shame among one's relatives as well.

Traditional Sex Roles

Traditionally, Asian women are supposed to be demure, docile, passive, and humble people who are reluctant to express themselves. Their self-worth is measured by marriage to a "good" husband, and femininity in terms of the accommodating role they assume with family members, while being subservient to their husbands (Uba, 1994).

However, this traditional characterization of accommodating Asian women is being eroded and challenged by the dominant culture, which places a high value on individualism, independence, and self-worth. Their traditional role is also challenged by economic factors, which force both the husband and wife to work, while the wife is expected to assume the added responsibilities of attending to household chores and cooking for the family. Many Asian husbands are trained to consider housework far more demeaning to perform than white husbands would.

Asian American women drink far less than Caucasian women. However, there seems to be an increasing rate of cigarette, alcohol, and tranquilizer abuse among Asian American women. One factor that cuts across Asian subcultural lines is rapidly changing attitudes on the part of Asian American women about their traditional roles and functions.

The traditional Asian male, in particular, the first born, inherits the responsibility of carrying on the family name by marrying and having sons. He must show respect to his parents, particularly his father. He is the role model for other siblings and owes his father absolute obedience. He is expected to support and nurture his parents as they grow old.

Like the characterization of the Asian female role, the traditional male role is also slowly being eroded with each successive generation of families. The more successive generations an Asian family has living in the United States will have a direct correlation with the erosion of the filial piety ideology.

The Elderly

The elderly are revered within most Asian populations and their long lives give them the wisdom to advise younger generations. The Japanese, for example, recognize the 60th birthday with an elaborate celebration. Elders symbolically pass family caretaking to the next generation, absolving themselves of adult responsibilities, and return to the joys of childhood and personal pursuits (Kagawa-Singer, 1994). They also have the assurance that they now will be cared for with respect and with appreciation for sacrifices made on behalf of their families (Doi, 1991). Even after death they are to be respected and worshipped. In many Asian homes, there is often a shrine in which a picture or artifact of the individual is placed, and every morning and every evening the family greets its ancestors.

It is the traditional responsibility of the children to care for the elderly when they are not able to care for themselves. However, depending on the individual Asian culture, many elderly prefer to live on their own, so as not to be a burden to others. However, when care is finally needed, to fail to care for elders brings shame to the family and some degree of censorship from the community.

The concept of nursing home care would be considered unacceptable, and someone within in the family would quit his or her job rather than place an elder in a nursing home (Richardson, 1990). Many Asian immigrants find it very difficult and stressful to meet the demands of economic responsibility and elderly care in the United States. If the husband and wife must both work and there are no relatives to share the responsibility, then the family may agree to place an elder in a nursing home. This is done only as a last resort and often with great guilt and shame.

Death and Grief

Because Buddhism is a common religion among many Asian populations, the belief in reincarnation is an important part of the death process. Death is accepted as a natural and inevitable part of life and is talked about freely by everyone, including children. Commemorative rituals and shrines that honor the deceased provide comfort for the surviving family. It is believed that death occurs when it is time for the person to die. In most Asian traditional cultures, the elderly or sick die at home. Family members care for the patient so that he or she can die peacefully, surrounded by family. Patients also prefer to die at home rather than in a hospital setting. It is important to recognize that funerary practices within Asian cultures vary significantly. For example, Vietnamese Buddhists express grief by loud crying, keening, and wailing from death until burial. Sometimes professional wailers are hired to indicate to the community how deeply loved the deceased was. Japanese Buddhists, however, are very solemn, audible crying is highly unusual, and tears seem to be restricted to the immediate family.

Even though death is accepted as a natural part of life, in many Asian cultures, the patient is often denied diagnosis and prognosis of his or her illness, especially if the prognosis is possible death. This is based on the belief that such information may be stressful or upsetting and that the patient's final days should be peaceful in thought (Lai and Kevin-Yue, 1990; Assanand et al., 1990). When a patient is aware that death is imminent, he or she will talk about it comfortably with family and friends.

After death the grieving process for the surviving families and friends is very open and expressive. Individuals will publicly cry and dramatically express their loss. To accept death serenely is usually not acceptable and is open to criticism (Dinh et al, 1990; Richardson, 1990). Cremation is the most common Buddhist funeral practice within these populations.

A wake is held before the cremation. Depending on the Buddhist practice, additional services are held on certain symbolic days after the death and special ceremonies are practiced on specially selected anniversary years after the death. It is common for families to maintain special altars in their homes where deceased members are made offerings on special occasions.

Different traditional Asian cultures have different beliefs and rituals before and after death. For example, a pregnant Chinese woman is not allowed to attend funerals for fear that sadness may harm her and her child's health (Lai and Kevin-Yue, 1990); Cambodians celebrate with festive gatherings and share food and drink for three days and nights before the cremation (Richardson, 1990); Japanese Buddhists sprinkle salt over those returning from the funeral as an act of purification (Okabe et al, 1990); many Asian cultures do not allow autopsies or postmortems of bodies because they are intrusive; some Asian cultures wash the deceased's body; a dying Hindu may touch clothing or other goods before they are distributed to the needy (this will help the dying person in his or her next life) (Assanand et al., 1990); in Vietnamese culture, the child or wife of the deceased person must wait three years to marry, and the husband must wait one year; and the Vietnamese will wear white for 14 days, followed afterward by the wearing of black armbands (Dinh et al., 1990).

REFERENCES

Assanand, S., Dias, M., Richardson, E., and Waxler-Morrison, N. The South Asians. In N. Waxler-Morisson, J. Anderson, and E. Richardson, (Eds.). *Cross-cultural caring: A handbook for health professionals.* Vancouver: UBC Press, 1990, pp. 141–180.

Attneave, C. American Indians and Alaska native families. In M. McGoldrick, J. Pearce, and J. Giordano (Eds.), *Ethnicity and family therapy* (pp. 58–83). New York: Guilford, 1982.

Billingsley, A. Black families in a changing society. In J. Dewart (Ed.), *The State of Black America.* New York: National Urban League, 1987, pp. 120–131.

Boyd-Franklin, N. *Black families in therapy.* New York: Guilford, 1989.

Brokenleg, M., and Middleton, D. Native Americans: Adapting, yet retaining. In D. Irish, D. Lundquist, and V. Jenkins-Nelsen. *Ethnic variations in dying, death, and grief.* Washington, DC: Francis & Taylor, 1993, pp. 101–112.

Champagne, D. *The Native North American almanac.* Detroit, MI: Gale Research, 1994.

Child Trends. Drop in teen birth rate nationally reflects changes in most states. *Facts at a Glance.* A publication by Charles Stewart Mott Foundation, 1996. http://www.kidscampaigns.org:80/New/teenbirthpr.html

Children's Defense Fund. *Teens and AIDS: Opportunities for prevention.* Washington DC: Author, 1988.

Cummings, J. Break up of black family imperils gains of decades. *New York Times* (November). 1983, p. 10.

Dinh, D., Ganesan, S., and Waxler-Morrison, N. The Vietnamese. In N. Waxler-Morisson, J. Anderson, and E. Richardson. (Eds.), *Cross-cultural caring: A handbook for health professionals.* Vancouver: UBC Press, 1990, pp. 181–213

Doi, M. L. *A transformation ritual: The Nisei 60th birthday. Journal of Cross-Cultural Gerontology,* 6, 153–163, 1991.

Edelman, M. The seas is so wide and my boat is so small: Problems facing black children today. In H. McAdoo and J. McAdoo (Eds.), *Black children: Social, educational and parental environments.* Newbury Park, CA: Sage, 1985, pp. 72–84

Fitzpatrick, J. The Puerto Rican Family. In C. Mindel and R. Havbenstein (Eds.), *Ethnic families in America* (pp. 271–286). New York: Elsevier, 1981.

Franklin, A. Therapeutic intervention with urban Black adolescents. In E. Jones (Ed.), *Minority mental health* (pp. 272–296). New York: Praeger, 1982.

Friedl, E. Society and sex roles. In J. Spradley and D. McCurdy (Eds.), *Conformity and conflict: Readings in cultural anthropology.* New York: Longman, 1997. 210–245.

Furstenberg, F., and Gellas, T. Adolescent mothers in later life. Cambridge, England: Cambridge University Press. In M. Ho (Ed.), (1992). *Minority children and adolescents in therapy.* Newbury Park: CA: Sage, 1987, p. 87.

Gary, L. (Ed.). *Black men.* Beverly Hills, CA: Sage, 1981.

Glaskow, J., and Adaskin, E. The West Indians. In N. Waxler-Morisson, J. Anderson, and E. Richardson (Eds.), *Cross-cultural caring: A handbook for health professionals.* Vancouver: UBC Press, 1990, pp. 214–244.

Greene, A. Social context differences in the relationship between self-system and self-concept during late adolescence. *Journal of Adolescent Research.* 1992 (April), vol. 7(2), 266–280.

Hanson, W. (1980). The urban Indian woman and her family. *Social Casework* 61, 476–484. In M. Ho (Ed.), *Minority children and adolescents in therapy.* Newbury Park: CA: Sage, 1992.

Hill, R. *Informal adoption among black families.* Washington, DC: National Urban League Research Department, 1977.

Hines, P., and Boyd-Franklin, N. Black families. In M. McGoldrick, J. Pearce, and J. Giordano (Eds.), *Eth-*

nicity and family therapy, (pp. 84–107). New York: Guilford, 1982.

Hippler, A. (1974). The North Alaska Eskimos: A culture and personality perspective. *American Ethnologist* 1, 449–469. In M. Ho (Ed.), *Minority children and adolescents in therapy.* Newbury Park: CA: Sage, 1992, p. 59.

Ho. M. (Ed.). *Minority children and adolescents in therapy.* Newbury Park: CA: Sage, 1992.

Irish, D., Lundquist, K., and Jensen-Nelsen, V. *Ethnic variations in dying, death, and grief.* Washington, DC: Taylor and Francis, 1993.

Jaynes, G., and Williams, R. (Eds.). *A common destiny: Blacks and American society.* Washington, DC: National Academy Press, 1989.

Kagawa-Singer, M. Diverse cultural beliefs and practices about death and dying in the elderly. In D. Wieland, D. Benton, B. Kramer, and G. Dawson (Eds.), *Cultural diversity and geriatric care.* New York: Haworth Press, 1994. 136–156.

Keefe, S., and Padilla, A. *Chicano ethnicity.* Albuquerque, NM: University of New Mexico Press, 1987.

Kennedy, T. *You gotta deal with it: Black family relations in a southern community.* New York: Oxford University Press, 1980.

Knox, D. Spirituality: A tool in the assessment and treatment of Black alcoholics and their families. *Alcoholism Treatment Quarterly* 2(3/4), 31–44, 1985.

Kramer, B. J. *Urban Indian aging. Journal of Cross-Cultural Gerontology* 6, 205–218, 1991.

Lai, M. and Kevin-Yue, K. The Chinese. In N. Waxler-Morisson, J. Anderson, and E. Richardson (Eds.), *Cross-cultural caring: A handbook for health professionals.* Vancouver: UBC Press, 1990, pp. 68–90.

Lindblad-Goldberg, M., and Dukes, J. Social support in black, low-income, single-parent families: Normative and dysfunctional patterns. *American Journal of Orthopsychiatry* 55, 42–58, 1985.

Martin, E. and Martin, J. The black extended family. Chicago: University of Chicago Press, 1978.

Moore, Facts on births to US teens. In M. Merger (Ed.), *Facts at a glance* (pp. 64–69). Washington, DC: Child Trends, 1986, pp. 64–69.

Moynihan, D. *The Negro family: The case for national action.* Washington, DC: U.S. Department of Labor, 1965.

Okabe, T., Takahashi, K., and Richardson, E. The Japanese. In N. Waxler-Morisson, J. Anderson, and E. Richardson (Eds.), *Cross-cultural caring: A handbook for health professionals.* Vancouver: UBC Press, 1990, pp. 116–140.

Ortiz, V. The diversity of Latino families." In R. Zambrana (Ed.), *Understanding Latino families: Scholarship,* *policy, and practice.* Thousand Oaks, CA: Sage, 1995. pp. 25–42.

Pepper, F. Teaching the American Indian child in mainstream settings. In R. Jones (Ed.), *Mainstreaming and the minority child.* Reston, VA: Council for Exceptional Children, 1976.

Ramirez, M. and Castaneda, A. *Cultural democracy, bicognitive development and education.* Orlando, FL: Academic Press, 1974.

Richardson, E. The Cambodians and Laotians. In N. Waxler-Morisson, J. Anderson, and E. Richardson (Eds.), *Cross-cultural caring: A handbook for health professionals.* Vancouver: UBC Press, 1990, pp. 11–35.

Rubin, R. Adult male absence and the self-attitudes of Black children. *Child Study Journal* 4, 33–44, 1974.

Scribner, S., and Cole, M. *The Psychology of Literacy.* Cambridge, MA: Harvard University Press, 1981.

Staples. R. The black American family. In C. H. Mindel, R. W. Haberstein, and W. R. Wright, Jr. (Eds.), *Ethnic families in America: Patterns and variations* (pp. 303–24). New York: Elsevier, 1988.

Strom, R., Park, S., and Daniels, S. Child rearing dilemmas of Korean immigrants to the United States. *International Journal of Experimental Research in Education* 24, 91–102, 1987.

Sutton, C., and Broken Nose, M. American Indian families: An overview. In E. McGoldrick, J. Giordano, and J. Pearce (Eds.), *Ethnicity and family therapy.* New York: Guilford, 1996), pp. 31–44.

Sweet, J., and Bumpass, L. *American families and households.* New York: Russell Sage, 1987.

Trakina, F. (1983). Clinical issues and techniques in working with Hispanic children. In M. Ho. *Minority Children and Adolescents in Therapy.* Newbury Park, CA: Sage Publications. 1992, p. 111.

Uba, L. *Asian Americans: Personality patterns, identity, and mental health.* New York: Guilford Press, 1994.

U.S. Commission on Civil Rights. *Social indicators of equality for minorities and women.* Washington, DC: Government Printing Office, 1978.

Vega, W. A. The study of Latino families: A point of departure. In R. E. Zambrana (Ed.), *Understanding Latino families: Scholarship, policy, and practice* (pp. 3–17). Thousand Oaks, CA: Sage, 1995.

Watson, W. Family care, economics and health. In Z. Harel, E. McKinney, and M. Williams (Eds.), *Understanding diversity and service needs* (pp. 50–68). Newbury Park, CA: Sage, 1990.

Wattleton, F. Reproduction rights and the challenge for African Americans. In R. Braithwaite and S. Taylor (Eds.), *Health issues in the black community* (pp. 301–14). San Francisco: Jossey-Bass, 1992.

Weyer, T. *Hispanic USA: Breaking the melting pot.* New York: Harper & Row, 1988.

Whitaker, C. (University of Minnesota Adolescent Health Program, Indian adolescent health survey). Unpublished raw data. In M. Ho (Ed.), *Minority children and adolescents in therapy.* Newbury Park, CA: Sage, 1989.

White, J. Towards a black psychology. In R. Jones (Ed.), *Black psychology.* New York: Harper & Row, 1972.

White, J., and Parham, T. *The psychology of Blacks: An African-American perspective.* Englewood Cliffs, NJ: Prentice-Hall, 1990.

Younoszai, B. Mexican American Perspectives Related to Death. In D. Irish, K. Lundquist, and V. Jensen-Nelsen (Eds.), *Ethnic variations in dying, death, and grief.* Washington, DC: Taylor and Francis, 1993.

CHAPTER

4 Stress and Culture

We must learn to appreciate diversity, not suppress it. How devastating to think of a world in which everyone is the same.
—Janice LaFountain (Crow Indian)

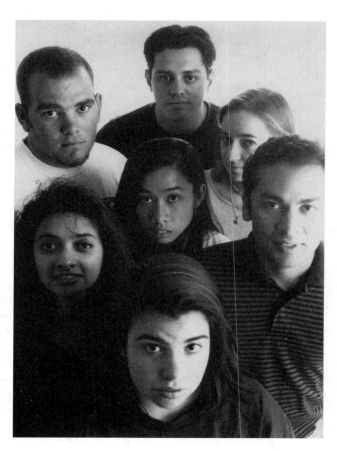

Photo by Aaron Peck, published in *Cultures* magazine, volume 3, issue 1

The Mind–Body Connection

Our body is a self-healing organism. It has developed the ability to make routine repairs and to defend us against injury and illness. If you scrape an elbow falling down, you can watch the healing process start almost immediately. Specialized mechanisms within the body start the healing process, and the small wound will quickly disappear. Catch the common cold and within a week to 10 days your immune system moves you back toward health. Each day our body routinely protects us from potential infections and disease. However, the human body is not invincible, and for reasons not always understood, infections and injuries can overwhelm the body. The expanding definitions of both health and wellness have forced doctors and patients to look beyond the issues of treatment and care. Illness is no longer viewed as something that passively happens to an individual; the patient plays an active role in the process.

Good health requires an integration of the dimensions of wellness described in Chapter 1, in particular, those dimensions related to the mind, such as emotions and spirit. In recent years, medicine has been paying more attention to the mind's ability to affect the body, realizing that the mind has the capacity both to cause and to heal disease. Most people understand instinctively that our emotions and spirit play some role in health, healing, and sickness. Such factors as stress, the will to live, fear, and worry can affect how well or how sick we become.

Researchers are finding that the human body is an indivisible whole and cannot be separated into mind and body. The mind and body are not separate entities but an integrated whole, and every thought is everywhere within the physical body. In a very real sense, every thought may be connected to every cell in the body. The mind and the body can work together to protect one's health or break down the barriers within the body that allow the disease process to take place. The mind influences our body through the brain and central nervous system. The autonomic nervous system is a branch of the peripheral nervous system that controls such vital unconscious functions as heart rate, digestion, breathing, and other body functions that are linked to the mind. You are reminded of it whenever you sweat because of nervousness or blush out of embarrassment.

Recent studies have also linked the mind to both the endocrine and immune systems, which help guard against infections and other illnesses. Arising from this biological research is a new science called psychoneuroimmunology (PNI) that postulates links or interactions between the mind, nervous system, and immune system that ultimately affect our health. In addition, psychological research has shown that our personalities, feelings, stresses, and beliefs may influence our health through mind–body connections. Many physicians have been skeptical about the role of the mind in medicine, but this skepticism is gradually eroding in the face of evidence. More and more physicians are acknowledging that the way the patient thinks and feels can be a powerful determinant of physical health.

A Brief Definition of Stress

Claude Bernard, a 19th-century pathologist, maintained that disease was resisted by a central equilibrium within the patient. He believed that illnesses hovered constantly about us but they did not enter the human body unless it was ready to receive them. The central equilibrium was, of course, related to the mind. The work of Hans Selye (1976) and Walter Cannon (1932) reintroduced to Western medicine Claude Bernard's concept of a central equilibrium. Cannon introduced the concept of homeostasis and the autonomic nervous system and the body's continual attempt to achieve internal balance in response to external change. Selye suggested that, if the changes were too great, the body might not adjust and disease might result.

Cannon formulated the chemical response to stress, the release of neurotransmitters and hormones from the endocrine system. Today, that response is known as the *fight-or-flight* mechanism. Selye built on Cannon's work and formalized the concept of stress and the "stress response," a set of physiological reactions to changing physical or emotional upsets. Both Selye and Cannon were important in showing how emotional distress can lead to disease through chemical mind–body connections.

Hans Selye (1976) defined stress as the body's nonspecific response to any demand made on it. Our bodies react to stress in the same way primitive individual's bodies reacted: A hormonal surge of epinephrine (adrenaline) enables the body to mobilize itself. The heart beats faster, breathing speeds up, palms sweat more, and blood flows to our brain. The body is ready for action.

A stressor is the emotional or physical event or condition that triggers the stress response. Final examinations, an embarrassing moment, a happy moment, an unexpected loud noise, participating in a ball game, or an argument with another person are examples of stressors. Some stressors last only a moment, while others may continually affect the person over a long period of time. For example, a salesperson who has to sell a certain number of units each week in order to provide for his or her family financially would be under continual stress.

What constitutes a pleasant or unpleasant stressor is based on the perception the individual has of the event or condition. Some people, for example, are exhilarated during a roller-coaster ride, while others are scared to death. A pleasant stressor creates *eustress,* an unpleasant stressor causes *distress.* Some events may be distressful to some individuals, while others perceive it as a neutral event that creates no stress for them.

The General Adaptation Syndrome

Regardless of whether the stress is distress or eustress, the stress response is the same for both. The stress response is a predictable series of physical reactions called the General Adaptation Response (GAS). The GAS is divided into three distinct states: the alarm stage, the resistance stage, and the exhaustion stage (see Figure 4.1).

1. *The alarm stage.* The alarm stage is the fight or flight reaction, the immediate response to a stressor. The nervous system, operating independently of conscious thought, sends messages throughout the body to trigger hormonal, muscular, cardiovascular, metabolic, respiratory, and other changes. Marks (1978) stated:

> The effects of strong fear and anxiety cause unpleasant feelings of terror; paleness of the skin; sweating; hair standing on end; dilation of the pupils; rapid pounding of the heart; rise in

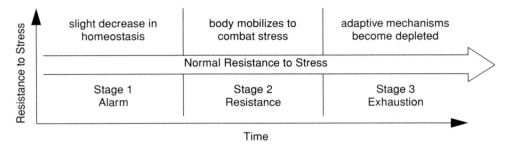

FIGURE 4.1   The General Adaptation Syndrome

blood pressure; tension in the muscles and increased blood flow through them; trembling; a readiness to be startled; dryness and tightness of the throat and mouth; constriction of the chest and rapid breathing; a sinking feeling in the stomach; nausea; desperation; contraction of the bladder and rectum leading to urges to pass urine and feces; irritability and a tendency to lash out; a strong desire to cry, run, or hide; difficulty in breathing; tingling in the hands and feet; feelings of being unreal or far away; paralyzing weakness of the limbs; and a sensation of faintness and falling. (p. 5)

2. *The resistance stage.* The resistance stage is when the body begins to return to some degree of normalcy. The internal activities that were activated in the alarm stage are returning to a homeostasis. At this point, the individual focuses more energy on the emotional aspect of the stressor instead of the physical. If the source of distress is a long-term situation, the body expends a considerable amount of energy to keep the body in homeostatsis. During this stage, many psychological problems may begin to appear if the person cannot find a reasonable way to deal with the continuous stress.

Rutter & Quinto (1976/1982), for example, addressed the link between childhood psychiatric disorders and the impact of inner-city stress factors on psychological development. They reported that children living in the inner city had twice the number of diagnosed emotional and conduct disorders as children living in rural areas. La Vietes (1979) observed that crowded housing exposes children to many negative stresses such as bed sharing, limited areas of play, lack of privacy, and a potentially excessive degree of body contact. In addition, Langner et al., (1979/1982) reported that high stress levels among children were associated with changes in residence, parental marital discord, and parental illnesses (both emotional and physical).

3. *Exhaustion.* If the stresses continue, eventually the body cannot maintain its resistance and depletes itself of the energy required to keep itself in homeostasis. As a result, the individual is more susceptible to disease and illness.

When people cannot deal with the chronic stress in their lives, their bodies may suffer continual wear and tear from the fight-or-flight response, If we do not learn to deal effectively with our stresses, we can develop headaches, backaches, gastrointestinal disorders, sleeplessness, ulcers, heart attacks, and a variety of other unhealthy symptoms and problems.

Social Stressors That Affect Minority Populations

The Commonwealth Fund survey (1994) reported that 36 percent of minority adults and 26 percent of white adults report having "high" levels of stress, based on a range of quality-of-life measures. The survey also reported that minority respondents describe more problems in life than white adults concerning money (25 percent versus 17 percent), their spouse/partner (11 percent versus 6 percent), and mistreatment of a family member for race or cultural reasons (5 percent versus less than one-half percent). Fear of crime or violence affects more minority adults (18 percent) than white adults (8 percent), and minority adults (12 percent) were more likely than white adults (9 percent) to have been physically assaulted in the past five years. The survey concluded that stress, fear of violence, and health behaviors add to the health problems of minority adults.

Numerous psychological studies have addressed the link between stress and psychological well-being, happiness, and physical well-being (Adler, 1981; Holmes & Rahe, 1967; Lazarus, 1966). Distress can contribute to unhappiness, physical illness, and mental disorders in anyone. Minority Americans have negative stressors facing them that the majority of white Americans do not, and these stressors may contribute to the development of physical and mental disorders in minority Americans.

Landrine and Klonoff (1996) designed an inventory to determine if racist events (stressors) were correlated to negative health practices or problems. Included in the inventory were such questions as:

How many times have you been treated unfairly by your employers, bosses, and supervisors?

How many times did you want to tell someone off for being racist but didn't say anything?

How many times have you been called a racist name?

Landrine and Klonoff suggested that the positive relationship between acculturation and smoking among African Americans is a function of racism; traditional African Americans experience more racial discrimination and smoke cigarettes, whereas their more acculturated counterparts experience significantly less discrimination and do not smoke. Likewise, being traditional also was related to increased hypertension. Smokers not only reported more frequent racist events but also found those events to be more stressful than did nonsmokers. Kreiger (1990) also reported a strong relationship between reports of racial discrimination and high blood pressure among African Americans. Landrine and Klonoff (1996) cited additional support from other studies that have found strong relationships among anger, rage, and hypertension.

The Landrine and Klonoff study is most intriguing because it has major implications for other racial groups and suggests the following problems:

Both acculturation and racism may play a role in the health status and behavior of ethnic minority Americans.

The level of acculturation is a predictor for the intensity of racism. The more traditional, the greater the racism. The more acculturated, the less racism.

Racism leads to smoking and hypertension and these, in turn, lead to stroke, heart attack, cancer, and all of the other diseases associated with these two health problems.

The emphasis in the following section is on sources of stress for minority Americans that are distinct from the sources of stress that face other Americans. At the core of most stress in minority Americans are racial discrimination and prejudice, which lead to other distressors, such as cultural conflicts, economic oppression, racial violence, racist law enforcement, and so on. There are a number of ways in which minority status can lead to psychosocial stress for minority Americans. Figure 4.2 depicts some of the stressors faced by ethnic minority populations.

Racial Prejudice

Racial prejudice is defined as any program or practice of discrimination, segregation, persecution, and domination based on race. Racial prejudice entails the belief that one's own race is superior to another. The group or individual who becomes the object of prejudice most often experiences a position of disadvantage. This belief is based on the erroneous assumption that physical attributes of a racial group determine their social behavior as well as their psychological and intellectual characteristics. Cose (1993) reported that the single life event that makes African Americans most angry is racism. In addition, the National

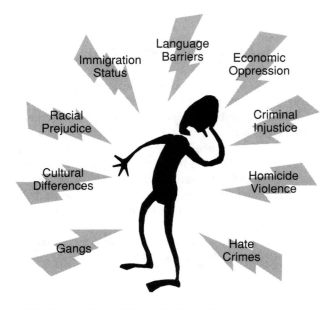

FIGURE 4.2   Ethnic Minority Stress Factors

Institute of Mental Health (1983) reported that the single most common problem reported by African Americans who seek psychotherapy is pent-up rage.

The potential to experience the social stressors of prejudice and discrimination exists for most minority children as they move into the broader society (Spurlock, 1986), especially when a change of residence relocates them into a predominantly nonminority community. Canino and Spurlock (1994) reported the following comments from children they know and children they have treated in their medical practice:

"My teacher says black people can't follow instructions; that's why I didn't do the right assignment."

"These black kids from the projects don't want to learn; they're dumb and might just as well drop out of school."

Despite the efforts of some professionals to eliminate disparaging images of minority group members in the mass media, there are still some who continue to report insensitive media coverage of minority groups and issues, leading to the perpetuation of negative stereotypes and prejudice. Reruns of old movies and television shows, in particular, continue to portray negative images of minority groups. For example, old Western movies usually portray Native Americans as savages and as a people who needed to be conquered; old

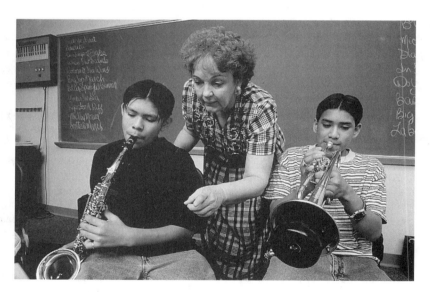

Photo by Will Hart.

I truly believe that someday, our White brothers, and Black brothers, our yellow brothers and our Brown brothers will recognize their charge that we must live in harmony within the Universe, one with another and that all rights be recognized and we treat our fellow man the same way we want to be treated.

—Jake L. Whitecrow, Jr. (Quapaw, Seneca)

war films portray the Japanese as sinister, stupid, and savage; and many old films portray African Americans as only criminals and drug users.

"Japan-bashing" occurred in the early 1990s because the media, politicians, and corporate spokespersons provided ammunition for a small percentage of Americans to justify their taunting, disrespect, and violence against Asian Americans. Uba (1994) observed that these actions were directed against all Asian Americans because most Americans make no effort to distinguish Japanese from Japanese Americans, Chinese, Chinese Americans, or any other Asian or Asian American group. Uba further states that there is a confluence of factors that lead to racism against Asian Americans, and this confluence is compounded by the tendency of many people to form stereotypes based on limited association with Asian Americans.

Racial prejudice affects the physical, social, economic, and psychological well-being of minority groups. It is also important to recognize that the majority of Americans are not racially prejudiced.

Cultural Conflict

Culture can protect against stress but it can also create it. Each society has expected standards of behavior. Each member will usually try to attain the standards or traditional goals that the culture expects of its members. Failure to reach these goals or standards can be very stressful and frustrating to some members. Cultural conflict arises whenever the norms, values, and behavior of one culture clash with those of another (Sue and Chin, 1983). Children from Southeast Asia, for example, are taught to be obedient, quiet, and respectful. This may clash with white American culture that often encourages independence, assertiveness, and expressiveness. White American culture encourages honesty regardless of the situation, while Asian people will often hide the truth to avoid embarrassment of themselves or others.

Cultural differences may also impair communication. Susan Irujo (1988) presented the following circumstances that elicit different emotional cultural responses:

> Not looking another person in the eye is a recognition of that person's authority for African Americans, while whites interpret this as shiftiness and unreliability.
>
> Differences in gaze behavior may cause some misunderstandings. Latinos interpret a direct gaze as having sexual connotations, and a steady stare with raised eyebrows as anger.
>
> Africans, Arabs, and Hispanic Americans touch a great deal in interpersonal relationships, whereas in Britain, Japan, and the United States there is very little touching. Touching in certain cultures causes embarrassment and discomfort. (pp. 142–150)

Some cultural beliefs can even be the direct cause of the stress, such as the belief that one has been "cursed" or "hexed" by a powerful person, against whom the "cursed" person believes she or he has little or no defense. Although this form of stress may seem absurd to members of another society, it is very real to the person who has been hexed. Landry (1977) has documented that individuals within certain societies who believe they have been marked for death by sorcery sicken and die within a short period, apparently of natural causes.

Acculturation and Immigration Status

Migration from one culture to another is a stressful experience, involving major disruptions in the individual's cultural values and life. Eitinger (1960) noted that the new immigrant has to deal with isolation, helplessness, and a feeling of insecurity in his or her surroundings, coupled with a flood of incomprehensible stimuli, language difficulties, hostility or indifference by the host population, and with new cultural practices that may be at variance with their religious beliefs. Earlier studies, reported by Helman (1986), indicated higher blood pressure, increased mental illness, and a higher rate of attempted suicide by immigrants when compared to the population of their country of origin.

Language barriers can negatively affect employment opportunities for many foreign-born minority Americans. Frequently, they have low-paying menial jobs. Consequently, many find little reward or fulfillment in their work and feel pessimistic about prospects for the future. These feelings are compounded by the fact that many immigrants were highly educated and respected professionals in their homeland but are unable to transfer their skills into the American economy because their education and employment history are devalued in the United States (Okamura and Agbayani, 1991).

Stress often occurs when foreign-born children adopt Western cultural ways more quickly than their parents. Not only do immigrants have to adjust to new social norms, but they also adjust to the changing social norms within their families. Children generally acculturate much quicker than their parents and become "Americanized" at a faster pace (Yu and Kim, 1983). This, of course, can be stressful because it affects the behavior norms and relationships within the family (Lee, 1988). The children struggle over appropriate behavior and values as they try to adhere to two, sometimes contrasting, sets of standards. In addition, as one acculturates, he or she may also lose some personal identity.

Economic Oppression

Unemployment among minority Americans is disproportionately high when compared to white Americans. Even community-based job development programs have minority Americans disproportionately represented in those courses geared toward low-wage, low-demand occupations, with little, if any, upward mobility. As the cost of living and inflation continue to rise, the parent(s) are forced to be out of the house earning income to support the family. Such situations often leave children alone or in inadequate day care for significant periods of time. This is just one of the many vicious cycles that develop from economic oppression.

Minority youth who come from poor families have a higher rate of mental illness, although not every child who comes from poor and highly stressed families is mentally ill. For those who are vulnerable to illness because of genetic or psychological factors, the added stress factors of poverty and homelessness can affect symptom manifestation, the course of an illness, and its prognosis (Canino and Spurlock, 1994). Rates of psychopathology are generally higher in inner-city and rural small communities. Therefore, the area of residence may serve as either a protective or a high-risk environment for children (Wolkind and Rutter, 1985). Inner-city living may present children and their parents with multiple stressors (lack of social cohesion and integration, overcrowded and unsafe buildings, and frequent environmental changes), which, if cumulative, may be more damaging to healthy functioning than a single acute stressor would be (Canino and Spurlock, 1994).

Even when minority Americans are successful, they face economic barriers of a different kind. Asian Americans, for example, are generally viewed as a successful minority group in America. Many Asian Americans are well educated and have high levels of income. However, Asian American workers receive smaller economic rewards for their education than white workers (Min, 1995). This means that Asian Americans need more education or work more hours to maintain economic parity with white Americans.

Minority Americans are also underrepresented in executive and managerial positions. Closely related to the underrepresentation of minority Americans in high-ranking executive and administrative positions is the "glass ceiling," a situation in which people cannot advance beyond a certain level in their careers. This barrier affects both women and minority members and, in particular, Asian Americans.

Criminal Injustice

Stress has also been generated when a number of police have engaged in racially discriminatory actions by stopping and harassing minority Americans driving through elite suburban neighborhoods, while ignoring white Americans. It is important to point out that most police are not racist and do not perform such acts. But many innocent minority Americans have, unfortunately, faced the humiliation of being arrested and having their pictures added to a mug book of "gang members" with no proof of such affiliation or probable cause to suspect that they are gang members (Uba, 1994). As a result, many Americans feel apprehensive about entering certain neighborhoods.

Hate Crimes

Crimes against individuals based on race, religion, and sexual orientation are referred to as *hate crimes*. Between 1983 and 1991, 62 percent of all hate crimes were racially motivated (Gall and Gall, 1993). Fifty-six percent of the race-related crimes were against African Americans, 29 percent were against European Americans, 10 percent were against Asian Americans, and 5 percent were against all other races. The stopping of hate crimes is one of the major issues facing all Americans today.

More Stressors for Minority Americans: Violence, Homicide, and Gangs

Homicide and Violence

Homicide (any killing of one person by another) is the leading cause of death for young black men and women. Blacks, who make up some 12 percent of the population in the country, account for 44 percent of all murder victims (Federal Bureau of Investigation, 1987).

Homicide was the 11th leading cause of death in the United States for all ages in 1987, accounting for more than 21,000 deaths per year, a rate of 8.6 deaths per 100,000 population (National Center for Health Statistics, 1990). The homicide rate in the United

States continues to be significantly higher than that of any other industrialized nation (Curtis, 1985).

In 1987, the homicide death rate among black males was nearly seven times the rate for white men. Black females have consistently higher homicide rates than white males and a much higher homicide rate than white females.

Within the United States, rates of homicide are highest in large cities and, in particular, in areas with high poverty and unemployment levels, physical deterioration, welfare dependency, racial and ethnic concentrations, broken homes, working mothers, low levels of education and vocational skills, overcrowded and substandard housing, low rates of home ownership or single-family dwellings, mixed land use, and high population density (The National Commission on the Causes and Prevention of Violence, 1969).

In addition, the chronic stresses, frustrations, violence, and the multiple losses that inner-city minority children and adolescents experience may predispose them to depressive symptoms and often to a presentation of dysthymic disorder or a depressive disorder not otherwise specified (Canino and Spurlock, 1994). Many have suffered the loss of their peers to violent death.

Homicidal Behavior and Prevention

Three categories of homicidal behavior have been identified:

> *Sociological* theory focuses on structural factors such as poverty, broken homes, and limited economic opportunities, which foster a subculture of violence filled with aggressive behaviors and high-risk destructive activities.

> *Psychological* theory attributes homicide rates to psychological scares inflicted by racism that cause feelings of low self-esteem, self-hatred, and rage that are conducive to violence against others (Poussaint, 1983).

> *Environmental* theory points to factors in the external environment—encompassing physical, historical, cultural, social, and economic factors—as producing high levels of stress and social pathology, which in turn provokes violence.

Violence in the Schools

Homicide is becoming one of the leading causes of death for teenagers and, in particular, it has reached epidemic proportions for African American youth in some cities. Hechinger (1992) cites the National Center for Health Statistics report that young black males face the most serious threat of harm to life and limb, and they are seven times more likely than white youths to die as a result of homicide. The rates for Native American and Hispanic American youths were about three to four times that of Western European Americans; that for Asians was virtually the same as Western European Americans. The following section discusses adolescent violence in our schools. In his book, *Fateful Choices,* Fred Hechinger (1992) wrote about adolescent death and violence and reported the following information:

1. In that same year, the FBI reported one of sixteen adolescents was a victim of violent crimes—a total of 1,728,120 young people.

2. Researchers at the University of Maryland's School of Medicine surveyed 168 teenagers who were visited at an inner-city clinic and reported that 24 percent had witnessed a murder and 72 percent knew somebody who had been shot.
3. Forty-one percent of juveniles held for violent crimes had used a weapon, most frequently a gun.
4. In California, from 1988 to June 1989, schools confiscated 10,569 weapons, an increase of 21 percent over the past year.
5. Each month, 300,000 high school students are physically attacked, many in, or on the way to, school.

Students can live in fear for only so long. The body and mind can endure only so much. Eventually, over time, students who feel personally victimized by continued physical or emotional assaults are likely to develop anxiety, depression, and helplessness and will live in fear, not knowing when the abuse will happen next. They will lose faith in the school and develop a persistent preoccupation with the problem. Some think that here is no escape except to quit. Others become preoccupied with revenge.

When fear stalks the halls of a school or the streets to and from school, education is also a victim. As a result of this epidemic, many schools have incorporated antiviolence programs. Schools have adopted programs that have included strict rules and regulations, safety classes, conflict resolution workshops, stronger counseling referral systems, primary intervention programs, and peer education and mentoring programs.

It is imperative that schools establish safety zones that are free of violence, weapons, and drugs. The goal for any school is to assure that children and youths are able to go to and from school without fear of bodily harm. Educators, administrators, community leaders, police authorities, the courts, parents, youth organizations, the media, and politicians must find avenues of true cooperation to stem the tide of adolescent violence. In addition, violations, such as possession of firearms, knives, and other weapons, and the sale or use of drugs, must be instantly and severely penalized through legal action.

Prevention of Violence

Prevention of violence requires primary, secondary, and tertiary prevention efforts. Primary prevention efforts need to be directed at cultural, social, technological, and legal aspects of the environment in the United States that facilitate the perpetuation of the nation's extraordinarily high homicide rate. Such preventive strategies include public education, professional education, community self-help, and interventions against mass media violence. Implementation of these strategies will require that health professionals join with others in an effort to eradicate factors that impair health.

Secondary prevention, early detection, and case-finding are the means by which future, more serious morbidity may be decreased. In the case of homicide, such case-finding requires identification of individuals manifesting early signs of behavioral and social problems that are logically and empirically related to increased risks for subsequent homicide (Shah and Roth, 1974). Adolescent and family violence, childhood aggression, and school truancy and dropout may be important focal points for efforts at secondary prevention of homicide.

The third type of prevention, tertiary prevention, is concerned with situations in which health problems are already well established. Aggravated assaults, spousal violence, police disturbance calls, and gang violence may be important focal points for tertiary prevention.

Gangs

The *Attorney General's Report on the Impact of Criminal Street Gangs on Crime and Violence in California by the year 2000* (1993) reported that criminal street gangs have become one of the most serious crime problems in California. Gang violence—particularly assaults, drive-by-shootings, homicides, and brutal home invasion robberies—accounts for one of the largest, single, personal threats to public safety in California.

The Department of Justice estimates there may be as many as 175,000 to 200,000 gang members in California (*Attorney General's Report,* 1993). The gangs in California include Hispanic gangs, African American gangs, Asian gangs, and white gangs. Of those, Hispanic gangs comprise the majority of the gang population in California. Asian gangs—especially Vietnamese, Cambodian, and Laotian gangs—are becoming one of the fastest growing crime problems in California.

Hispanic Gangs.   The Department of Justice estimates there could be as many as 95,000 Hispanic gang members in California today (*Attorney General's Report,* 1993). Their criminal activities now range from robberies, burglaries, grand thefts, vehicle thefts, and receiving stolen property to assaults, batteries, drive-by-shootings, and murder. They are becoming involved as entrepreneurs in the selling of narcotics—particularly PCP, Mexican tar heroin, methamphetamine, and marijuana. The gangs' arsenals have expanded to large-caliber handguns, shotguns, and automatic weapons, and their crimes are becoming more violent.

Asian Gangs.   The Department of Justice estimates there could be as many as 15,000 Asian gang members in California today (*Attorney General's Report,* 1993). They are still principally comprised of Vietnamese, Laotian, and Cambodian gangs that continue to terrorize and prey on their communities with violent crimes, which occasionally result in murder. They have increased their traveling patterns, and their growing level of mobility and violence has made them a national crime problem. One of the most frightening aspects of Asian gangs is their brutal home invasion robberies. In a typical home invasion, gang members enter a home, tie up the inhabitants, then terrorize, torture, beat, rob, and, at times, kill them. Extortion, burglarizing, ransacking, and vandalism of businesses are also common.

African American Gangs.   The Department of Justice estimates there could be as many as 65,000 African American gang members in California today (*Attorney General's Report,* 1993). The majority of them are still Crips and Bloods gang members. The Crips and Bloods continue to control the distribution of crack cocaine in several California cities and other states. Besides crack cocaine, African American gang members also sell marijuana and PCP. Federal and state law enforcement authorities report Crips and Bloods gang members in 33 states and 123 cities. Their use of weapons has evolved to high-powered, large-caliber handguns and automatic and semi-automatic weapons, including AK-47 assault rifles and Mac-10s with multiple-round magazines, and they sometimes wear police-type body armor. In Los Angeles, during 1990, there were 135 homicides, 1,416 assaults and batteries, and 775 robberies attributed to Crips and Bloods gang members.

Coping with Stress

Coping is defined as "efforts we make to manage situations we have appraised as potentially harmful or stressful" (Kleinke, 1991). In other words, it is the process of trying to keep our composure when faced with life challenges and working out an appropriate course of action. There are seven skills that can help you cope with stress.

Seven Steps for Coping with Stress

1. Maintain a strong support system. Family and friends are important support systems in our lives. They provide emotional support. If it turns out that they cannot provide the support you need, seek professional health care professionals. Seeking professional help is a competent coping skill and should not be viewed as a sign of weakness.

2. Be a problem solver. Problem-solving is a four-step procedure that includes (1) the self-perception or belief that you can solve the problem, (2) the ability to clearly define the problem, (3) brainstorming and listing options or alternative plans, and (4) choosing the best alternative and carrying out the selected course of action.

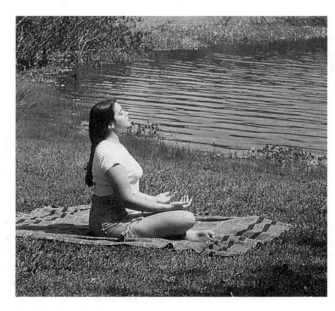

Natural forces within us are the true healers of disease.
—Hippocrates

Photo by Tony Nesti.

A. *Develop self-perception.* A person must believe that "I can solve the problem." The first step in successful problem-solving is for the person to develop the belief that he or she is a problem solver and can negotiate a fair and honest solution. A problem solver accepts the fact that problem situations are a normal part of life and that it is important to face such challenges calmly and rationally, not impulsively.

Some people, for example, despise personal conflict and make concessions to try to reach quick and amicable resolutions that leave them feeling exploited and angry. A true problem solver knows that he or she can rely on his or her problem-solving skills to decide on a reasonable and fair course of action.

In addition, some people have attitudes at the opposite extreme. They feel that "Someone has to suffer," "This can't make a difference," "You really can't trust anyone," or "I can't let you win, so I'm going to argue." These are examples of negative beliefs that obstruct progress in finding a solution. "It is possible to make a difference," "It is possible for everyone to win," and "It is possible to learn to trust ourselves and others" are examples of positive beliefs that can lead to fair solutions.

B. *Identify the problem or situation to be improved.* The first thing to do when faced with a challenge or conflict is to understand exactly what is happening by defining the problem. The process of identifying the true problem is extremely important because your emotions often distort objective thinking.

Unfortunately, many people try to argue or defend their position rather than focusing on the underlying concerns of all parties. Consequently, reaching a fair solution is unlikely, and less satisfactory decisions are usually made.

If, for example, the problem is a conflict with another person, avoid taking a position. A simple process is to have each party write in one sentence, on a separate sheet of paper, what he or she thinks the problem is. This simple procedure will often solve the problem without any further steps. Viewing the problem from the other person's perspective often creates an immediate understanding of the situation. Seeing the problem from the other person's point of view puts the problem into a mutual perspective. Then, together, describe the situation on one single sheet of paper.

C. *Brainstorm to generate options to improve the situation.* The procedures for brainstorming are:

    (1) List all options that could be taken to improve the situation. All ideas are valid and welcomed. They are not judged, criticized, or commented on. Write down each option on a blackboard or large sheet of paper so that all concerned can see.

    (2) Whenever appropriate, consolidate ideas by joining or combining one with another. After viewing them, mark the most promising ideas that may be worth developing further.

    (3) Select a plan of action. Become selective by evaluating each of the ideas. Through a process of discussion without criticism, choose the best of the listed options. Be willing to invent ways to make some of the more promising ideas better or more realistic. If more than one option is going to be used, make a rank-order list of what you will do first.

D. *This final step is to choose and carry out the appropriate option(s) to improve the situation.* The selected option is then evaluated after a predetermined period of time to determine whether it is working. If it is not working, the brainstorming process is started over.

The process of problem-solving is consistent, and the basic steps do not change. Problem-solving can be used whether there are one or several issues and whether there are two or more individuals.

3. Practice relaxation techniques. Many ancient Asian cultures have long known something that modern medicine is just beginning to incorporate into its treatments: Meditation can reduce stress and alter specific bodily processes. Ancient practitioners assumed that the mind had a degree of influence on bodily processes that modern-day technology has only recently been able to measure. At the same time that scientists were measuring the effects of the fight-or-flight response to stress, other scientists were studying how that response might be switched off to restore relaxation and calm.

Herbert Benson (1975) reported that transcendental meditation, or TM, one of many forms of Eastern Asian meditation, could cause a relaxation response. This announcement was a rediscovery of ancient and widely held beliefs about healing. Meditation has long been a part of Eastern religious traditions in which practitioners believed that it helped heal not only physical but emotional and spiritual stress.

There are a number of techniques, such as meditation, biofeedback, and visualization, that can be utilized to help reduce stress. Each has value in its ability to cause a relaxation response. A simple method of meditation is described below.

Meditation is an ancient technique that has a long history in various Asian religions. It includes a *mantra,* the use of a single, unchanging word, chant, or prayer. This single focus helps to dissipate the continual chatter that goes on in our minds. By quieting the mind, meditation helps relax the body. There are many ways of meditating, but they all have certain things in common.

A mantra is a sound, word, or phrase that is repeated to yourself. It can be spoken aloud, as a chant, or silently, as in meditation. Pick a focus word or short phrase that is firmly rooted in your personal belief system. Most people think the best mantras are sounds that have no clear meaning. If you do not already know of a good mantra, a commonly used one is *hamsa.* This is a natural mantra. It is the sound that one makes when breathing, with *ham* (h-ah-m) on inhalation and *sa* (s-ah) on exhalation. If you are using a single word, repeat it as you exhale.

> Sit comfortably, not cross-legged. If that is comfortable for you, you can meditate in that position. However, sitting in a chair with your feet flat on the floor is also acceptable. Do not lie down.

> Close your eyes, breathe naturally, and gaze straight ahead in a relaxed and alert manner. Watch whatever space you perceive after closing your eyes. Sit for about one minute before you begin thinking the mantra to allow your heart and breathing to slow down.

> Slowly bring your attention to your breathing and begin to think the mantra, gently and easily. Just let it come, don't force it. Think *ham* as you inhale and *sa* as you exhale. Allow yourself to be absorbed in it.

Allow your thoughts and feelings to come and go. If other thoughts come to mind, just accept them and do not try to control them. Gently return to your mantra.

Meditate for about 10 to 20 minutes. It is okay to occasionally glance at a clock to time the mediation. Do not use an alarm timer.

When finished, take about one minute to slowly return to normal awareness.

Not all meditation sessions will be equally peaceful and relaxing. Some will be fretful, uncomfortable, and full of obsessive thought. Regardless, daily meditation will have a positive effect on your life. Try to meditate for at least 10 minutes in the morning and 10 minutes in the evening and enjoy the results.

In health care settings, relaxation and meditation exercises are utilized to reduce stress and anxiety, reduce pain, and cleanse the mind of tension. However, meditation should not be used for these purposes only; it should be used as a life skill to bring about a sense of calm, focus, self-mastery, and inner control.

4. Keep control of your own life. The concept of locus of control means that a person believes he or she has control over his or her life. Researchers have shown that people with a sense of mastery or control over their lives suffer fewer symptoms of physical and psychological stress than those who feel much of their life is beyond their control (Peterson and Bossio, 1993). Having control over your own life is beneficial to your health.

People who take responsibility for both the positive and negative things that happen in their lives have an *internal locus of control*. They believe that their personal actions affect the outcome of their life's events. Therefore, they believe that the events in their lives can be potentially controlled. Those who believe that most of what happens to them is beyond their control are said to have an *external locus of control*. These individuals believe that the things that happen to them are unrelated to their own behavior and, therefore, beyond their control. It is important to point out that an individual's locus of control is developed through learning and experiences through life. More importantly, our locus of control is based on life perceptions and can be continually reevaluated and changed.

Although developing an internal locus of control is ideal, you don't want to push yourself beyond reality. There are many things that occur in our lives that we can't control, such as accidents and disasters. It is foolish to blame yourself for things you cannot control. Part of your coping mechanism is to accept the things that you cannot change and use your internal locus of control to come up with the most adaptive way to adjust to them.

5. Talk yourself through challenges. It is not unusual for a person to talk to himself or herself when faced with a difficult situation or challenge. If somebody is willing to take risk, he or she can use the following three techniques to help himself or herself go beyond self-talk and deal more effectively with the challenge or difficult situation.

A. *Prepare for the challenge.* Use the problem-solving techniques discussed above to help get through the challenge. Use social support systems in preparing your plan. Picture yourself going through the situation as you use your problem-solving skills to cope when things become stressful. If you get angry or anxious while rehearsing this challenge, use your relaxation techniques to calm yourself down. Practice going over the challenge until you feel in control.

B. *Confront the challenge.* Be confident. Believe that you can handle the situation and that you will survive. Remind yourself not to get caught up in anxiety and anger. Try to remain calm and stick to your plan. Most importantly, be willing to make mistakes. Do not force yourself to be perfect.

C. *Reflect on what you have learned.* When the challenge is over, take some time to reflect on what you have learned. It is okay to notice your mistakes. Remember, mistakes are wonderful opportunities for learning. Ask yourself what you did right and ask yourself how you can improve. Do not be too critical. Reflect on the situation and picture yourself going through it again and remind yourself that you survived and that you did pretty well and that you will be even better the next time.

6. Keep a sense of humor. Science is beginning to recognize something that you probably already knew: Laughter is an important part of your life. Scientists who study laughter have discovered that play, fun, and humor are essential to health (Rose, 1990). Norman Cousins, former editor of the *Saturday Review,* intrigued the medical profession when he applied his own special brand of therapy: laughter therapy and vitamin C. Given little chance of recovery from a degenerative illness, Cousins watched *Candid Camera* shows and Marx Brothers movies. His sedimentation rate (a measure of inflammation or infection) dropped by five points during laughter. Cousins (1976) also reported that 10 minutes of belly laughter gave him two hours of pain-free sleep without medication. In addition, he believed he recovered because of the healing emotions of love, hope, faith, and laughter. Studies have shown that laughter increases S-IgA antibodies, which helps the body fight off colds, flus, and respiratory infections (Dillon et al., 1986), stimulates the Beta-endorphins that produce natural highs in humans, and decreases mood disturbances, such as depression and anger, during and after stressful events (Martin and Lefcourt, 1983).

A good belly laugh gives a hearty workout to practically every organ in the body. It is a sort of "inner jogging." Laughter is therapeutic for painful and stressful events. It can distract you from worry and help banish gloomy thoughts. It can lighten stress, anxiety, depression, and pain. Laughter, like love, heals.

7. Exercise regularly. Exercise is a useful skill for coping with stress and reducing anxiety, while at the same time enhancing physical fitness (Brown and Siegel, 1988; Long and Haney, 1988). Exercise also has positive effects on one's self-concept and mood. It requires a real commitment (internal locus of control) that leads to feeling physically better and developing a well-functioning body (King et al., 1989).

A regular exercise program will provide the following benefits: lower blood pressure, more efficient heart and lungs, stronger bones, increased collateral blood vessels to the heart, increased HDL's and decreased LDL's, a reduction of body fat, stronger muscles, fewer infections, bone growth, self-esteem, and much, much more.

Conclusion

The effect of stress on the body and mind cannot be underestimated, nor can the importance of stress management. Stress management must be a part of everyone's lifestyle. Remember: When you handle stress better, there is less stress to handle.

REFERENCES

Adler, R. *Psychoneuroimmunology.* New York: Academic Press, 1981.

Attorney general's report on the impact of criminal street gangs on crime and violence in California by the year 2000. 1993. http://electric.ss.uci.…ica/Gangs2000/open.html

Benson, H. *The relaxation response.* New York: Morrow, 1975.

Brown, J., and Siegel, J. (1988). Exercise as a buffer of life stress: A prospective study of adolescent health. *Health Psychology,* 7, 341–353.

Canino, I., and Spurlock, J. *Culturally diverse children and adolescents.* New York: Guilford, 1994.

Cannon, W. *The wisdom of the body.* New York: W. W. Norton, 1932.

Centers for Disease Control, National Center for Health Statistics. *Vital statistics of the U.S.,* vol. 2, PHS. Washington, DC: U.S. Government Printing Office, 1992.

The Commonwealth Fund. *A comparative survey of minority health.* New York: The Commonwealth Fund. hppt://www.cmwf.org:80/minhlth.html

Cose, E. *The rage of the privileged class,* New York: Harper Collins, 1993.

Cousins, N. Anatomy of an illness as perceived by the patient. *New England Journal of Medicine,* 295 (1976), 1458–1463.

Curtis, L. *Violence, race, and culture.* Lexington, MA: D. C. Heath, 1985.

Dillon, K., Minchoff, B., and Baker, K. Positive emotional states and enhancement of the immune system. *International Journal of Psychiatry in Medicine,* 15 (1986), 13–18.

Eitinger, L. The symptomatology of mental illness among refugees in Norway." *Journal Mental Science,* 106 (1960), 947–966.

Federal Bureau of Investigation. *Uniform crime reports. Crime in the United States: 1986.* Washington, DC: U.S. Department of Justice, 1987.

Gall, S., and Gall, T. (Eds.) *Statistical Record of Asian Americans.* Detroit: Gale Research, 1993.

Hechinger, F., and the Carnegie Council on Adolescent Development. *Fateful choices: Healthy youth for the 21st century.* New York: Carnegie Corporation of New York, 1992.

Helman, C. *Culture, health and illness.* Bristol, England: John Wright and Sons. 1986.

Holmes, T., and Rahe, R. The social readjustment rating scale. *Journal of Psychosomatic Research,* 11 (1967), 213–218.

Irujo, Suzzane. An introduction to intercultural differences and similarities in nonverbal communication.

In J. Wurzel (Ed.), *Toward multiculturalism.* Yarmouth: Intercultural Press, 1988, pp. 142–150.

King, A., Taylor, C., Haskell, W., and DeBusk, R. Influence of regular aerobic exercise on psychological health: A randomized, controlled trial of healthy middle-aged adults. *Health Psychology,* 8 (1989), 305–324.

Kleinke, C. *Coping with life challenges.* Pacific Grove, CA: Brooks/Cole, 1991.

Kreiger, N. Racial and gender discrimination: Risk factors for high blood pressure?" *Social Science and Medicine,* 30 (1990), 1273–1281.

Landrine, H., and Klonoff, E. *African American acculturation: Deconstructing race and reviving culture.* Thousand Oaks, CA: Sage, 1996.

Landry, D. (Ed.). Culture, disease and healing: Studies in medical anthropology. New York: Macmillan, 1977.

Langner, T. S., Gersten, J. C., Eisenberg, J. G. Approaches to measurement and definition in the epidemiology of behavior disorders: Ethnic background and child behavior. *Inter Journal of Health Services,* 4 (1979) 483–500. In R. Bacerra, M. Karno, and J. Escobar (Eds.), *Mental health and Hispanic Americans: Clinical perspectives.* New York: Grune & Stratton, 1982. p. 161.

La Vietes, R. The Puerto Rican child. In R. Bacerra, M., Karno, J., and Escobar. *Mental health and Hispanic American: Clinical perspectives.* New York: Grune & Stratton, 1982, p. 161.

Lazarus, R. *Psychological stress and the coping process,* New York: McGraw-Hill, 1966.

Lee, E. Cultural factors in working with Southeast Asian refugee adolescents. *Journal of Adolescence,* 11 (1988), 167–179.

Long, B. and Haney, C. Coping strategies for working women: Aerobic exercise and relaxation interventions. *Behavior Therapy,* 19 (1988), 75–83.

Marks, I. *Living with fear: Understanding and coping with anxiety.* New York: McGaw-Hill, 1978.

Martin, R., and Lefcourt, H. Sense of humor as a moderator of the relation between stressors and moods. *Journal of Personality and Social Psychology,* 45 (1983), 1313–1324.

Min, P. G. *Major issues relating to Asian American experiences in Asian Americans: Contemporary Trends and Issues.* Newbury Park, CA: Sage Focus Editions, Vol 174, pp. 38–57.

National Center for Health Statistics, Division of Vital Statistics. *Vital statistics of the United States: 1990.* Washington, DC: Government Printing Office, 1991.

National Commission on the Causes and Prevention of Violence. *Crimes of violence, vol. 12: A staff report.*

Washington, DC: U.S. Government Printing Office, 1969.

National Institute of Mental Health. *Research highlights; Extramural research,* Washington, DC: Government Printing Office, 1983.

Okamura, J., and Agbayani, A. Filipino Americans. In Noreen Mokuau (Ed.), *Handbook of social services for Asian and Pacific Islanders* (pp. 97–115). New York: Greenwood Press, 1991.

Peterson, C., and Bossio, L. Healthy attitudes: Optimism, hope, and control. In D. Goleman and J. Gurin (Eds.), *Mind body medicine.* Yonkers, NY: Consumer Reports Books, pp. 351–366.

Poussaint, E. Special techniques for management of hypertension in blacks. In W. D. Hall, E. Saunders, and N. Shulman (Eds.), *Hypertension in blacks: Epidemiology, pathophysiology, and treatment* (pp. 209–236). Chicago: Year Book, 1983.

Rose, J. Psychologic health of women: A phenomenologic study of women's inner strength. *Advancements in Nursing Science,* 12, 2 (1990) 56.

Rutter, M., and Quinto, D. Psychiatric disorders: Ecological factors and concepts of causation. In H. McGurk (Ed), Ecological factors in human development. Amsterdam: North Holland, in R. Bacerra, M.

Karno, J. Escobar. (Eds.), 1976; *Mental health and Hispanic Americans: Clinical perspectives.* New York: Grune & Stratton, 1982. p. 121–140.

Selye, H. *The stress of life (*rev. ed.). New York: Harper Collins, 1976.

Shah, S., and Roth, L. Some considerations pertaining to prevention. In D. Glaser (Ed.), *Handbook of criminality.* Chicago: Rand-McNally, 1974.

Spurlock, J. Development of self-concept in Afro-American children. *Hospital and Community Psychiatry,* 37, 1 (1986) 66–70.

Sue, S., and Chin, R. The mental health of Chinese-American children: Stressors and resources. In Gloria Powell (Ed.), *The psychosocial development of minority group children* (pp. 358–397). New York: Brunner/Mazel, 1983.

Uba, L. *Asian Americans: Personality patterns, identity, and mental health.* New York: Guilford, 1994.

Wolkind, S., and Rutter, M. *Sociocultural factors in child and adolescent psychiatry.* Boston: Blackwell Scientific, 1985.

Yu, K., and Kim, L. The growth and development of Korean American children. In G. Powell (Ed.), *The psychosocial development of minority group children* (pp. 147–158). New York: Brunner/Mazel, 1983.

CHAPTER

5 Culture and Mental Health

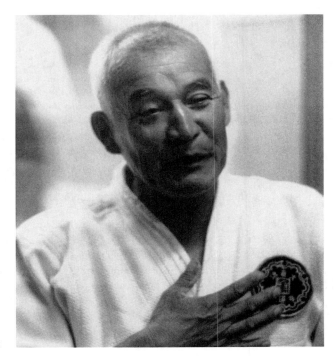

If we are to achieve richer culture, rich in contrasting values, we must recognize the whole gamut of human potentials, and so weave a less arbitrary fabric, one in which each diverse human gift will find a fitting place.

—Margaret Mead

Photo by Marcy Israel, published in *Cultures* magazine, volume 2, issue 1.

The Importance of Healthy Self-Esteem

Emotional health is related to your feelings and moods. You may feel happy, sad, fearful, or angry. Emotionally healthy individuals are aware of their feelings and can express them in constructive ways. Emotional health is also subjective because only you know your own feelings. How you are able to cope with stress, maintain flexibility with change, assess your values, interact with others, and compromise to resolve conflict are all part of being emotionally healthy. People who consistently try to improve their emotional health have a better chance of leading happier and healthier lives. Emotionally healthy people are more likely to have a positive picture of themselves and are more likely to develop higher levels of self-esteem.

Self-esteem is a composite picture of perceived self-value. It's the disposition to experience yourself as worthy of happiness, health and wellness, respect, friendship, love, achievement, and success (Youngs, 1991). Self-esteem is the most important variable in regard to human development and maturation. It is the master key that can open the door to the actualization of an individual's potential.

Youngs (1991) states that

> self-esteem is central to what we make of our lives—the loyalty we have to developing our-
> selves and to caring about others, and it is at the heart of what we will achieve in the course
> of our lifetime. Perhaps nothing affects health and energy, peace of mind, the goals we set
> and achieve, our inner happiness, the quality of our relationships, our competence, perfor-
> mance, and productivity, quite as much as the health of our self-esteem. (p. 2)

Self-efficacy and *self-respect* are the dual pillars of healthy self-esteem. If either one is absent, self-esteem is impaired (Brandon, 1969). How people view themselves and how much self-worth they possess will affect their health, relationships, competence, goals that are set and achieved, performance, and happiness. This self-image or inner picture will influence how people will treat themselves or others.

> *Self-efficacy* means confidence in your ability to think and in the process by which you
> judge, choose, and decide. It's knowing and understanding your interests and needs. It
> incorporates self-trust and self-reliance (Brandon, 1969). It is your perception of your abil-
> ity to take on and complete tasks successfully. This belief stems from your past experiences.
> For example, practicing diligently on the piano has helped you successfully play a difficult
> musical piece; therefore, you believe that more diligent practice will do the same for you
> with future musical pieces.
>   *Self-respect* means assurance of your values. It's an affirmative attitude toward the
> right to live and be happy, toward freedom to assert your thoughts, wants, needs, and joys.
> The experience of self-respect allows for mutual regard of others and makes possible a non-
> neurotic sense of fellowship with them. (Youngs, 1991, p. 8)

Everyone has a self-image of her- or himself that is based on her or his self-esteem. Every person perceives himself or herself in some positive or negative way—pretty, ugly, overweight, skinny, athletic, clumsy, or different. Everyone has adjectives that describe themselves.

DeBoer (1984), for example, did a study on how high school females perceived their science abilities when compared to the male students. DeBoer found that female high school students rated their science ability lower than male students even though their actual performance was generally better. DeBoer hypothesized that this negative self-perception in science ability is an important issue and one of the reasons why women have reduced participation in science courses and careers. Allen (1986) found that male students outnumber female students by 2 to 1 in computer programming courses and that more female students perceive computer programming as too difficult, partly because computer courses are usually based within the mathematics department.

Your self-image is a result of the kinds of reinforcements you receive from your parents, peers, relatives, friends, and other important community members. Of all the judgments and beliefs that you have, none is more important than the one you have about yourself.

Self-esteem is part of a person's personality. Personality is extremely complex and consists of many variables or traits. Our self-esteem is developed from the sum of the many variables that make up our personality. Each of us possesses some personality traits and lacks others and it is the combination of these traits that helps define who we are and how we think about ourselves at any particular moment. Because we all have the ability to improve or acquire personality variables, we are all subject to change. Thus, our personality and self-esteem are not static but constantly changing as we learn to adjust to life events.

It is important to discuss personality theories because they are the basis for our self-esteem. A number of individuals have studied personality development and many theories have been discussed over the years. Two opposite personality theories will be discussed in relation to ethnic minority populations and self-esteem: humanistic psychology and behavioral psychology. The humanistic model is based on subjective interpretations of experience while the behavioral model is based on external forces.

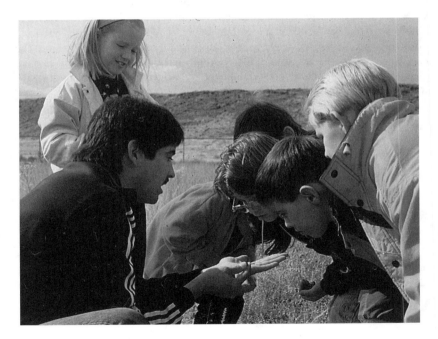

Photo by Stephen Marks.

Tell me, and I'll forget. Show me and I may not remember. Involve me, and I'll understand.

—Native American saying

Humanistic Theories of Personality:
Building Healthy Self-Esteem by Meeting
a Person's Basic Emotional Needs

The works of Abraham Maslow, Carl Rogers, Rudolf Dreikurs, Alfred Adler, and William Glasser have all supported the theory that, if given the opportunity and appropriate encouragement, individuals will grow in positive ways. Individuals are basically made up of the total of their individual experiences. The following discussion is based on the blending of common traits found in the basic humanistic theories of personality development and self-esteem.

People, like plants, have basic needs. Plants need soil, water, and sunshine to grow. If one neglects the needs of a plant, it may never grow to its fullest potential. If one neglects the needs of people, they may never grow into their fullest potential. What are the basic human needs? The following list of basic needs was developed by blending the works of humanistic theorists such as Maslow (1983), (Rogers, 1951), Dreikurs (1964), Glasser (1969), Youngs (1991), and Glenn & Nelsen (1989). *Also, for the sake of consistency and continuity, the following basic needs model will focus on student populations.* However, this model can be applied to any population and is depicted in Figure 5.1.

1. ***The need to be accepted and to belong.*** Acceptance and belonging—being connected to those you care for—are essential elements in building self-esteem. Nothing contributes to one's self-esteem more than being accepted by others. Without acceptance, people will perish just as surely as if you deprive them of food and water. The concept of acceptance is based on respect, affirmation, caring, empathy, fairness, sensitivity, and warmth. Acceptance is recognizing and appreciating another person's intrinsic worth. It is unconditional, not contingent on anything particular about the individual. A person does

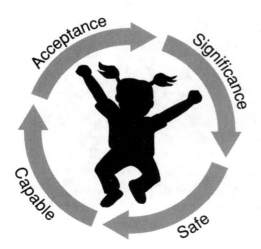

FIGURE 5.1   Basic Emotional Needs

B O X **5.1**

A Simple Gesture

The following excerpt was written by Glenn Van Eckeren (1988). Although this story is related to sports, its implications apply to life in general.

History was made in the baseball world in 1947. It was in that year that Jackie Robinson became the first black baseball player to play in the major leagues. The Brooklyn Dodgers' owner, Branch Rickey, told Robinson, "It'll be tough. You are going to take abuse, be ridiculed, and take more verbal punishment than you ever thought possible. But I'm willing to back you all the way if you have the determination to make it work."

In short order, Robinson experienced Rickey's prediction. He was abused verbally and physically as players intentionally ran him over. The crowd was vociferous with their racial slurs and digging comments. Opponents ridiculed Robinson as well as the Dodger players.

Around mid-season, Robinson was having a particularly bad day. He had fumbled grounders, overthrown first base, and had an equally disastrous day at the plate. The crowd was celebrative in their boos. Then something special happened. In front of this critical crowd, Pee Wee Reese walked over from his shortstop position, put his arm around Jackie Robinson, and indicated his acceptance of the major league's first black baseball player.

Robinson later reflected, "That gesture saved my career. Pee Wee made me feel as if I belonged."

Consider the number of newcomers who happen in our lives every week. They too are awaiting for the displayed acceptance from the crowd. But more important, they need to feel as if they belong in our world and are considered an important contributor. We have a significant impact on the lives of others by simply letting them know we accept them.

not have to accomplish anything to receive this acceptance. Each person has inherent value, and so acceptance is not something to be earned (Nakamura, 1996).

Many minority students, however, do not feel that they are really accepted, but only tolerated, by mainstream American society. This lack of acceptance is reinforced early in life by the fact that schools, for example, have not traditionally valued either their ethnicity, their history and heritage, or their language. Even their cultural mannerisms in talking, behaving, moving, and living are perceived as unacceptable or inferior.

Minority students, in particular, need to feel that there is some meaning to their existence in the classroom. The research on school dropouts indicates that being unaffiliated—not belonging—is one of the leading causes of dropping out of school. McKay (1988) reported that Hispanic Americans are far more likely to drop out of school than are members of any other ethnic group. Nationally, at least one-half of Mexican American and Puerto Rican youth leave school without a high school diploma. Hispanic Americans not only have higher dropout rates, but they also tend to leave school earlier than do blacks or whites. It has been estimated that about 40 percent of Hispanic American dropouts leave high school before the spring semester of their sophomore year. In addition, Seller (1989) reported that perhaps most troubling is that in the mid-1980s, the high school dropout rate of Hispanic women was more than double that of whites or blacks…and the high school dropout rate of teenage mothers suggests that needs of these young women were not being met in traditional schools.

2. *The need to feel significant.* All people need to feel that they are important, that their participation in school, work, family, and society has meaning and purpose, and that their existence matters (Nakamura, 1996). People need to feel that their contributions are appreciated and necessary. Individuals will give up or lose their motivation to compete or progress when they believe that they are not important.

The need to feel needed can be more powerful than the need to live. People have even committed suicide when they felt that their lives had no meaning or significance. Wehlage (1989) reported that teenagers who feel alienated from family, school, or the community are more likely to abuse drugs, get pregnant or father a child, fail in school, commit vandalism, develop depression, or commit suicide. Wehlage stated,

> The challenge clearly for these social institutions—and especially for the schools—is to engage youth by providing them opportunities to participate in meaningful, valued activities and roles, those involving problem-solving, decision-making, planning, goal-setting, and helping others. (p. 4)

Bernard (1991) reinforced Wehlage by stating,

> Once again, the operating dynamic reflects the fundamental human need to bond, to participate, to belong, to have some power or control over one's life. When schools ignore these basic human needs, they become ineffective and alienating places. (p. 4)

Sarason (1990) summarized it well by saying,

> When one has no stake in the way things are, when one's needs or opinions are provided no forum, when one sees oneself as the object of unilateral actions, it takes no particular wisdom to suggest that one would rather be elsewhere. (p. 2)

A simple test to determine the social climate of a school is to answer the following questions:

1. Which students traditionally receive most of the social rewards of the school? How many were minority students? Are certain students from within the majority population excluded?
2. Are minority students actively involved in activities such as cheerleading, the debate team, the school play, or other similar activities?
3. How many minority students are in leadership positions?
4. Who is in charge of the minority student clubs or activities? Are they members of the majority group?
5. Are minority students chosen to represent the school in school social functions such as "open house" or escorting important guests?
6. Does the school's sports program equally support both men and women?

Historically, the curricula in most schools have had a Western European-American focus that denies the importance of other multicultural populations. Fortunately, in recent years, schools have been making efforts to encourage a multicultural perspective in the curricula. Hopefully, in the near future, this will be completely accomplished. The things that most culturally diverse students know as a result of their experiences outside of school (home, community, and culture), are very different from the things a typical white American teacher might expect them to know. As a consequence, what is presented in class can be meaningless to culturally diverse students, resulting in their feeling that their significance in the classroom is at best peripheral, or at worst an unwelcome intrusion. Because the materials are often irrelevant to them, many minority students reciprocate by not participating. This creates a cyclic effect in which they are not expected to participate and ends with the students feeling that their contributions are not important.

On the other side of this issue is the fact that many children from the macroculture come to school with preconceived negative attitudes toward people who are different from them (Lasker, 1970). As a consequence, teachers must work to change these negative attitudes and develop strategies that encourage positive attitudes about economic, cultural, and racial differences.

Minority students, in particular, are motivated when materials are relevant to them and their culture or gender. When educators incorporate teaching materials that include the perspectives and the experiences of culturally diverse populations, minority students respond with greater enthusiasm. James Love (1985) stated that "knowledge must have a special relationship with the learner if it is to be learned." Learning about one's culture within the concepts basic to each discipline reinforces the student's importance or significance.

Gordon, Miller, and Rollock (1990) noted that African Americans and other students of color are asked to learn and relate to material that:

1. has not been often reproduced in their community or culture;
2. is not presented from their perspective;
3. tends to ignore their existence and often demeans their personal characteristics;
4. may distort or misinterpret data; and
5. makes unwarranted generalizations that differences are deficits.

The curricula in some schools do not reflect a diverse society. A mainstream Western European-American focus with a male orientation is one of the reasons why racism and sexism are reinforced and perpetuated in both our schools and society. It creates an atmosphere in which mainstream white American male students may come to believe that they are superior to women and other racial and ethnic groups. It denies both mainstream white American students and minority students the opportunity to study and benefit from the knowledge, perspectives, and experiences of other cultures and groups. In addition, there is a serious cultural gap in most present-day textbooks. It has only been within the past few years that authors have become sensitive to diversity issues. This gap, of course, has contributed greatly to the ignorance, stereotyping, and underestimation of many ethnic minority groups and women. As a result, teachers must evaluate their textbooks, other learning materials, and lessons for bias. Teachers must then supplement learning activities with additional materials to redress bias.

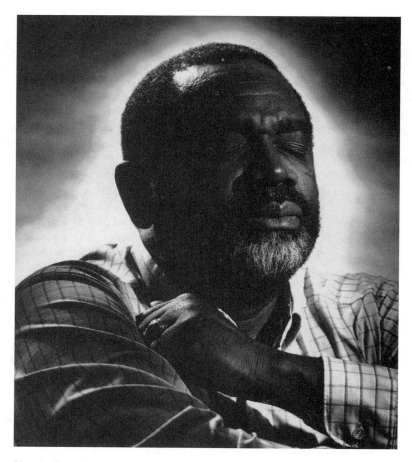

Photo by Everado Martinez-Inzunza, published in *Cultures* magazine, volume 1, issue 2.

The bug disease kills more people than any other disease in the world, and that
is why it is important not to let anything bug you.

—Duke Ellington, *Music Is My Mistress,* 1973

The mainstream Eurocentric curriculum diminishes the minority students' experiences and culture and creates a mirror that does not reflect their aspirations and hopes. If the curriculum undermines the minority students' capacity for full intellectual development and their lives are not matters for serious attention or concern, this will limit their professional success. Also, if limited views of minority students are overtly or subtly communicated by teachers, some students will experience a reinforcement of their own negative views about minority students, especially because such views are confirmed by people of knowledge and status. This, of course, hampers a student's ability to relate to minority students as equals and work with them in collaborative situations.

Minority students are more highly motivated when the school curriculum reflects their cultures, experiences, and visions. The curriculum should be organized around the basic concepts of each discipline, but must begin to draw from the experiences and perspectives of both men and women and the many different cultural groups. This is essential as we move into the global era of interdependence, as people of various nations and cultures move closer together. No one culture must dominate the curriculum, and students must be encouraged to study issues from diverse viewpoints.

3. *The need to feel capable or competent.* People need to feel that they can take on responsibility and that they are skilled and can do things well. Teachers and students who feel capable know that they can learn to do things. They are challenged by tasks even though they face difficult odds (Nakamura, 1996).

If people view themselves as incapable and their environment continues to reinforce that view, they may eventually come to believe it. Somebody, for example, who is continually treated as inferior by people will eventually perceive him- or herself as inferior. Once the perception of inferiority is established, it becomes the foundation out of which that person acts. Such a person will act inferior in relation to others, and other people will reciprocate by treating the person as inferior.

The historical Rosenthal and Jacobson's (1968) study, "Pygmalion in the Classroom," reported that, when children were "stereotyped" as being exceptionally bright and treated by the teachers in such a manner (positive facial expressions, tone of voice, supportive statements, and behaviors of acceptance), they reciprocated by assuming that role. The following list includes some of their findings.

1. The general climate factor that consisted of the overall warmth a teacher exhibits was shown more to high expectancy students.
2. Students for whom high expectations are held received more praise for doing something right than do students for whom low expectations are held.
3. High expectancy students are taught more than low expectancy students.
4. Students for whom the teacher has higher expectations are called on more often and are given more chances to reply, as well as more frequent and more difficult questions.

Rosenthal and Jacobson's original study was eventually criticized for its methodological weaknesses (Brophy and Good, 1974), but further research has continued to support the general principles of the study.

Unfortunately, some teachers expect less of some minority students, so these students produce less. The U.S. Commission on Civil Rights (1973) conducted a study of 429 classrooms to determine if Mexican American students were treated less favorably than the Anglo students. The term *Anglo* was used instead of *Western European-American* in this study. The study concluded that many teachers:

1. Unconsciously assumed that Mexican American students were more unruly and consequently needed more discipline. As a result of this assumption, Mexican Americans were scolded more often than Anglo students; consequently, the interactions between Mexican American students were less favorable and resulted in less interaction with the teachers. Teachers spoke more frequently with Anglo students than Mexican American students.

2. Unconsciously assumed that Mexican American students were less bright, which resulted in the teachers asking more difficult questions of the Anglo students. As a result of this, Anglo students were praised more and challenged intellectually more than were Mexican Americans.
3. Favor Anglo students, over Mexican American students, as shown by the quality of verbal and nonverbal interactions.

These teachers unconsciously assumed that Mexican Americans were more violent, less intelligent, and experience more difficulty with the English language. As a result they treated the students according to their expectations, and the self-fulfilling prophecy held true.

Garcia (1982) concluded that teacher expectations are more influenced by negative information about pupil characteristics than positive data. As a result:

1. Teachers who do not have high academic expectations for minority students ask them low-level memory, recall, and convergent questions, do not praise or encourage them as often as Anglo students, user lower standards of judging the quality of their work, and do not call on them as frequently and feed them academic pabulum.
2. Counselors who do not believe minority students can master math and science skills do not schedule them into these classes.
3. Special purpose instruction for minorities tends to be remediation and for Anglo students it tends to be enrichment.
4. Presumed high-achieving Anglo students who do not live up to teachers' expectations are described as underachievers. These attitudes and expectations cause great disparities in how educators interact with Anglo and minority students in the day-to-day operations of schools and, thereby, perpetuate educational inequalities among them.
5. Schools use culturally biased tests and procedures to diagnose student needs and to evaluate their performance. For instance, tests may require skills in scenarios about situations that are not relevant to the cultural backgrounds and life experiences of minorities. Thus, minority students are placed at a disadvantage because they may know the skill or subject matter but be unfamiliar with the contextual scenario.
6. Many minority students are "tracked" into lower level academic groups, which perpetuates the stereotypical image of an incapable ethnic minority student and reinforces the feeling of superiority of the majority group. This process also leads to isolating students along cultural, racial, or economic lines and thereby perpetuating in-school segregation.

In addition to Garcia's study, Simpson and Erickson (1983) reported that white American teachers gave white American male students more verbal and nonverbal praise while using more nonverbal criticisms of African American males. Sadker and Sadker (1985) also reported that teachers would accept incorrect answers from African American students with a verbal "okay." As a result of this behavior, African American students were denied useful information about the quality of their performance. Natriello, McDill, and Pallas (1990) reported that teachers have lower academic expectations of poor children.

Lowered expectations frequently reinforce themselves, and children will often internalize what the teacher believes.

In relation to gender issues, Campbell (1984) concluded that teachers give males more feedback and check their work more often. When males answered questions incorrectly, they were encouraged to try harder. When females answered incorrectly, they were praised for trying. Bossert (1981) reported that teachers called on males to perform tasks that involved manual skills while females were more likely to be requested to conduct housekeeping chores and secretarial tasks. Fennema and Peterson (1986) reported that, in high-level math achievement, male students were given more feedback than female students. Female students were given no feedback more often than male students.

Stereotypes and prejudices relative to low-income minorities adversely affect their self-concepts and feelings of inadequacy. Minority women, in particular, may experience a double disadvantage in living in a society that values both maleness and whiteness and, therefore, are more vulnerable to mental disorders as a result of prejudices and discriminatory practices.

4. *The need to feel safe.* Physical and emotional safety means that people feel they are in control of their own selves within their environment, that they have mastery over their being. Without a feeling of physical and emotional safety, people find it difficult to move beyond strong fear and anxiety and to be willing to enthusiastically explore new challenges (Nakamura, 1996). Strong fear and anxiety limit people, sometimes in small ways, sometimes in ways so large that they become imprisoned by them. Intense fear or anxiety can affect thinking, remembering, behavior, and physical performance.

People must see their daily environment as a place (1) where all precautions have been taken to ensure their physical safety, and (2) where their emotional well-being is not being violated (Nakamura, 1996). Would most people stay on a job if they were afraid for their own physical or emotional safety? Probably not. How long adults stay on a job is determined largely by whether or not they consider the environment to be safe and orderly. This perception is also related to their level of performance and productivity, how much trust they have in their fellow workers, and how much they support their boss. Employees who do not feel safe while at work suffer more depression and mood swings and have the highest absenteeism and quitting rates.

When people are forced to live in unsafe environments because of poverty, lack of employment, and social injustices, they become victims of fear and anxiety. Individuals who perceive their living environment to be unsafe are less likely to invest positive energies in their community.

Unfair Discipline Practices in Schools and Their Influence on Multicultural Children. According to the annual Gallop Poll of Public Attitudes toward Education (Carter 1987) the lack of discipline was the number one problem in the public schools. Teachers from the United States and Canada list classroom management or the control of students as their greatest concern. Each individual teacher sets different behavior standards as well as disciplinary actions. For example, a teacher may ask the student to leave the room, call a parent, send the student to the principal's office, add more homework, or make a student stay after school. However, a teacher's decision about how and whom to discipline is not always based solely on the misbehavior.

Consistently, racial or ethnic minority students, especially African Americans, receive harsher reprimands than Western European-American students when measured by school suspension records. Dearman and Plisko (1981) reported that African Americans were twice as likely to be disciplined than Western European-Americans. Meier and Stewart (1991) reported that: (1) Hispanic students are more likely to receive corporal punishment than Anglo students; (2) Puerto Rican students are 43 percent overrepresented among students expelled from school; (3) as the African American suspension rate increases, the relative level of suspension among Hispanics decreases; (4) African American students are suspended for offenses that are often permitted of Anglo students; (5) dress codes are more rigidly enforced against Hispanic students than Anglo students.

Discipline based on cultural biases is one of the most devastating forms of discrimination in the education system. It reinforces existing stereotypes and creates a situation in which one group receives preferential treatment over another. In addition, these punishment trends can discourage students from attending school or encourage them to rebel against school policies, procedures, and adults in authority.

The Basic Needs Model Applied to Minority Student Stressors

Salanda (1995) developed a Minority Student Stressors Inventory. The respondents were to indicate which of the items described in the inventory were considered stressful. The purpose of this section is not to discuss the specific results of the inventory but to relate the inventory items to the previous discussion of the four basic human needs of feeling accepted, significant, capable, and physically and emotionally safe. Although it was not the intent of the inventory to categorize the concerns according to the four basic needs, every concern was related to a basic need. Table 5.1 is a partial list of some of the inventory items, or stressors, listed on the survey and the need(s) that it affects.

TABLE 5.1   Minority Student Stressors

Scale and Item	The Need
Scale 1: Academic concerns	
Not enough professors of my ethnic group	Significance
Anglo student and faculty expecting poor academic performance from students of my ethnic group.	Capability
Tense relationships between Anglos and minorities at this university	Safety
Scale 2: Ethnic–nonethnic group concerns	
Having to live around mostly Anglo people	Acceptance
Scale 3: Discrimination concerns	
Being treated rudely or unfairly because of my ethnicity	Safety

The Basic Needs Model Applied to Gang Participation

The Gangs 2000: A Call to Action report (The Attorney General, 1993) determined that seven major factors are involved in why youth, especially high-risk youth, join gangs. A close investigation of the factors reveals that all seven are related to the basic needs discussed earlier.

1. Gangs provide them with a sense of friendship, camaraderie, and family, things that they are not receiving at home or school. This factor is related to acceptance and belonging.
2. They experience a kind of success in gangs, whereas, they experience failure at school and in the home. This factor is related to feeling capable and significant.
3. There is nothing else to do; they have no hope and see no alternative but to join a gang. This factor is related to feeling capable and significant.
4. They feel their survival may depend on joining a neighborhood gang. They fear for their safety and believe that being in a gang gives them protection. This factor is related to feeling safe.
5. They have not developed the skills to express feelings of anger and rage constructively. This factor is related to feeling capable.
6. It is a way to gain respect and money. Gangs can provide lucrative economic opportunities, status, and prestige, especially for youths who do not believe they have employment opportunities, or who have no job skills. This factor is related to feeling capable and significant.

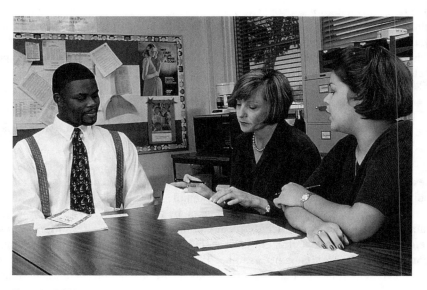

Photo by Will Hart.

No one can make us feel inferior without our permission.

—Eleanor Roosevelt

7. Some youths grow up in families in which parents and relatives are active gang members, and joining a gang is part of family tradition. In Hispanic neighborhoods, for instance, gangs have been an integral part of the barrio for generations. This factor is related to acceptance and belonging.

To counter these seven factors we must develop strategies to fulfill the basic needs in a healthier way by providing a reason and means for young people to get out of gangs and to empower individuals, families, schools, and communities so that they can take action to solve problems associated with gangs.

Behavioral Psychology

Behavioral psychology is based on the theory that one's behavior is the result of external stimuli or forces that prompt responses. It is the opposite of humanistic theory, which believes that behavior is based on the internal thought processes of the mind. Another name for behavioral psychology is *behavior modification.* Behavior modification has its roots in the works of B. F. Skinner, who theorized that all behavior is in response to stimuli (external forces) that prompt responses. Behavioral psychology is an extremely complex science and a complete discussion of the subject is beyond the scope of this book. Only a superficial overview is presented below.

Behaviorists theorize that external stimuli are reinforcers that either increase or maintain a behavior. If a behavior decreases in frequency, it is not being reinforced. The contingent presentation of a stimulus that increases or maintains a response is called *positive reinforcement.* Some people also refer to reinforcers as *rewards.* Parents may reward a child with a piece of candy (stimulus, S) if the child behaves (response, R) appropriately. A verbal "thank you" (the stimulus or reinforcer) keeps a student in his or her seat (response) while the teacher attends to other matters. A person lights up a cigarette (response) and gets a nicotine fix (stimulus). These two reinforcing events are diagrammed below:

R $\longrightarrow$ S	R $\longrightarrow$ S
Child stays in seat "thank you"	Lights up cigarette nicotine fix

There are two different types of reinforcers: *primary* reinforcers (e.g., water, food, sex), which reduce physiological needs, and *secondary* reinforcers, which increase the probability of obtaining primary reinforcers. Examples of secondary reinforcers include *social* reinforcers (e.g., a smile or compliment given by others); *token* reinforcers (e.g., accumulating points for academic achievement can be cashed in for a reward); and *contingency* reinforcement (e.g., a contract or agreement in which a behavior is allowed contingent on completion of an assignment). Another type of reinforcer is a *cue.* A *cue* is something within the environment that triggers a response. For example, the smells (cue) coming from a bakery may cause someone to buy a sweet roll whether she or he is hungry or not. Eating food may be a response to boredom (cue), and the time of day (afternoon break time at work) may cause someone to eat whether he or she is hungry or not. Reinforcers are specific to each individual. Not all people respond to the same reinforcers. For example, money is not a reinforcer for all people to work. If a stimulus does not maintain or increase the behavior, it is not a reinforcer.

Behavior can be shaped by the application of reinforcers. This is referred to as *conditioning.* Unfortunately, many individuals are conditioned into engaging in unhealthy behaviors. For example, eating lots of ice cream (response) because it tastes good (stimulus) is not a healthy behavior. Continued behavior of this type can lead to weight management problems. A college student may binge drink on weekends because it leads to acceptance by certain peer groups or because the student thinks it is fun. Some reinforcers, in reality, may not be fun, but as long as the individual believes they are, then the behavior will continue to be reinforced. For example, an alcoholic may say that he drinks because it is relaxing and it increases his sociability. However, in reality, the alcoholic is irritable and aggressive when drinking. As long as he believes he is relaxed and sociable, he will continue to be reinforced.

Negative reinforcement is an aversive stimulus that maintains or increases a behavior. For example, a parent nags (aversive stimulus) her daughter to wear a certain dress. If the child finally relents and wears the dress, than the nagging is a negative reinforcer. If she chooses to wear another dress, nagging is not a reinforcer. Using a drug to avoid the effects of withdrawal is another example of negative reinforcement. Cultural expectations may act as negative reinforcers for some ethnic groups. For example, Asian American parents may use shame or guilt (negative reinforcement) to get their children to study (response) a certain number of hours each night. Guilt and shame are common strategies used by Asian American adults.

It is important not to confuse negative reinforcement with punishment. Negative reinforcement maintains or increases a behavior, while punishment decreases a behavior. Punishment is not a reinforcer. Spanking a child to make her stop swearing is punishment if the behavior stops. In some cultures it is acceptable to use physical punishment to decrease certain behaviors of children.

Peer pressure is a strong social reinforcer. Children usually start drinking alcohol or smoking cigarettes in response to peer pressure. Cultural pressures are also strong social reinforcers because they condition people to behave in certain ways. For example, consumption of high-fat fried foods is part of the cultural heritage of African Americans from the southern states. This diet of high-fat foods, unfortunately, has contributed to increased risk of heart disease and diabetes in African Americans. The media (television, magazines, etc.) have reinforced the image of extremely thin white American women, which has led to a higher rate of anorexia and bulimia among young white American females. Smoking of cigarettes is socially reinforced among the male immigrants living in Laotian communities. Health professionals who work with patients must be aware of the cultural reinforcers and influences. For example, to educate patients about the harmful effects of smoking is not enough because the social reinforcers of acceptance and camaraderie within the Laotian community are stronger reinforcers than the knowledge of the dangers of smoking.

Many peer and cultural reinforcers also lead to positive healthful behaviors. Smoking among Hispanic women is not culturally supported and has resulted in low smoking rates within this group. Encouragement and support from family, friends, and community can reinforce healthful behaviors and motivate people to pursue healthier lifestyles.

The use of behavioral psychology strategies is extremely common in the health field. School health educators often utilize contracts (contingency reinforcement) to get students to perform certain healthy behaviors. Worksite health promotion programs often give rewards (e.g., T-shirts, free dinners, and other prizes) when employees participate in employer-sponsored health programs. Weight-reduction programs help clients identify and remove cues within the environment that reinforce unnecessary eating.

Depression

Somatization as an Expression of Psychological Disorders

Feeling anxious or down is a normal response to the ordinary challenges in life. We have all felt emotionally distressed over unexpected things occurring in our lives. But when emotions are strong enough to interfere with one's normal functioning, they can be regarded as symptoms of a psychological disorder. One of the most interesting concepts in the analysis of culture and psychological disorder is that people learn to express symptoms of their distress in ways acceptable to others of the same culture. As part of the socialization process, people learn to express psychological disorders in three ways: (1) the expressions are acceptable within their culture, (2) they are expressed in ways that will be understood, and (3) they are expressed in ways that will evoke a response, such as sympathy, from others.

Somatization refers to the patient's reported physical symptoms that are experienced during psychological stress. For example, a college student might feel homesick and report gastrointestinal problems, a shortness of breath, or menstrual irregularities. Further, no identifiable organic or physical causes can be found even though they are very real and troublesome to the patient. Hispanic Americans often exhibit symptoms of headache, heart palpitations, a sense of heat in the chest, generalized body pain, trouble sleeping, faintness, and persistent worrying due to *nervios* (nerves) and *ataques de nervios* (attack of nerves) (Guarnaccia et al., 1990). *Nervios* refers to chronic feelings of stress that result from bad marriages, a death of a loved one, finding employment, and other life challenges.

Some cultures reinforce the concept that complaints about anxieties, worries, and depression are signs of weakness and that people who exhibit these symptoms are "sick in the head." As a result, people from these cultures find more acceptance by reporting physical symptoms rather than emotional ones. In many African American and Asian American homes, emotional illness is considered a weakness, and individuals are reluctant to seek mental health services. Tseng and Hsu (1980) reported that Latin groups in Europe and America generally tended toward somatization, as did North Africans, while English-speaking populations expressed their distress to a greater extent through anxiety and depression.

The benefit of understanding cultural somatization is that researchers will be better able to interpret and diagnose psychological disorders. Because many minority populations tend to underutilize mental health facilities, many are misdiagnosed and misprescribed when the physician is unaware of the differences in cultural somatization. An Asian American student, for example, who is having problems with grades may somatize the problem into physical symptoms, such as complaints about body aches and pains. A physician unaware of cultural somatization symptoms may prescribe painkillers instead of stress-reducing activities.

It is also important to recognize that all people within a culture will not exhibit the same behavior and symptoms. There are many differences among the people of every culture. Still, if professionals (teachers, physicians, counselors, etc.) are aware of possible cultural differences, they will be better prepared to intervene in the early stages of a client's psychological concerns. Unfortunately, research in the area of cultural somatization is limited, and cultural-general and cultural-specific symptoms for various psychological disorders need to be explored. However, cultural somatization in depression disorder has been investigated and is providing some new information. Studies in this area will provide researchers with a better perspective on the mental health problems in minority populations.

Depression as a Model for Understanding Somatization

One of the main psychological disorders that interfere with people's everyday functioning is depression. Depression is the most common expression of mood disorder. The chances of developing depression are about 12 percent for men and 20 percent for women (Wing & Bebbington, 1985) regardless of the culture one comes from (Fugita and Crittenden, 1990). Fugita and Crittenden also reported that women are more likely to express depressive symptoms than men. There is no widely accepted single reason for this difference, and most researchers would suggest that the cause of depression among women is multifaceted, including biological and social factors.

Many minorities, regardless of site or social variables, also suffer special added stress as a result of threatened, perceived, and actual racism. For example, the reported subdued expressiveness of emotionality of some Asian American groups does not mean that they do not suffer from depression. Kuo (1984) reported that Asian Americans (Chinese, Japanese, Filipino, and Korean) had higher average scores for depression than did whites. Kuo further reported that about 19 percent of the Asian Americans studied were identified as potential cases of depression. Depression is found in all cultures and has been analyzed in terms of cultural-general and cultural-specific concepts.

Cultural-general refers to symptoms that are core to all individuals regardless of race, ethnicity, or culture. The following cultural-general depression symptoms have been suggested by the World Health Organization (1983) and Escobar, Gomez, & Tuason (1983):

1. Sadness and hopelessness
2. Loss of enjoyment or pleasure in doing usual activities
3. Anxiety or the state of emotional tenseness and distress resulting from fear
4. Inability to concentrate on tasks necessary for daily living
5. Lethargy or the lack of energy to accomplish simple goals
6. Escobar et al., (1990) listed less commonly reported cultural-general symptoms such as loss of weight, sexual interest, and appetite; hopelessness; and self-guilt.

Hopelessness is a state in which individuals experience a feeling of futility, lose hope, and feel powerless to intercede. Hopelessness can grow from repeated experiences of failure. For many minorities, isolation, lack of economic resources, disenfranchisement, and limited opportunities contribute to the feeling of hopelessness. From a clinical perspective, hopelessness is significantly associated with depression. A feeling of hopelessness can lead to substance abuse and self-destructive behavior, including suicide.

Family dissolution has been the most damaging to the mental health of many minority families. This can be seen especially in Native American culture, in which traditional roles have been eroded by federal government control over time. As a result of their loss of independence, many Native Americans have lost their sense of purpose, which has led to feelings of despair and, resentment and, ultimately, depression.

Cultural-specific symptoms are symptoms that go beyond the general core. Kleinman (1982), for example, reported that Chinese generally tend to somatisize their depression while white Americans learn to focus more on psychological symptoms, such as sadness and listless. Somatization of depression was also observed in other Asian groups (Yamamoto, 1982). Diekstra (1989) reported that suicide is often associated with depressive behavior in China. However, suicide is not usually associated with Chinese Americans. Although suicide can occur with depression, it is not part of the cultural-general core. Although suicide can happen unpredictably and even in the absence of depression, its risk increases with severe depression. Suicide among minority populations is discussed in the next section of this chapter.

Suicidal Behavior among Minority Youth

Across ethnic groups, adolescent suicide has increased over the years. Suicidal behavior is a serious health problem for adolescents, second to accidents as the leading cause of death among young people.

Native Americans

Native Americans, one of the most impoverished ethnic groups, often live without adequate nutrition, shelter, and sanitation. They suffer from a high rate of mental illness, which stems from feelings of hopelessness, desperation, and family dissolution, all of which are related to a history of poverty, harsh living, social injustices, and discrimination. As a result, Native Americans suffer from depression, anxiety, violence, substance abuse, and family conflicts. Native Americans have the highest rate of completed suicide of any ethnic group in the United States, even though the rate is decreasing (McIntosh, 1990). Alcohol abuse is a critical risk factor associated with suicidal behavior; 80 percent of American Indians who attempt suicide also have alcohol abuse problems (Young, 1988). Table 5.2 reports suicide mortality rates by age and sex for Native Americans in 1987.

Age is also a risk factor. High rates of suicide are found primarily among young American Indians from 15 to 34 years, the age group that makes up the largest proportion of the population.

African Americans

Suicide is the third leading cause of death among African American youth aged 15 to 24, after homicides and accidents (Gibbs, 1988). African American males between the ages of 15 and 19 have a suicide rate of 8.2 per 100,000 and African American males between the

TABLE 5.2   Suicide Mortality Rates, by Age and Sex

Age Group	Indian and Alaskan Native			U.S. All Races			Nonwhite		
	Both Sexes	Male	Female	Both	Male	Female	Both	Male	Female
5–14	1.7	2.9	0.6	0.7	1.1	0.3	0.5	0.7	0.2
15–24	23.5	40.7	6.5	12.9	21.3	4.3	8.7	14.4	3.0
25–34	28.7	49.6	8.3	15.4	24.8	5.9	11.7	20.1	4.0
35–44	19.6	30.3	9.3	15.0	22.9	7.2	9.5	16.4	3.6
45–54	13.1	21.7	5.0	15.9	23.8	8.5	7.6	12.7	3.3

Rates per 100,000 population for American Indians, Alaskan Natives, 1986–1988, and U.S., all races, 1987.

Source: Trends in Indian Health, 1991, U.S. Department of Health and Human Services, Public health Service, Indian Health Service, p. 46.

ages of 20 and 24 have a rate of 18.5 per 100,000 (USDHHS, 1985). The suicide rate for African American males is lower than white American males at all ages. This also applies to African American females in comparison to white American females.

Hispanic Americans

Wyche and Rotheram-Borus (1990) concluded that there are few studies reporting the suicide rates among Hispanic adolescents, and substantial discrepancies appear in the data that are reported. Recorded suicide rates from Mexican Americans have varied from 1.8 to 10.5 per 100,000 persons (Hope and Martin, 1986).

Asian Americans

Statistics are limited on all Asian American populations, but the rate of suicide among Chinese and Japanese Americans has been reported and is lower than white Americans. However, Yu, Chang, Liu, and Fernandez (1989) reported that, even though suicide rates are lower, the proportion of suicide deaths accounts for a larger portion of the deaths when compared to white Americans (see Table 5.3).

TABLE 5.3   Percentage of All Deaths Attributed to Suicide, 15–24 years old

	Chinese Americans	Japanese Americans	White Americans
Males	15.1%	21.3%	12.9%
Females	20.8%	14.0%	8.8%
Total	16.8%	19.0%	11.9%

Percentages are based on an analysis by Yu, Chang, Liu, and Fernandez (1989).

Suicide by Gender and Age

The U.S. Bureau of Health and Human Services (1991) reported that, until boys and girls are 9. their suicide rates are identical; from 10 to 14, the boys' rate is twice as high as the girls'; from 15 to 19, four times as high; and from 20 to 24, six times as high. However, the highest rate for both genders is in the 80- to 84-year age group (five to six times more prevalent than among teens). Women are twice as likely to attempt suicide, but men have a higher completion rate (National Institute of Mental Health Report, 1992). Men are more likely to use more violent means, like a gunshot to the head. Women are more likely to take an overdose and then can be saved. Those who complete the suicide also have a higher rate of substance abuse. Alcohol plus other substances like marijuana or cocaine increases the risk by ten times (Delphi Communications, 1996). Combining a mental disorder, such as severe depression or schizophrenia, and substance abuse has a synergistic effect that significantly increases the chances of successful suicide.

Delphi Communications (1996) stated that the National Institute of Mental Heath reported the following eight risk factors for teen suicide:

- Family history of suicide
- Family history of mental or substance abuse disorder
- Family violence, including emotional, physical, or sexual abuse
- Separation or divorce
- Prior suicide attempt
- Firearm in the home
- Incarceration
- Exposure to suicidal behaviors of others, including family members and/or peers

Mental Health and Help-Seeking Behavioral Patterns of Minority Americans

Contemporary mental health service delivery models in more recent year have shifted away from hospitalization and institutionalization to more outpatient and community mental health center facilities. Despite this transition, ethnic minorities are still underrepresented and underserved. Minority Americans do not generally turn to mental health facilities and services despite their need for them. Mental health disturbances among minority populations is a very serious issue. However, the issue of underuse of mental health services is a more serious one. Several barriers have been identified to explain this lack of utilization.

Asian Americans

There is very little literature that focuses on the mental and psychological problems of Asian Americans. One reason for this void is that Asian Americans underuse mental health services and are underrepresented as mental health patients (Snowden and Cheung, 1990). Based on these data, Min (1995) wrote that policy makers and non-Asian social scientists assume that Asian Americans have lower rates of mental disturbance than the U.S. general population. An assumption that Min (1995) clearly disagrees with. Low demand, as reflected in low utilization, should not be misconstrued as an absence of need. Sue and Morishima (1980) reported that moderately disturbed Asian Americans are reluctant to seek help from mental health services. Cultural values play a major role in this reluctance. Mental illness in many Asian American cultures is considered shameful to both the individual and his or her family (Tsai, Teng, and Sue, 1975).

Miranda and Kitano (1976) identified the following barriers for Asian American Clients: (a) fragmentation of services that shifts the patient from one practitioner to another, (2) cultural differences between the professional and that of the client, (3) inaccessibility of services, and (d) the primary focus of the professional on being accountable to fellow professionals rather than to the ethnic community.

Native Americans

American Indians have underutilized mental health and social services for several reasons. Wise (1979) listed the following: (a) Not all Indian reservations or medical communities have medical clinics or hospitals, and those that do have small and outdated facilities, (b) Many Indian communities are located on isolated reservations with access only by primitive roads, and, as a rule, many American Indians do not have appropriate transportation, (c) Because of the high unemployment rate among Native Americans, many cannot afford to purchase health care outside of the Indian Health Service, (d) Policies and procedures are highly impersonal and require a great deal of motivation and knowledge in filling out complicated forms, (e) There is a mistrust of the dominant culture, (f) The value systems and therapeutic approaches employed by these agencies are frequently inappropriate and conflict with an Indian's view of the world, and (g) By utilizing these public services, they fear that they may lose their traditional culture and ethnic and spiritual identity.

African Americans

African Americans are more likely to rely first on traditional support networks (relatives, extended families, ministers, grandmothers) before seeking professional help (White & Parham, 1990). Mindel, Habenstein, and Wright (1988) found that the family support systems were much more important for African Americans than for European Americans, among whom the family support system is used to supplement formal services, not as an alternative. Unfortunately, when family members offer inappropriate lay solutions to problems, service providers may see clients who are more debilitated because the amount of time between the presenting problem and therapeutic intervention is apt to be longer. Many African Americans do not use mental health services for the following reasons: (a) Many African Americans still view mental health service as strange and think of it as a process for "strange" or "crazy" people only (Ho, 1992), (b) Reliance on the family support system produces fewer feelings of defeat, humiliation, and powerlessness, (c) The probability of working with a non-African American therapist is high, and having to entrust one's feelings and pain to a non-African American is difficult. This creates a greater sense of fear and anxiety in the patient. This last point is important because many of the mental health problems of African Americans stem from racism and discrimination. Therapists must be sensitive to the relationship between racism and discrimination and ill health (Mays et al., 1996).

Hispanic Americans

Like African Americans, Hispanic Americans also rely on the family and extended family network for mental health care and treatment. Ghali (1977/1992) reported that Hispanic Americans often make use of mental health services or social agencies as a last resort; instead, they are more likely to seek assistance from family, friends, or people with some special expertise who are known informally through their social networks, not as in institutional representatives. Acosta et al. (1982) reported the following reasons for underutilization of health and mental services: (a) language and communication differences, (b) cultural and social class differences between practitioner and Hispanic American patients, (c) lack of mental health facilities in Hispanic American communities, and (d) many Hispanic Americans are simply not aware of the services available.

REFERENCES

Acosta, F., Yamamoto, J., and Evans, J. *Effective psychotherapy for low-income and minority patients.* New York: Plenum, 1982.

Allen, J. Gender equity in computer education. *Association for Educational Data Systems Monitor* 24, 10–23, 26. (January–February, 1986).

American Council on Education. *One-third of a nation.* Washington DC: ACE, 1988.

Attorney General's Report on the Impact of Criminal Street Gangs on Crime and Violence in California by the year 2000. *Gangs 2000: A Call to Action.* California Department of Justice, Division of Law Enforcement, Bureau of Investigation, 1993. http://electric.ss.uci....ica/Gangs2000/open.html

Bernard, B. *Fostering resiliency in kids.* A paper prepared for the Western Regional Center for Drug Free Schools and Communities, 1991.

Bossert, S. Understanding sex differences in children's classroom experiences. *The Elementary Journal* 81 (1981), 95.

Brandon, N. *The psychology of self-esteem.* New York: Nash, 1969.

Brophy, J. E., and Good, T. L. *Teacher-student relationships: Causes and consequences,* New York: Holt, Rinehart & Winston, 1974.

Campbell, P. Girls, boys and educational excellence. A paper presented at the annual meeting of the American Education Research Association, New Orleans, LA: 1984.

Carter, M. A model for effective school discipline. Bloomington, IN. *The Phi Delta Kappa Foundation,* 1987.

Dearman, N. B., and Plisko, V. W. *The condition of education.* Washington, DC: U.S. Government Printing Office, 1981.

DeBoer, G. Sense and competence in science as a factor in the career decisions of men and women. Paper presented at the annual meeting of the National Association for Research in Science Teaching, New Orleans, LA., 1974.

Delphi Communications. *Statistics and cites on suicide.* Men's Health, 1996. http://www.vix.compub/men/health/stat/suicide.html

Diekstra, R., Suicidal behavior and depressive disorders in adolescents and young adults. *Neuropsychobiology* 22 (1989), 194–207.

Draguns, J. Applications of cross-cultural psychology in the field of mental health. In R. Brislin (Ed.), *Applied cross-cultural psychology* (pp. 302–324). Newbury Park, CA: Sage, 1990.

Dreikurs, R. *Children: The challenge,* New York: Penguin Books, 1964.

Escobar, J., Gomez, J., and Tuason, V. Depressive phenomenology in North and South American patients. *American Journal of Psychiatry* 140 (1983), 47–51.

Fennema, E., and Peterson, P. Teacher-student interactions and sex-related differences in learning mathematics." *Teaching and Teacher Education* 2, 3, 19–42. (1986).

Fugita, S., and Crittenden, K. Towards culture- and population-specific norms for self-reported depressive symptomatology (Korea, the Philippines, Taiwan, and the United States). *The International Journal of Social Psychiatry* 36 (1990), 83–92.

Garcia, Ricardo. *Teaching in a pluralistic society: Concepts, models, strategies.* New York: Harper & Row, 1982.

Ghali, B. Ethnic America. New York: Basic Books, 1977. In Ho, M. (Ed.), *Children and adolescents in therapy.* Newbury Park, CA: Sage, 1992.

Gibbs, J. Conceptual, methodological and sociocultural issues in black youth surveyed: Implications for assessment and early intervention. *Suicide and Life Threatening Behavior* 19 (1988), 17–29. In A. Stiffman and L. Davis (Eds.), *Ethnic issues in adolescent mental health.* Newbury Park: CA: Sage, 1990.

Glasser, W. *Schools without failure.* New York: Harper & Row, 1969.

Glenn, H. S., and Nelsen, J. *Raising self-reliant children in a self-indulgent world.* Rocklin, CA: Prima Publishing & Communication, 1989.

Gordon, E., Miller, M., and Rollock, D. Coping with communicentric bias in knowledge production in the social sciences. *Educational Researcher* 19 (1990), p. 58–63.

Guarnaccia, P., Good, B., and Kleinman, A. A critical review of epidemiological studies of Puerto Rican mental health. *American Journal of Psychiatry* 147 (1990), 1449–1456.

Ho, M. *Minority children and adolescents in therapy.* Newbury Park, CA: Sage, 1992.

Hope, S., and Martin, H. Patterns of suicide among Mexican Americans and Anglos, 1960–1980. *Social Psychiatry* 21 (1986), 83–88.

Kleinman, A. Neurasthenia and depression: A study of somatization and culture in China. *Culture, Medicine, and Psychiatry* 6 (1982), 117–190.

Kuo, W. H. Prevalence of depression among Asian Americans. *Journal of Nervous and Mental Disease* 172 (1984), 449–457.

Lasker, B. *Race attitudes in children.* New York: American Library, 1970.

Love, James. Knowledge transfer and utilization in education. In Edmund W. Gordon, (Ed.), *Review of Research in Education,* Vol. 12. Washington, DC: American Educational Research Association, 1985.

Maslow, A. H. *The farthest reaches of human nature,* Magnolia, MA: Peter Smith, 1983.

Mays, V. M., Coleman, L. M., and Jackson, J. S. Perceived discrimination, employment status, and job stress in a national sample of black women. In H. Neighbors, and J. Jackson (Eds.). *Mental health in Black America.* Thousand Oaks, CA: Sage, 1996.

McIntosh, J. Suicide among native Americans: Further tribal data and considerations. *Omega* 14, 3, 219–229. In A. Stiffman and L. Davis (Eds.). *Ethnic issues in adolescent mental health,* Newbury Park: CA: Sage, 1990.

McKay, E. G. *Changing Hispanic demographics.* Washington DC; Policy Analysis Center, National Council of La Raza, 1988.

Meier, K., and Stewart, J. *The politics of Hispanic education: UN paso palante y dos patras.* Albany, NY: State University of New York Press, 1991.

Min, G. *Asian Americans: Contemporary trends and issues.* Thousand Oaks, CA: Sage, 1995.

Mindel, C., Habenstein, R., and Wright, C. (Eds.). *Ethnic families in America: Patterns and variations.* New York: Elsevier, 1988.

Miranda, M., and Kitano, H. Barriers to mental health: A Japanese and Mexican dilemma. In N. Hernandez (Ed.), *Chicanos: Social psychological perspectives* (pp. 212–328). St. Louis, MO: C. V. Mosby, 1976.

Nakamura, R. *The power of positive coaching.* Boston, MA: Jones and Bartlett, 1996.

National Institute of Mental Health Report. *Suicide facts.* Washington, DC: Author, 1992.

Natriello, G., McDill, E., and Pallas, A. *Schooling disadvantaged children: Racing against catastrophe.* New York: Teachers College Press, 1990.

Rogers, C. *Client-centered therapy: Its current practice, implications, and theory.* Boston: Houghton Mifflin, 1951.

Rosenthal, R., and Jacobson, L. *Pygmalion in the classroom,* New York: Holt, Rinehart & Winston, 1968.

Sadker, D., and Sadker, M. Is the O.K. classroom O.K.? *Phi Delta Kappan* 66 (January 1985), 358–61.

Salanda, D. Acculturative: Minority status and distress. In A. Padilla (Ed.), *Hispanic psychology: Critical issues in theory and research.* Thousand Oaks, CA: Sage, 1995.

Sarason, S. *The predictable failure of educational reform.* San Francisco: Jossey-Bass, 1990.

Seller, M. The United States. In G. Kelley (Ed.), *International handbook of women's education.* New York: Greenwork, 1989.

Simpson, A. W., and Erickson, M. Teachers' verbal and non-verbal communication patterns as a function of teacher race, student gender and student race. *American Educational Research Journal* 20 (Summer 1983), 183–98.

Snowden, L. R., and Cheung, F. K. Use of inpatient mental health services by members of ethnic minority groups. *American Psychologist* 45 (1990), 347–355.

Sue, S., and Morishima, J. *The mental health of Asian Americans.* San Francisco: Jossey-Bass, 1980.

Trends in Indian Health. U.S. Department of Health and Human Services, Public Health Service, Indian Health Service, Washington, DC: Government Printing Office, 1991.

Tsai, M., Teng, L., and Sue, S. Mental status of Chinese in the United States. *American Journal of Orthopsychiatry* 45 (1975), 111–118.

Tseng, W., and Hsu, J. Minor psychological disturbances of everyday life. In Triandis and J. Draguns (Eds.), *Handbook of cross-cultural psychology,* vol. 6: *Psychopathology* (pp. 61–97). Boston: Allyn & Bacon, 1980.

U.S. Bureau of Health and Human Services, National Center for Health Statistics, *Vital Statistics of the United States* (Washington D.C. USGPO, 1991), vol. 2, Part A "Mortality," page 51, tables 1–9: Death Rates for 72 Selected Causes by 5-Year Age Groups, Race, and Sex: U.S., 1988.

U.S. Commission on Civil Rights. *Teachers and students, Report V,* Washington DC: U.S. Government Printing Office, 1973.

U.S. Department of Health and Human Services. *Vital statistics of the U.S.: Vol. II. Mortality.* Washington DC: U.S. Government Printing Office, 1985.

Van Eckeren, G. *The speaker's sourcebook: Quotes and stories.* Englewood Cliffs, NJ: Prentice-Hall, 1988.

Wehlage, G. (Ed.). *Reducing the risk: Schools as communities of support.* Philadelphia, PA: Falmer Press, 1989.

White, J. L., and Parham, T. A. *The psychology of Blacks: An African American Perspective.* Englewood Cliffs, NJ: Prentice-Hall, 1990.

Wise, B. The health of American Indian children. *Health Service Report* 87 (1979), 872–876.

World Health Organization. *Depressive disorders in different cultures: Report of the WHO collaborative study of standardized assessment of depressive disorders.* Geneva, Switzerland: Author, 1983.

Wyche, K., and Rotheram-Borus, M. Suicidal behavior among minority youth in the United States. In A. Stiffman, and L. Davis (Eds.). *Ethnic issues in adolescent mental health,* Newbury Park, CA: Sage, 1990. pp. 323–338.

Yamamoto, J. Japanese-Americans. In A. Gaw (Ed.), *Cross-cultural psychiatry* (pp. 31–53). Boston: John Wright, 1982.

Young, T. Substance use and abuse among Native Americans. *Clinical Psychology Review,* 1988, vol 8(2), 125–138.

Youngs, Bette. *The 6 vital ingredients of self-esteem and how to develop them in your child.* New York: Rawson Associates, 1991.

Yu, E., Chang, C., Liu, W., and Fernandez, M. (1989). Suicide among Asian American youth. In L. Uba, *Asian Americans: Personality patterns, identity, and mental health.* New York: The Guilford Press, 1994, p. 184.

6 Culture, Food, and Unhealthy Eating Behaviors

What I most remember was an abiding sense of comfort and security. I got plenty of mothering not only from Pop and my brothers and sisters when they were home, but from the whole of our closeknit community.

—Paul Robeson,
Here I Stand, 1958

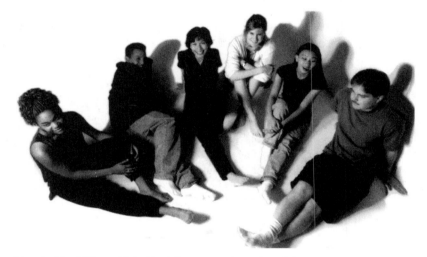

Photo by Kim Miller, published in *Cultures* magazine, volume 2, issue 1.

What is the typical American diet? No one can really answer that question because of the many different ethnic and cultural groups that make up America. The diversity of different ethnic and cultural groups is more than just a physical blend but a religious and spiritual blending as well. Food and food habits are a part of this mix.

Diets are influenced by biological, environmental, and cultural factors. People eat what is available and what tastes good to them. In the past, people primarily relied on foods produced close to home. Culture also plays an important role in influencing what people will eat. For example, Americans do not usually eat insects, frogs, armadillos, or rattlesnake. Culture also determines how foods are prepared, how often one eats, and when to eat.

Food goes beyond simple nutrition. Humans use foods symbolically, and it is this symbolic use of food that is important to each cultural group. Food is often related to religious and cultural behaviors as well as a means of maintaining cultural identity. Culturally based food habits are one of the few cultural characteristics that most people retain to some degree, regardless of how acculturated they become to a new society. This is especially true during cultural celebrations and festivals.

In U.S. society, very few people eat only their own traditional foods. In the United States, food is transported, refrigerated, processed by technology, and packaged so that almost every variety of food is readily available. Food choices in America are almost unlimited. Eating and trying different ethnic foods has become a favorite pastime for many Americans. As a result, most food patterns in various cultures have changed considerably as families have adapted to the "melting pot" customs of American society.

The following section will first describe the United States Department of Agriculture's Food Guide Pyramid, followed by some of the traditional eating customs of Native Americans, African Americans, Hispanic Americans, and Asian Americans. The reader must remember that most minority Americans do not eat traditionally all of the time but have made many adaptations to their diets through the acculturation process.

The USDA's Food Guide Pyramid: A Guide to Daily Food Choices

The goal of any nutritious diet is to get adequate amounts of nutrients by eating from a variety of foods. The United States Department of Agriculture (USDA) has developed a plan to help people eat a nutritionally balanced diet by eating a wide variety of foods from different food groups. The USDA developed a Food Guide Pyramid that consists of five food groups and one miscellaneous group that makes little contribution to nutrient intake, for a total of six groups. In addition, the guide recommends the number of daily servings that should be eaten from each of the groups. The Food Guide Pyramid was also designed to meet the recommended dietary allowances (RDA's) for calories, protein, 11 vitamins, and 7 minerals. The fundamental principles of this food guide are moderation, variety, and balance for most people. Individuals with specific health problems or susceptibilities to developing such problems as high serum cholesterol, high blood pressure, obesity, cancer, and other health problems should consult a physician and nutritionist to determine how these guidelines should be applied. The latest version of the food group plan of the USDA's Food Guide Pyramid is found in Figure 6.1.

The food groups and the number of daily servings within the Food Guide Pyramid are as follows:

Food Group 1: Bread, cereal, rice, and pasta (6–11 daily servings)

Some of the major contributions from this food group include complex carbohydrates, B-complex vitamins, protein, iron, and fiber.

A *serving* equals 1 slice of bread, 1/2 c. cooked cereal, rice, or pasta; 1/2 bagel, small roll, biscuit, or muffin; 2 large crackers.

Food Group 2: Vegetables (3–5 daily servings)

Some of the major contributions from this food group include Vitamins A and C, complex carbohydrates, fiber, and potassium. Vegetables also lack fat and cholesterol.

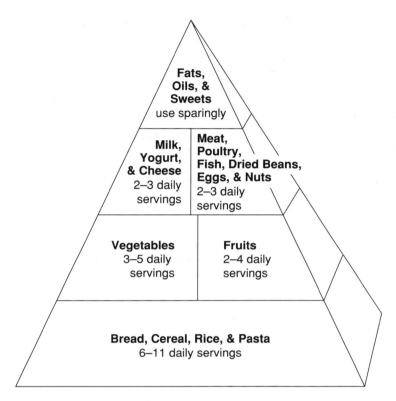

FIGURE 6.1   The Food Guide Pyramid

U.S. Department of Agriculture

A *serving* equals 1/2 c. cooked or raw vegetables, 1 c. leafy raw vegetables, 1/2 c. cooked legumes, 3/4 c. vegetable juice.

Food Group 3: Fruits (2–4 daily servings)

Some of the major contributions from this food group includes Vitamins A and C, complex carbohydrates, fiber, and potassium. Fruits also lack sodium, fat, and cholesterol.

A *serving* equals a medium-sized apple, orange, or banana, 3/4 c. fruit juice, 1 melon wedge, 1/2 c. berries, or canned or dried fruit.

Food Group 4: Milk, yogurt, and cheese (2–3 daily servings)

Some of the major contributions from this food group include proteins, calcium, vitamins B_{12}, and, when fortified, Vitamins A and D.

A *serving* equals 1 c. milk or yogurt, 1 1/2 ounce of cheese or 2 ounces of processed cheese.

Food Group 5: Meat, poultry, fish, dried beans, eggs, and nuts (2–3 servings)

Some of the major contributions from this food group include protein, iron, B vitamins, zinc, magnesium, niacin, and thiamin.

A *serving* equals 2–3 ounces of lean cooked meat, poultry, or fish, 1 egg, 1/2 c. cooked legumes, or 2 tbs. peanut butter.

Food Group 6: Fats, oils, and sweets (use sparingly)

Foods such as butter, candy, soft drinks, potato and corn pastries, donuts, coffee, beer, cookies, salad dressings, cream cheeses, pretzels, pickles, salt, wine, and other miscellaneous foods in this category should only be used sparingly. Most of the items mentioned do not contribute to healthful nutrition and provide additional calories and large amounts of salt and fat.

Foods from each of the five major food groups are all important and are needed. Each group includes a large number of foods that allows for substitution. For example, milk products, such as yogurt and cheese, can be substituted for milk. In addition, serving portions vary within each of the categories depending on the specific needs of the individual.

In summary, the Food Guide Pyramid provides a strategy that allows an individual to:

1. Eat from a wide variety of foods;
2. Maintain healthy weight;
3. Choose a diet low in fat, saturated fat, and cholesterol;
4. Choose a diet with plenty of vegetables, fruits, and grain products;
5. Limit sugar, salt, and alcohol intake.

Each of these, of course, is important in helping each individual develop positive dietary guidelines for himself or herself.

Ethnic Diets and the Food Pyramid

Traditional African American Foods

The diets of African slaves in the United States largely depended on the slave owners and what they provided for them. When allowed to grow gardens, the slaves planted a variety of plants, corn, okra, peas, sweet potatoes, turnips, and leafy vegetables, such as cabbage, collard greens, kale, spinach, and mustard greens. Whatever wild life (rabbits, opossums, squirrels, etc.) and fish (catfish and other freshwater fish) they were able to kill or catch provided meat.

When the slave masters slaughtered the pigs, many of the discarded parts, such as the snouts, hocks, ears, feet, intestines (called *chitterlings* or *chitlins*), and stomach lining (called *maw*) were sometimes given to the slaves. If they were discarded, many of the slaves rummaged through the garbage to gather these parts. The slaves would boil or fry their meats, vegetables, and legumes in pork fat (lard) (Kittler & Sucher, 1995). Even when boiling foods such as vegetables, the water was flavored with salt pork, fatback, bacon, or ham. Corn was used as cornmeal, grits, and hominy. One-dish stews were popular meals as well as fried corn, sweet potatoes (*pone*), and cornmeal cakes. Most foods were flavored with a variety of spices and often served with pork gravy (Quick-Tilley, 1996).

The slaves who worked and cooked in the homes of the slave owners enjoyed the luxury of a variety of poultry, meats, and fish. The culinary abilities of the African American slaves popularized southern fried chicken and fried fish (Kittler and Sucher, 1995).

The African American pyramid of foods (Figure 6.2) has a foundation of biscuits, corn (corn breads, grits, hominy), pasta, and rice. In urban communities, store-bought breads have replaced biscuits. Vegetables (green leafy vegetables—chard, collard, kale, mustard greens—corn, okra, sweet potatoes, yams), and fruits (apples, bananas, berries, peaches, watermelon) make up the middle of the pyramid. Fruit consumption by today's African Americans is considered low when compared to other groups. Pork (chitterlings, intestines, ham hocks, sausages) remains the primary protein source, and frying is still the most popular way of preparing foods. Fruit drinks and tea are the drinks of choice over milk (consumed in puddings and ice cream).

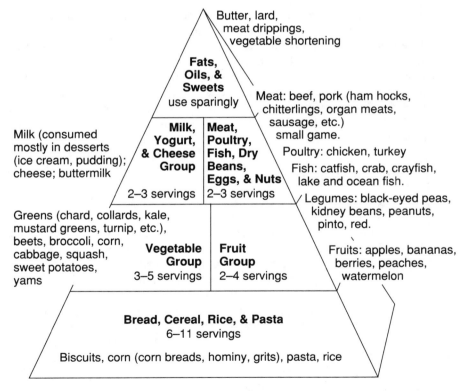

FIGURE 6.2   Traditional African American Foods (Southern United States) Placed in the Food Pyramid Guide Developed by the U.S. Department of Agriculture, 1993

Source: Kittler and Sucher, 1995; Quick-Tilley, 1996; Harris, 1995.

Some precautions should be taken when eating traditional southern African American food. Many of the pork meals are high in fat, and green leafy vegetables are often mixed with ham, salt pork, or bacon. Gravy from animal drippings is extremely popular and is often poured over most of the meals. Broiled fish and chicken, beans, corn breads, and steamed vegetables are better choices.

The African American diet still stresses the consumption of meat (particularly pork), fried foods, and eggs (Kittler & Sucher, 1989), and, as a result, is high in cholesterol and saturated fats. African American diets also tend to be low in foods that are good sources of complex carbohydrates and dietary fiber, namely whole-grain products and fresh fruits and vegetables. Additionally, from 60 to 95 percent of adult African Americans are lactose intolerant, and many of these individuals habitually avoid milk and milk products (Kumanyika & Adams-Campbell, 1991). African Americans who live in or near poverty level consume diets that are marginal in vitamins A, C, D, B-complex, calcium, magnesium, iron, and zinc (Blocker, 1994).

Muslim Food Practices

Muslims follow dietary laws laid down in the Quran that forbid the eating of pork in any form or eating the blood of any animal. Special methods of slaughtering are used to produce meat that is *halal* (meat that can be eaten). Non-*halal* meat is forbidden. Only fish with fins or scales are allowed; shellfish are not permissible. Alcohol is forbidden. Each year, all post-adolescent Muslims observe the month-long fast of Ramadan when no food or beverage is consumed from sunrise to sunset. Muslim dietary law allows young children, the sick, journeying people, and women who are menstruating, pregnant, or breast feeding an exemption during Ramadan but they are expected to make a compensatory fast at another time (Cott, 1977).

Traditional Mexican Food

In recent years, Mexican dishes, like fried chimichangas, lard-based refried beans, fried tacos, fried chile rellenos, and fried taquitos have been highlighted by various nutrition organizations as being extremely unhealthy. Although the frying of food is popular in traditional Mexican cooking, these foods are not truly representative of Mexican foods, just as fast-food pizza is not representative of Italian cuisine.

The Mexican food pyramid (Figure 6.3) has a foundation of corn-based recipes such as tortillas and tamales. Although these foods are still popular, wheat tortillas and store-bought breads are also popular today. Unfortunately, acculturated Mexican Americans are consuming great quantities of sweets, such as donuts, cake, and cookies. In addition, sugared breakfast cereals are become a breakfast staple. Vegetables (especially squash, pumpkin, tomatoes, garlic, chile peppers, chayote, and greens) and fruits (especially exotic fruits such as mango, papaya, pineapples, and many types of bananas) are an integral part of Mexican cuisine and make up the middle of the pyramid. Fruits remain popular as dessert and snack items for acculturated Mexican Americans. Mexicans eat only small portions of meat and rely primarily on beans for protein. Beans (*frijoles*) are the staple of Mexican cooking and are eaten in large amounts. Cheeses, such as fresh goat cheese and lower-fat

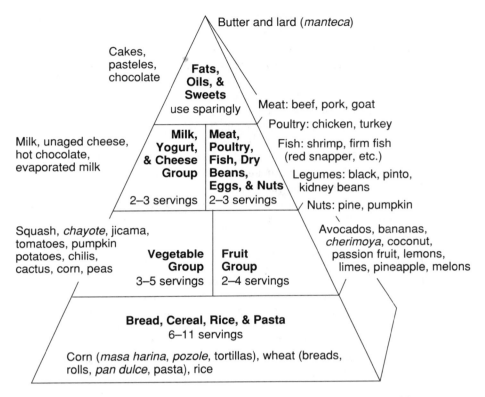

FIGURE 6.3   Traditional Mexican Foods Placed in the Food Guide Pyramid Developed by the U.S. Department of Agriculture, 1993

Source: Kittler and Sucher, 1995; Higuera-McMahan, 1994; Sanjur, 1995; Fergusson, 1973; Kennedy, 1989; Warner, 1992.

crumbly queso ranchero, are used in small amounts to act as the finishing touch for such dishes as enchiladas and dishes of beans. Pureed fruits are often used as beverages. Unfortunately, there has been increased consumption of Kool-Aid and soft drinks among young Hispanic Americans.

The traditional Mexican diet is high in complex carbohydrates and is semivegetarian. Corn is one of the most important staples in Mexican cooking and, as many Mexican cooks would say, "it is never just right unless it is hulled and ground in the old way with the proper blending of spices, which requires long and gentle simmering." Corn is also used to make one of the staples of the Mexican diet, ground maize to make tortillas and tamales. Beans, chiles, tomato verde, and squash are also quite popular.

The addition of lime juice in the preparation of maize significantly enhances the calcium and niacin intake. In addition, when corns and beans are eaten together, they provide an excellent source of protein. The combination of rice and beans is also an excellent source of protein.

One of the weaknesses of Mexican cooking, of course, is frying. In Mexican cooking, meat, *menudo* or *mondongo* (tripe), and other organ meats, beans, tortillas, rice, green and ripe plantains, potatoes, and many other foods are liked best when fried. In addition, generous toppings of Mexican cream on traditional dishes (such as enchiladas) and as spreads in Mexican sandwiches (tortas), is a major concern (Sanjur, 1995). Another weakness of the Mexican diet is a preference for high-fat meats, including *chorizos* (sausages), *chicharron* (fried pork skin), *cabeza de puerco* (pig's head), *patitas de puerco* (pig's feet), and several other organ meats (Sanjur, 1995).

Some precautions should be taken when eating Mexican food. Avoid foods fried in fat, such as fried tortillas, tacos, chimichangas, flautas, and fried chile rellenos. Avoid refried beans fried in fat. Although meats are generally served in small portions, many are deep fried and should be eaten sparingly. Also be aware of the heavy cheese toppings placed on many dishes. Beans, rice, and vegetables are better choices. Fajitas are also generally lower in fat. Many Mexican nonfried chicken meals are also available.

Traditional Caribbean Food

The Caribbean, with its necklace of islands in their turquoise seas, has long been a culinary marvel. Indians brought southern American ingredients with them as they migrated through the islands. Successive waves of new arrivals—settlers and missionaries, slaves and immigrants, pirates and peasants—brought with them the tastes of Spain, England, France, the Netherlands, Africa, North and South Asia, and the United States. Caribbean cooking is a patchwork quilt of colors, textures, and flavors. It is a multiethnic tapestry woven from the cuisines of many countries. Each island has its own unique culinary traditions, spices, and tastes. The pyramid discussed below focuses only on the foods most available on the many islands.

The traditional Caribbean Islander pyramid of foods (Figure 6.4) has a foundation of cassava bread, cornmeal (fried breads), oatmeal, and rice. Vegetables (black-eyed peas, pigeon peas, fiery chilis, broccoli, cabbage, taro leaves, corn, okra, squash, sweet potatoes) and fruits (coconut, plantain, passion and other exotic fruits, banana, avocado, guava, pineapple, sugar cane, citrus fruit) make up the middle of the pyramid. Tropical fruit jams and jellies, rum punches, fruit cheeses, fruit curds, and coconut candies are popular Western Indian sweets. Today, there is less consumption of fruits and vegetables among Caribbean Islanders. Fish, such as snapper, barracuda, and dolphin were once often consumed but in recent years, meat (pork and goat) has become increasingly popular. Cow's milk and coffees are popular drinks.

The traditional Caribbean diet tends to be high in starches and features foods such as roti (flat bread wrapped around a curried meat and potato stew), plantain (a starchy banana-type fruit used as a vegetable), peas and rice (a complete protein combination), breadfruit, cassava root, and so on (Glaskow & Adaskin, 1990). Meat dishes include highly seasoned curries made from chicken, beef, and goat.

Traditional Asian and Pacific Islander Foods

Traditional Chinese Food.   A well-prepared Chinese dish is expected to appeal to more senses than taste. It is colorful, uniformly shaped, and fragrant. There are contrasting tastes

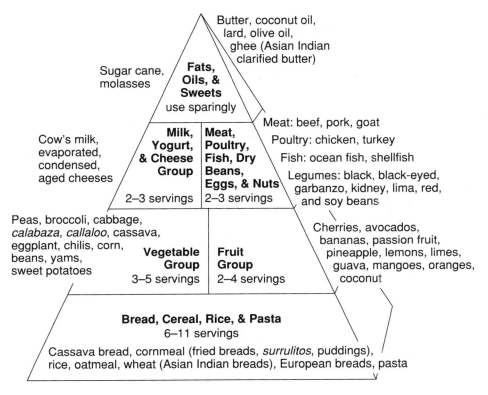

FIGURE 6.4   Traditional Caribbean Foods Placed in the Food Guide Pyramid Developed by the U.S. Department of Agriculture, 1993

Source: Kittler and Sucher, 1995; Raichlen, 1995; and Harris, 1996.

and textures within the meal; if one ingredient is crisp, it is offset by one that is smooth. A bland dish is accompanied by a spiced one. Balance is important. "Hot" and "cold" foods are also an important part of the balancing process because both are important to the Yin and Yang concept (Bley-Miller, 1966). Yin foods are cold and include such things as green vegetables, beans, fish, and shellfish. Grains are neutral. Yang foods include red meats, oily foods, hot seasonings, and ginger. Thus, ginger is served with fish and meat with green vegetables. People with a hot disease often balance their diet with cold foods, and vice versa. Soup broth is a vital home remedy and is often taken on a daily basis to maintain good health (Lai & Kevin-Yue, 1990). Food also has important social meaning for families and is the main occasion for the family to come together. Feasts occur on special occasions such as birthdays, weddings, or family births.

Meals are also balanced on the basis of five distinct tastes: sweet (sugar, honey, fruits, vegetables), sour (vinegars, citrus fruit, pickled vegetables), hot (chilis, ginger), bitterness (turnips, cabbage), and salt (soy sauce, soybean paste, pickled vegetables).

The Chinese diet relies heavily on grains and fresh vegetables. It naturally provides plenty of complex carbohydrates, and meat is used sparingly. Fats are used in the diet primarily for flavor and texture. Butterfat, of course, is unknown in the Chinese diet. Milk is almost absent from the traditional Chinese diet because it is disliked and because many Chinese are intolerant to lactose (Lai & Kevin-Yue, 1990). Rice is considered a necessity for every meal; a person has not eaten well without rice.

The Chinese pyramid of foods (Figure 6.5) has a foundation of rice and noodles. Vegetables and fruits (apples, bananas, litchi, plums, persimmons, peaches, melons) make up the middle of the pyramid. Beef, lamb, poultry, and numerous varieties of fish and shell-fish are important staples in Chinese meals. Cow's milk and buffalo milk are consumed but tea and soups are the most popular beverages. Sugar consumption among Chinese Americans has increased, mainly because of increased consumption of soft drinks, candy, and American desserts.

Some precautions are necessary when eating Chinese food. Fried foods, such as fried rice, egg and spring rolls, and crispy noodles are high in fat. Monosodium glutamate (MSG) should be avoided by some people and Chinese soy sauce is extremely high in salt. Cholesterol-conscious individuals may choose to avoid the many egg dishes. Healthier

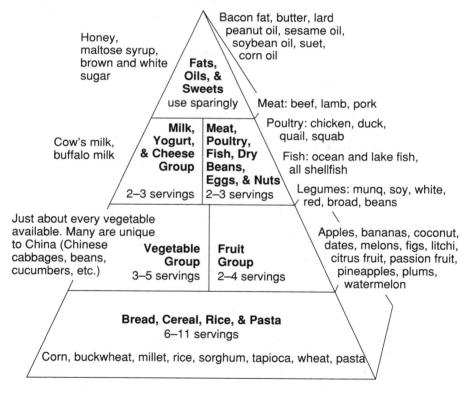

FIGURE 6.5   Traditional Chinese Foods Placed in the Food Guide Pyramid Developed by the U.S. Department of Agriculture, 1993

Source: Kittler and Sucher, 1995; Lai and Kevin-Yue, 1990; Warner, 1993, Lo, 1979; Bley-Miller, 1966.

choices can be selected from a wide variety of steamed or stir-fried vegetables and, of course, rice. There are also a variety of healthy soups to select from.

Traditional Japanese Food. Japanese food, of course, is much more than raw fish and has a wide range of ingredients. The one common staple of all Japanese cuisine is, of course, rice. Rice is the basis of nearly every meal. It is eaten for breakfast, lunch, and dinner. Japanese mothers ladle out bowl after bowl of steaming hot rice at just about every meal. No matter how many other dishes are eaten, most Japanese feel that they have not really eaten until they have had their rice. Rice is almost always eaten plain with pickled vegetables and miso soup. Rice is also the source of saki, a rich sweet wine that is frequently served with meals and is splashed liberally on some dishes.

Japanese diets are extremely healthy because they are low in high-cholesterol items like red meat, dairy products, and saturated oils, and high in seafoods and seaweeds, which are full of minerals. Available fish include: bonito, salmon, cod, flounder, tuna, mackerel, shark, whale, eel, red snapper, and many others. Other kinds of marine life eaten as food includes: prawns, shrimp, crab, squid, cuttlefish, oysters, abalone, scallops, clams, blowfish, and seaweed.

Vegetables are equally abundant and come in an endless variety. There are also many distinctive Japanese vegetables: *negi,* or leeks; *daikon,* or white radish; bamboo sprouts; *gobo,* or burdock; *wasabi,* similar to horseradish; *shoga,* or ginger; *nasu,* or eggplant; *shitake,* or black mushrooms; and *moyashi,* or bean sprouts. Noodles, such as soba (buckwheat noodles) and *udon* (macaroni), are also quite popular as well as *tofu,* bean curd. As evidence of their good health, Japanese have a longer life span than most other nations and a startlingly low incidence of heart disease. Conversely, they have a rather high level of salt-related diseases because of items like soy sauce and miso.

From soybeans comes soy sauce, one of the most important flavors in Japanese cookery. Soybeans are also the source of the more earthy and powerful flavors from which miso is derived. Miso is a salty paste made from fermented soybeans, used daily in miso soup. Another of the main flavoring elements is *dashi,* the basic stock that finds its way into most dishes. It is made from *kombu* (kelp) and dried shavings of the bonito fish.

The typical Japanese meal consists of a variety of tiny delicate portions as opposed to larger portions of a few foods. When Japanese eat Western food, they usually complain about the size of portions and the lack of variety. Each tiny delicate portion of food is chosen for its distinct taste and freshness and is usually served with hot tea. In addition, the food is arranged for the pleasure of the "eye." Home cooks arrange each dish as beautifully as possible so that looking at it can be as pleasurable an experience as eating it. There is no dessert in a traditional Japanese meal, but fresh fruit is sometimes offered.

The Japanese pyramid of foods (Figure 6.6) has a foundation of rice and noodles. Vegetables (all varieties) and fruits (apples, bananas, dates, cherries, citrus, pears, peaches, mandarin oranges) make up the middle of the pyramid. Fish, like rice, is the staple of the traditional Japanese diet. However, Japanese Americans eat more poultry and meat than fish. Tea (black and green), sake, coffee, and beer are popular beverages. Japanese Americans, however, drink less tea and more milk, coffee, and carbonated beverages. Sweets made with honey or sugar are very popular. Japanese Americans are consuming more fats and oils because of increased use of Western foods and cooking methods.

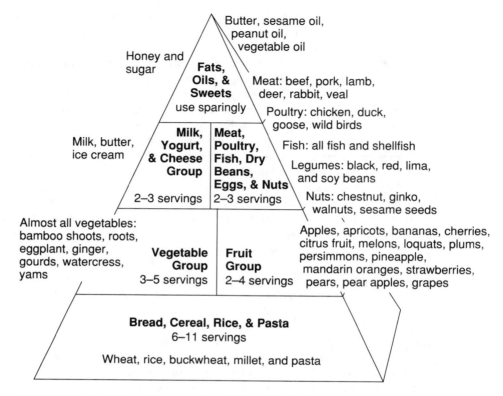

FIGURE 6.6   Traditional Japanese Foods Placed in the Food Pyramid Guide Developed by the U.S. Department of Agriculture, 1993.

Source: Rudzinski, 1969; Downer, 1993; Kittler and Sucher, 1995; and Okabe et al., 1990.

Spices, sauces, and flavorings are most important to Japanese cooking. Foremost of these is *shoyu,* or soy sauce, made from wheat or barley, soybeans, salt, and water. Some precautions are necessary when eating Japanese food. Soy sauces and miso are extremely high in sodium and fried rice dishes and tempura are high in fat. Although tasty, *sashimi* and *sushi* (raw fish) may carry harmful bacteria and parasites. Caution is suggested. Rice, vegetables, tofu, and broiled or steamed fish and chicken are healthy alternatives.

Southeast Asian Foods.   Southeast Asian food is colorful, fragrant, flavorful, and healthful. From the simplest noodle soup to an elaborate curry dish or a fiery chili sauce, Southeast Asian food is thoroughly satisfying. Rice is the staple carbohydrate with noodles a close second. Coconuts and coconut milk are nearly as essential as rice to authentic Southeast Asian cooking. Grating the meat of a mature coconut and squeezing out the liquid produces a milk that flavors curries, soups, sauces, and desserts. Southeast Asian recipes utilize a variety of spices and herbs. Typical spices include pepper, cloves, nutmeg, cinnamon, cardamom, coriander, cumin, and chili peppers. Herbs include mint, basil, and lemongrass.

Fish and shellfish are the major sources of protein. However, chicken, duck, beef, pigs, and goats (among Muslims who don't eat pork) are also quite popular but are eaten in modest portions. Soybeans, in the form of tofu and tempeh, are eaten. The Southeast Asian Diet is very healthy because it is based largely on complex carbohydrates such as rice, vegetables, and fruits.

The phrase *Southeast Asian,* of course, refers to many different cultures. The following Filipino pyramid of foods is just one of many. The Filipino pyramid of foods (Figure 6.7) has a foundation of rice and noodles. Vegetables (all types) and fruits (over 100 varieties of bananas, coconut, exotic and passion fruits, melons, persimmons) make up the middle of the pyramid. Traditional Filipino cuisine consisted of a lot of fish, shellfish, pork, and some poultry. Tea, soy milk, and coffee with milk are popular beverages. Sweets made of brown sugar, coconut, and honey are also popular.

Some precautions are necessary when eating Filipino food. Coconut milk, peanut drippings and sauces, and deep fried foods are high in fat. Steamed dishes and clear broth foods are recommended.

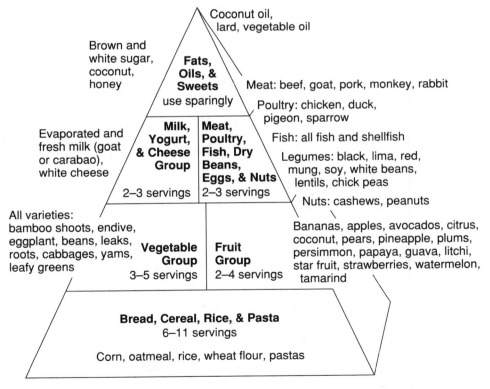

FIGURE 6.7   Traditional Filipino Food Placed in the Good Guide Pyramid Developed by the U.S. Department of Agriculture, 1993

Source: Kittler and Sucher, 1995; and Solomon, 1992.

Hindu Food Practices.   Strict Hindus abstain from meat and fish. In more orthodox Hindu practices, the cow is sacred and any form of beef is prohibited, but dairy products are acceptable. Pork is considered unclean, and any Hindu practitioner would not consider eating food that has been touched by meat or utensils that have been touched by meat.

Traditional Native American Foods

The great diversity of the Native American tribes has resulted in a great variety of cuisines. Traditional Native American foods were determined primarily by geography and weather. Each tribe was forced to adapt to their living conditions. Each tribe had local ingredients and foods, but staple foods, such as beans, corn, and squash, were common to most.

Food also has symbolic meaning in Native American culture. Sharing food is an integral part of Native American societies. It is considered a gift of nature and, therefore, is to be shared with others. Many tribes have elaborate ceremonies to enhance the growth of

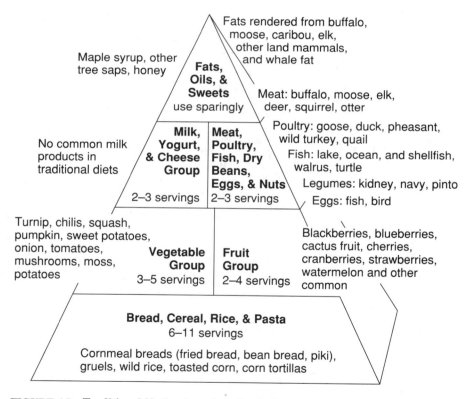

FIGURE 6.8   Traditional Native American Foods Placed in the Food Guide Pyramid Developed by the U.S. Department of Agriculture, 1993

Source: Kittler and Sucher, 1995; Champagne, 1994; and Cox and Jacobs, 1991.

their crops. Food is freely offered to guests and extended family and is often prepared to be shared communally. Community pot luck meals are part of Native American life. In the Southwest, food is considered a valuable gift from a woman to a man or a woman to a woman. Males usually bring clothing, game, or firewood as gifts to women.

The Native American pyramid of foods (Figure 6.8) has a foundation of corn-based breads, toasted corn, and wild rice. Unfortunately, in recent years, store-bought wheat (breads and sugared cereals) has widely replaced corn. Cakes, cookies, and pastries are also very popular. Vegetables (pumpkin, squash, potatoes, sweet potatoes, corn) and fruit (berries of all sorts, grapes, cactus fruit, melons) make up the middle of the pyramid. In modern times, Native Americans are eating more canned fruits and fresh fruits common to most other Americans such as apples, bananas, and oranges. Meats remain a favorite of Native Americans but wild game is now rarely eaten. Beef, lamb, and pork have become the meat staples in modern American Indian society. Milk products were not part of the traditional diets, but powdered milk and evaporated milk are now typical commodities. Fruits and syrups were part of the traditional diet but have been replaced by candy, jams, and jellies.

The Vegetarian Pyramid

A vegetarian is a person who does not eat meat, poultry, and fish. The diet of a vegetarian consists primarily of plant products: fruits, vegetables, legumes, grains, seeds, and nuts. Some vegetarians include some restricted intake of animal protein by consuming eggs, dairy products, or both. The dietary practices of vegetarians fall into three broad categories:

> **Vegan or strict vegetarian,** which means that no animals or animal products of any kind are included in the diet. Meat, fish, poultry, eggs, milk, and other dairy products are not eaten.
>
> **Lactovegetarian,** which means that limited dairy (*lacto*) products are consumed, but no other animal products, such as eggs, are.
>
> **Lacto-ovovegetarian,** which means eggs (*ovo*) and dairy (*lacto*) products are consumed in the vegetarian diet. Most vegetarians in the United States are lacto-ovovegetarian.

The reasons for becoming a vegetarian are numerous. Some of the reasons include health, economic and religious concerns, dislike of taste, compassion for animals, and a belief in nonviolence. Whatever the reason, there are some positive health benefits of vegetarianism. Vegetarians generally have lower blood pressures, and lower rates of death from coronary artery disease and certain types of cancer. Vegetarians are at lower risk for Type II diabetes and are more likely to be at or near their desirable weights. Vegetarians may also have a lower risk of osteoporosis, kidney stones, gallstones, and breast cancer. The reasons for these health benefits, of course, are because vegetarian diets generally are low in fat and high in fiber. High-fat and low-fiber diets are linked to many of the diseases mentioned above.

Vegetarian diets, if properly planned, provide all the nutrients that are necessary for a healthy diet. Eating a wide variety of plant foods will provide adequate protein, calcium, iron, vitamin B_{12}, vitamin D, and other nutrients. It is a myth that vegetarians do not get enough protein of good quality. As long as a person is taking enough calories to maintain his or her weight, a mixture of proteins (e.g., legumes, peas, potatoes, bread, pasta, tofu, and nuts) throughout the day will provide enough amino acids. It is not necessary to plan combinations of "complementary protein" as once advised. The body will make its own proteins if a variety of plant foods are eaten.

A concern about the "vegan" diet is that it lacks vitamin B_{12} and vitamin D. The adult recommendation for Vitamin B_{12} is very low, about three micrograms per day. Many foods, such as Nutri-Grain and Cheerios, are fortified with B_{12}. Check labels to discover other products that contain B_{12}. To be on the safe side, a vitamin B_{12} supplement should be taken if dairy products, eggs, or fortified foods are not eaten regularly. Few foods are naturally high in vitamin D. Dairy products are reinforced with vitamin D, and the human body can produce it when exposed to sunlight. A vegetarian that does not consume dairy products should get at least 20 to 30 minutes of direct sunlight at least two to three times weekly or take a vitamin D supplement. The vegetarian food pyramid is shown in Figure 6.9.

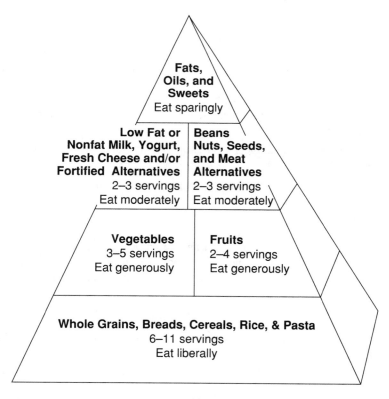

FIGURE 6.9   The Vegetarian Food Pyramid Developed by the Seventh-Day Adventist Dietetic Association

Vegetarian diets are healthy for anyone at any age. However, there are certain times when vegetarians must take precautions. Pregnant or breast-feeding women must consume a reasonable variety of foods and enough calories to sustain the body's greater demands. Calcium needs can met by eating at least four servings of calcium-rich (e.g., collard greens, kale, broccoli, low-fat dairy products, turnip greens, yogurt, tofu prepared with calcium, and fortified soy milk) foods a day. Vegans should include a source of vitamin B_{12} through fortified breakfast cereals or a vitamin B_{12} supplement. A vitamin D supplement should also be taken if the woman does not get at least 20 to 30 minutes of direct sunlight on at least her hands and face two to three times weekly. For all infants and growing young children, a registered dietician or pediatrician should be consulted to be sure they are getting adequate calories and nutrients.

Unhealthy Eating Behaviors

Obesity

If genetic adjustments take hundreds of generations to unfold, how do they keep pace with an environment that changes as rapidly as that found in modern industrialized societies? Unfortunately they don't. Industrialized society is providing an unlimited supply of calories and fat to a society that lives a relatively inactive lifestyle. As a result, the United States is among the most obese populations in the world. Common factors among most Americans include high fat intake, high refined sugar intake, low fiber intake, and a sedentary lifestyle.

One certain fact is that excess fat is the end result of consuming more calories than the number expended to sustain daily activities. Unfortunately, obesity is not just simply a problem of overeating. If it were, most dieters would be successful in their efforts to lose weight and obesity could be eliminated as a major health concern. There are obviously other factors that include genetic, psychological, cultural, social, environmental, and behavioral (overeating, unhealthy eating habits, lack of exercise) influences. All of these factors influence the balance between energy intake and output. As a result, there is no singular theory that has emerged to explain why some people become too fat, while others remain relatively thin despite an apparently large caloric intake. Another certain fact is that no two obese individuals will have gained their excessive weight in exactly the same manner.

The following topics related to obesity will be discussed: (1) definition of *obesity;* (2) medical and health aspects of obesity; (3) treatment of obesity; and (4) obesity and selected minority populations.

Definition of Obesity.   Even though obesity is recognized as a major health problem, it is still difficult to define precisely. In general terms, *obesity* can be defined as an excessive enlargement or storage of the body's total quantity of fat. The line of demarcation between normal levels of body fat and obesity is somewhat arbitrary because the normal range of body fat is based on sex and age. Researchers have not fully agreed on what is considered a normal percentage of body fat. For example, McArdle, Katch, and Katch (1996) state that the standards for overweight increase with age.

Hales (1994) reported that, according to the National Institutes of Health Technology Assessment Conference Panel's 1992 report, one quarter to one third of all Americans are 20 percent or more overweight. Mild obesity refers to a body weight that is 20–40 percent above the ideal weight; moderate obesity, to a body weight that is 41–100 percent above the ideal weight; and severe obesity, to a body weight that is 100 percent or more above the ideal weight for a person of that height and gender. Whitney and Rolfes (1993) say that the standard for normal body fat is between 12–18 percent for adult males and 18–24 percent for adult females. Within these statistical boundaries, overweight would correspond to percentage of body fat that exceeds the average value for fatness for a particular age and sex. There are also gradations of obesity that progress from the upper limits of normal, moderate obesity, excessive obesity, and massive obesity. There is disagreement as to where on the weight spectrum increased health risks begin. In general, however, researchers agree that the health risks of obesity increase with its severity.

In addition to total percent of body fat, scientists have also proposed that the size, number, and location of fat cells need to be considered when determining what is normal and abnormal with regard to body fatness. Some individuals have been genetically programmed to have a greater number of fat cells. Should these hypercellular individuals be considered obese even though their fat cells are of normal size? Are different races programmed with more or less fat cells? Do all races and nationalities fit into the normal body fatness range? These, of course, are questions that need to be researched. There is also a greater risk of health problems for people who carry their body fat in their trunk and abdomen as opposed to those who carry fat in their hips, thighs, and buttocks. The accumulation of excess body fat, particularly when distributed on the upper body, increases the risk of hypertension, coronary heart disease, noninsulin-dependent diabetes mellitus (Type II), gallbladder disease, sleep apnea, gout, osteoarthritis, and certain types of cancer (e.g., prostate cancer) (USDHHS, 1988; Medical Sciences Bulletin, n.d.).

Finally, to add to the complexity of the problem, there is controversy over whether obesity adversely affects health independently of other risk factors, such as smoking and diabetes. In other words, does obesity by itself, independently of other factors, constitute a health problem?

The Medical and Health Aspects of Obesity.   It is well established that chronic disease is more prevalent in obese individuals than individuals of normal body fat. Katch and McArdle (1983) and Byer and Shainberg (1995) listed the following medical and health problems associated with obesity:

1. hypertension and increased risk of stroke
2. renal disease
3. gallbladder disease
4. diabetes mellitus
5. pulmonary diseases and lowered respiratory capacity
6. problems with anesthesia during surgery and postsurgical complications
7. osteoarthritis, joint diseases, and gout
8. breast and endometrial cancer
9. abnormal plasma lipid and lipoprotein concentrations

10. impairment of cardiac function due to an increase in the heart's mechanical work
11. menstrual irregularities, toxemia of pregnancy, possible prolonged and more difficult labor, and higher infant mortality rates
12. psychological trauma
13. flat feet and intertrigious dermatitis (infection in skin folds)
14. organ compression by adipose tissue
15. impaired heat tolerance
16. atherosclerosis
17. abdominal hernias

Aside from all of the physical health problems associated with obesity, obese individuals often face discrimination. Our society is very image-conscious. All too often, advertisements tell us that to be lean and slim is to be more attractive, romantic, and popular. As a result, obese individuals are often the subject of cruel jokes and unkind words. Many obese individuals, especially children, develop negative self-images of themselves.

In many cultures, however, plumpness is seen as desirable because the rich are fat and the poor are thin. Being rotund is still a sign of prosperity, prestige, and/or fertility among Hawaiians and other Polynesians. Hawaiians view rotund women and men as being physically attractive and desirable.

Treatment of Obesity. Before discussing an appropriate plan of action for treating obesity, a brief survey of questionable practices will be listed. The weight loss industry has become a haven for quick-fix methods, gimmicks, and quackery. The following strategies should be approached with great caution and research and thoroughly discussed with a physician and nutritionist before consideration. Most should be completely avoided.

Fad diets and quick weight loss books: Although a few diet books offer useful advice and tips for motivation, most make promises they can't fulfill. Accept books that advocate a balanced approach to diet plus exercise and sound nutritional advice.

Diet supplements: Commercial supplements, especially those that constitute whole meals, provide only short-term relief. Dietary supplements teach reliance on commercial products, not on sound lifelong eating habits. After a time they become monotonous. And, although weight loss can be rapid, most weight is regained once the individual returns to his or her normal eating patterns. Dietary supplements should also be monitored by a reputable physician and nutritionist.

Diet pills and aids: Diet pills, whether they are over-the-counter or prescription, are limited in effectiveness and many are considered unsafe and hazardous. Diet drugs have side effects that may be harmful to the consumer. Amphetamines cause nervousness, insomnia, headaches, nausea, and increased blood pressure. Phenyl propanolamine hydrochloride (PPA), found in many over-the-counter diet pills, causes dizziness, headaches, rapid pulse, palpitations, sleeplessness, and hypertension. Although popular, diuretics or water pills do not cause people to lose fat. Diuretics can lead to dehydration. Diet gums and candies contain benzocaine, which numbs the taste buds on the tongue, thus reducing the sense of taste. No scientific evidence indicates that it works as a long-term diet aid. The Mayo Clinic and the U.S. government have reported that the most recent controversial prescription diet drug combination, known as fen-phen (a combination of fenfluramine and phentermine), may cause serious heart and lung damage.

Medical and surgical procedures: Any surgical or medical procedure, stapling the stomach (gastroplasty), shortening of the small intestines (gastroresection), wiring the jaw shut, and liposuction, is expensive and always associated with some risk. The success of these procedures over the long term will be determined by the dietary and exercise changes that the patient makes after the procedure.

Selecting a weight reduction program is difficult because there is no one single program for everyone. However, successful weight-control techniques do have certain things in common. The most successful programs are based on the integration of the following three approaches:

A low-calorie diet in relation to daily caloric expenditure: In order to develop long-term control of one's weight, the individual must develop an "eating plan" that (1) is based on permanent changes in one's lifelong negative eating habits and (2) balances energy input (calories consumed) with energy output (calories expended). To reduce weight, the individual must expend more calories then he or she consumes. An eating plan is more successful if it allows more calories per day and provides you with more adequate nutrition rather than a plan that drastically reduces calories and leaves you feeling starved and deprived. Weight reduction should be based on a gradual weight loss plan as opposed to a quick loss plan. It is also important that the eating plan provide nutritional adequacy.

Aerobic exercise: The amount of energy used increases as physical exercise increases. Obviously, the number of calories used up in a given exercise is dependent on the type, duration, and intensity of the exercise. Exercise also leads to an increased metabolic rate both during and after exercise. One's basal metabolism remains elevated for several hours after intense and prolonged exercise. In addition, as muscle mass increases from exercise, the lean muscle tissue is more metabolically active than fat tissue, so more calories are burned. Exercise also helps control appetite as well as providing an activity that replaces boredom. Some people cope with boredom through eating. Most importantly, the chosen exercise should be fun and something that you want to do and enjoy on a regular basis.

Behavior modification: Most eating patterns are learned behavior. For example, most Americans eat three meals a day. The British usually eat four times a day, while some people from European countries eat five to six times a day. Some African and Australian tribes are accustomed to eating only once a day. Some individuals eat when they are bored or stressed and others respond to cues in the environment such as time, smell, place, and people. The four basic steps in applying the principles of the eating behavior to be modified are: (1) description of the eating behavior to be modified, (2) replacement of established patterns of behavior with more desirable behaviors, (3) development of techniques to control behaviors, and (4) positive reinforcement or reward for maintaining or modifying the undesirable eating behavior.

After considering the above three factors, you must narrow your options and take into consideration your needs and preferences. Each of the three factors is different and you may find that you need to approach each one differently. For example, you may prefer a group or medical supervision to individual care when it comes to developing your "eating plan" or behavior modification program, but you may prefer an individual exercise program as opposed to a supervised one. Choosing the program that is best for you and your lifestyle will increase your chances for success.

Obesity in Minority Populations. Obesity in minority populations in the United States is part of this growing trend. The prevalence of obesity in some minority groups is generally higher than in the majority population. Minorities have not only increased in obesity but they have borne a heavier burden of obesity-related diseases than the rest of the majority population.

African American Women. African American women in the United States have an increased prevalence and incidence of obesity compared with white American women (Kumanyika, 1987; Williamson et al., 1991). Kumanyika (1987) pointed out that the difference in obesity between African American and white American women emerges only after adolescence.

In women aged 30–55 years, African American women are 50 percent more likely to gain 10 or more kilograms than white American women and 60 percent more likely to become obese over a 10-year period (Williamson et al., 1991). Additionally, they found that 16 percent of African American women and 10 percent of white women who were not obese at the beginning became obese during the ten-year duration of the study.

Kahn and Williamson (1991) determined that this difference in weight gain was not based on race factors but was associated with low income, low educational status, and marriage. Low income was a major factor. They reported a 70 percent increase in the risk of major weight gain in African American women who had low family incomes. They also speculated that, on marrying, an individual's eating pattern may change. The marriage results were similar for men and women.

Hispanic Americans. The Hispanic Health and Nutritional Examination Survey (HHANES) (1982–1984) showed that Hispanic Americans have higher levels of overweight and obesity than do white Americans (Center for Disease Control, 1989). Pawson and colleagues (1991) reported male adult prevalence rates were 10.6 percent (obesity) and 33.5 percent (overweight) for Mexican Americans, 9.6 percent (obesity) and 31.3 (overweight) for Puerto Ricans, and 9.0 percent (obesity) and 34 percent (overweight) for Cubans. In female adults prevalence values were, respectively, 15.1 percent (obesity) and 42.3 percent (overweight) for Mexican Americans, 7.8 percent (obesity) and 40.7 percent (overweight) for Puerto Ricans, and 15 percent (obesity) and 38.2 percent (overweight) for Cubans. Obesity and overweight were defined as a body mass index in excess of the 95th and 85th percentiles, respectively, of U.S. reference standards.

The San Antonio Heart Study (SAHS) (Stern et al., 1994) collected data between 1979 and 1988 on obesity and body fat distribution on Mexican Americans residing in San Antonio, Texas. The SAHS reported that Mexican Americans in San Antonio are more obese than Mexican Americans in the southwestern United States (based on data from HHANES) and that there has been a marked increase in overall obesity between 1982 and 1988, particularly in Mexican American women. The SAHS reported that the percentage of overweight ranged from 45 percent to 53 percent in men and from 35 percent to 65 percent in women, whereas the percentage of those severely overweight ranged from 14 percent to 35 percent in men and from 12 percent to 35 percent in women.

The role of socioeconomic factors in the etiology of obesity in Mexican Americans has been studied. Pawson and colleagues (1991) reported that increased socioeconomic status was significantly associated with obesity in Mexican Americans, independently of gender. However, Hazuda and colleagues (1991) reported that socioeconomic status (SES) and cultural assimilation are related. SES and assimilation are associated with lower overall obesity and more favorable body fat distribution. Acculturation was associated with a significant linear decline in both obesity and diabetes. This suggests that levels of fatness in some Hispanic groups may reflect cultural preferences and individuals may consciously seek to attain a certain level of fatness in keeping with culturally perceived norms (Massara, 1989).

American Indians. There is a scarcity of obesity research on American Indians, so the magnitude of the obesity problem in American Indians is not well understood or documented. A few studies have suggested that some American Indian tribes have higher rates of obesity when compared to other U.S. populations (Story et al., 1986; Terry & Bass 1984; Wolfe & Sanjur, 1988). Broussard and colleagues (1991) used self-reported information and surveys to determine that the prevalence of obesity in American Indians was higher than the U.S. population in all age groups. They reported obesity rates of 13.7 percent for men and 16.5 percent for women, which was higher than the U.S. rates of 9.1 percent and 8.2 percent, respectively. Obesity rates in American Indian adolescents and preschool children were higher than the respective rates for U.S. people combined. Twenty-four and one-half percent of adolescent Indian males and 25 percent of adolescent American Indian females were overweight. Obesity was 11.1 percent and 7.3 percent, respectively, for adolescent males and females.

Obesity has become a major health problem in Native Americans only in the past one or two generations. It was in 1968 that the television program, "Hunger in America," reported that malnutrition was a serious health problem in American Indian and Native Alaskan communities. Following that program, the government provided abundant food programs that were high-fat and low-fiber diets. At the same time, the government program led to sedentary lifestyle habits. Thus, the problem of malnutrition was solved and replaced by the problem of obesity and its consequences.

In conjunction with the increased prevalence of obesity over the past few decades, there has been an epidemic of diabetes, increased coronary heart disease, hypertension, and poor survival rates for breast cancer for American Indians and Native Alaskans.

Japanese Americans. Curb and Marcus (1991) utilized the data from the Honolulu Heart Program and determined that the mean body mass index (BMI; weight in kilogram divided by height in centimeter squared) was substantially higher among Japanese men in Hawaii and California than those in Japan. This study, at the time, was the only standardized collected data for the Asian populations that form substantial minority groups in the United States. Because there are many Asian populations, caution should be used in making generalizations about all Asians. In general, the trend illustrated in these largely first- and second-generation Japanese immigrants is toward a greater prevalence of obesity and central body fatness, both of which have been associated with detrimental changes in cardiovascular risk and events (Feinleib, 1985). It appears that the adoption of more Western lifestyles and diet by the Japanese in the United States has been negatively associated with risks and increased cardiovascular events. Curb and Marcus (1991) also reported that for Japanese females the mean values are similar in Japan and California for most ages. Mean values for Japanese females in Hawaii tend to be higher for ages six to seven but thereafter tend to be similar to the other two populations.

Native Hawaiians.   Native Hawaiians, the indigenous people of the Hawaii Islands, have the highest prevalence of obesity of the many Asian and Pacific Islander Americans living in the state of Hawaii (Hispanic Health and Nutritional Examination Survey, 1987). The Native Hawaiian rate for overweight was 3.3 times higher than the overall rate for the state. Native Hawaiians, in particular, full-blooded Native Hawaiians, are likely to have the highest mortality rates from heart disease in the nation. Native Hawaiians also have the highest mortality rates among the five major ethnic groups (Caucasian, Japanese, Native Hawaiian, Chinese, and Filipinos) living in the state (U.S. Congress, Office of Technology Assessment, 1987). However, to date no comprehensive population-based study of risk factors in Native Hawaiians has been conducted. Aluli (1991) reported that, of 257 Native Hawaiian adults, 63.8 percent of the women and 65.5 percent of the men were 20 percent or more overweight. Thirty-four percent of the women and 47 percent of the men were *severely* overweight. Women aged 45–54 were heaviest and men aged 25–34 were heaviest.

Aluli (1991) reported that the diet of all residents of Hawaii has changed significantly over the past few decades to include more processed, prepared, and fast-service foods. For the Native Hawaiian, polished white rice has replaced the traditional staple food of taro, a starchy tuber. Furthermore, Aluli reported that local people have a preference for canned meats, fatty snack foods and salad dressings, sweet drinks, and high-calorie sweets. In sharp contrast, the traditional diet was very low in fat and cholesterol, high in fiber, and high in complex carbohydrates, such as fruits and vegetables, and fish was the main source of protein.

Anorexia and Bulimia

While many Americans are struggling with concerns about being overweight, a number of Americans are in a struggle of another kind. Eating disorders have become a serious problem for some Americans, in particular young women. An eating disorder is a bizarre and dangerous pattern of food consumption. As a result of the cultural emphasis on thinness, two disorders have received much attention over the last 20 years: anorexia nervosa and bulimia nervosa. In both disorders, individuals feel "too fat," which may not be the case at all. As a result of those feelings, they engage in destructive eating patterns to control their weight. This intense desire for thinness becomes an obsession and requires intensive intervention.

Bulimia Nervosa (bulimia, for short) is characterized by binge-eating and purging. Binge-eating is uncontrolled consumption of large quantities of food followed by purging. Bingeing may last from a few minutes to several hours. The binger will often consume "forbidden" foods, such as sweets or starches, and is not concerned about the nutritional value of the food. Purging is done by self-induced vomiting, diuretics, laxatives, or all three. People with bulimia will also engage in other activities, such as enemas, fasting, severe diets, and vigorous exercise, in order to control their weight. Overall, most of them manage to maintain near normal weight.

Anorexia nervosa (anorexia, for short) is characterized by self-imposed starvation. Anorexia is primarily a disturbance in the person's perception of himself or herself. People with anorexia often report feelings of low self-esteem and powerlessness. Individuals with anorexia refuse to eat enough food to maintain normal body weight. This leads to severe weight loss, malnutrition, and possibly to death. It is not uncommon for people with anorexia to resort to many of the purging activities of a bulimic patient. Of all anorexics, 90–95 percent are female and typically are between the ages of 15 and 30, although the condition has been documented in middle-aged women and children under the age of 10.

Both anorexia and bulimia can lead to serious medical problems. Purging can upset the body's electrolyte balance and lead to abnormal heart rhythms and injury to the kidneys. The violence of repeated vomiting can ulcerate and rupture the esophagus and stomach and cause internal bleeding. Sore throats and swelling of the parotid glands are also common. The residual wash of the gastric juices can lead to serious damage to the enamel of the teeth. Extreme loss of body weight can lead to multiple problems, such as amenorrhea (loss of menstrual cycle), lowered blood pressure and body temperature, weakened bones, growth of downy hair over the body, depression, constipation, dry skin and hair, cold hands and feet, and death.

Both bulimia and anorexia are difficult to treat because the causes are psychologically, biologically, and culturally based. Victims of both disorders generally have low self-esteem and their eating behaviors are obsessive in nature. The earlier the treatment begins, the greater the chance of success. The sooner the treatment begins, the better the chances for a full recovery. The complete description, diagnosis, and treatment for both of these disorders is complex and beyond the scope of this book. This brief discussion is not a substitute for an informed discussion between a patient and his or her physician.

Eating Disorders and Minority Populations.   The research on the prevalence of eating disorders is limited because it is a "secretive" disorder. Of those identified and in therapy, the typical profile is a young white female from a middle or upper-middle socioeconomic group. The research on minority populations and eating disorders is limited. It was not until the mid 1980s that some limited research on minority populations in the United States was published, but it was limited to African American females. Most early studies indicated that disordered eating attitudes and behaviors exist among previously underreported minority populations. Researchers now realize that the disturbed eating behaviors of anorexia nervosa and, in particular, bulimia are not restricted to white, middle-class, college-aged females. Smith and Krejci (1991) administered an eating disorder inventory and bulimia test to Hispanic, Native American, and white youths. They reported that Native Americans consistently scored the highest on each of seven items, representing disturbed eating behaviors and attitudes. Native Americans scored significantly higher on self-induced vomiting and binge-eating, but did not show clinical symptoms of bulimia. They concluded that the rate of disturbed eating patterns among Native American as well as Hispanic youth is at least comparable to that of white adolescents. The greatest concern of the minority subjects was extreme fear of weight gain and body dissatisfaction. Excessive dieting or fasting was reported by half of the females and 19.8 percent of the males in the study. The fact that so many individuals responded to weight concerns with severe dieting is alarming, given the evidence that restrictive dieting frequently precedes the onset of bulimic symptoms.

Similar studies (Snow & Harris, 1989; Pumariega, 1986) have reported similar results. In terms of eating disorders, minorities have joined the majority.

REFERENCES

Aluli, N. E. Prevalence of obesity in a Native Hawaiian population. *American Journal of Clinical Nutrition* 53 (1991): 1556–60S.

Bley-Miller, G. *The thousand recipe chinese cookbook.* New York: Fireside, 1966.

Blocker, D. Nutrition concerns of black Americans. In I. Livingston (Ed.), *Handbook of black American health.* Westport, CT: Greenwood Press, 1994, p. 269–281.

Brossard, B., Johnson, A., Himes, J., Story, M., Fichtner, R., Hauck, F., Bachman-Carter, K., Hayes, J., Frohlich, K., Gray, N., Valway, S., and Gohdes, D. Prevalence of obesity in American Indians and Alaska Natives. *Journal of Clinical Nutrition* 53 (1991):153–162.

Byer, C., and Shainberg, L. *Living well: Health in your hands.* New York: Harper Collins, 1995.

Centers for Disease Control. Prevalence of overweight for Hispanics—United States, 1982–1984. MMWR 38 (1989): 838–42.

Champagne, D. (Ed.). *The Native North American almanac.* Detroit, MI: Gale Research, 1994.

Cott, A. *Fasting is a way of life.* New York: Bantam Books, 1977.

Cox, B., and Jacobs, M. *Spirit of the harvest: North American Indian cooking.* New York: Stewart Tabori & Chang, 1991.

Curb, J. D., and Marcus, E. B. Body fat and obesity in Japanese Americans. *American Journal of Clinical Nutrition* 53 (1991): 1552–555.

Downer, L. *At the Japanese table.* San Francisco: Chronicle Books, 1993.

Feinleib, M. Epidemiology of obesity in relation to health hazards. *Annual Internal Medicine* 103 (1985): 1019–24.

Fergusson, E. *Mexican cookbook.* Albuquerque: University of New Mexico Press, 1973.

Glaskow, J., and Adaskin, J. The West Indians. In N. Waxler-Morrison, J. Anderson, and E. Richardson (Eds.), *Cross-cultural caring: A handbook for health professionals.* Vancouver: UBC Press, 1990, p. 214–244.

Hales, D. *An invitation to health.* Redwood City, CA: Benjamin/Cummings, 1994.

Harris, J. *The welcome table: African American heritage cookbook.* New York: Simon & Shuster, 1995.

Harris, J. The culinary Caribbean. *Islands* 16, 6 (November/December, 1996), 118–182.

Hawaii State Department of Health (HHRBS). *Hawaii's health risk behaviors, 1987.* Honolulu: Hawaii State Department of Health, 1988.

Hazuda, H., Mitchell, B., Haffner, S., and Stern, M. Obesity in Mexican American subgroups: Findings from the San Antonio Heart Study. *Journal of Clinical Nutrition* 53 (1991): 1529S-34S.

Higuera-McMahan, J. *Healthy Mexican cookbook.* Lake Hughes, CA: Olive Press, 1994.

Kahn, H. S., and Williamson, D. F. Is race associated with weight change in U.S. adults after adjustment for income, education, and marital factors? *American Journal of Clinical Nutrition* 53 (1991): 1566–70S.

Katch, F., and McArdle, W. *Nutrition, weight control, and exercise.* Philadelphia: Lea & Febiger, 1983.

Kennedy, D. *The art of Mexican cooking.* New York: Bantam, 1989.

Kittler, P., and Sucher, K. *Food and culture in America.* New York: Van Nostrand Reinhold, 1989.

Kittler, P., and Sucher, K. *Food and culture in America.* (3rd ed). New York: West, 1995.

Kumanyika, S. Obesity in black women. *Epidemiological Review* 9 (1987): 31–50.

Kumanyika, S., and Adams-Campbell, L. Obesity, diet, and psychosocial factors contributing to cardiovascular disease in blacks. *Cardiovascular Clinics* 21 (1991), 47–73.

Lai, M., and Kevin-Yue, K. The Chinese. In N. Waxler-Morrison, J. Anderson, and E. Richardson (Eds.), *Cross-cultural caring: A handbook for health professionals.* Vancouver: UBC Press, 1990, pp. 68–90.

Lo, K. *Encyclopedia of Chinese cooking.* New York: Bristol Park, 1979.

Massara, E. B. *Que gordita! A study of weight among women in a Puerto Rican community.* New York: AMS Press, 1989.

McArdle, W., Katch, V., and Katch, W. *Exercise physiology: Energy, nutrition, and human performance* (4th ed.). Baltimore, MD: Williams & Wilkins, 1996.

Medical Sciences Bulletin. *Focus on obesity.* Pharmaceutical Information Associates, Ltd., n.d. http://pharmoinfo.com/pubs/msb/obesity.html

Okabe, T., Takahashi, K., and Richardson, E. The Japanese. In N. Waxler-Morrison, J. Anderson, and E. Richardson *Cross-cultural caring: A handbook for health professionals.* Vancouver: UBC Press, 1990, pp. 116–140.

Pawson, I., Martorell, R. and Mendoza, F. Prevalence of overweight and obesity in U.S. Hispanic populations. *American Journal of Clinical Nutrition* 53 (1991):1552–8.

Pumariega, A. Acculturation and eating attitudes in adolescent girls: A comparative and correlational study. *Journal of American Academy of Child Psychiatry* 25 (1986), 276–279.

Quick-Tilley, C. *African American heritage cookbook.* Secaucus, NJ: Birch Lane Press, 1996.

Raichlen, S. *The Caribbean pantry cookbook.* New York: Artisen, 1995.

Rudzinski, R. *Japanese country cookbook.* San Francisco: Nitty Gritty Productions, 1969.

Sanjur, D. *Hispanic foodways, nutrition, and health.* Boston, MA: Allyn & Bacon, 1995.

Seventh-Day Adventist Dietetic Association. *The vegetarian food pyramid.* Loma Linda, CA: Seventh-Day Adventist Dietetic Association, n. d.

Smith, J. and Krejci, J. Minorities join the majority: Eating disturbances among Hispanic and Native American youth. *International Journal of Eating Disorders* 10, 2 (1991): 179–186.

Snow, J. and Harris, M. Disordered eating in southwestern Pueblo Indians and Hispanics. *Journal of Adolescence* 12 (1989), 329–336.

Solomon, C. *The complete Asian cookbook.* Rutland, VT: Charles E. Tuttle, 1992.

Stern, M., Rosenthal, M., Haffner, S., Hazuda, H., and Franco, L. Sex difference in the effects of sociocultural status on diabetes and cardiovascular risk factors in Mexican Americans and non-Hispanic whites: The San Antonio Heart Study. *American Journal of Epidemiology* 120 (1994): 834–51.

Story, M., Tompkins, R., Bass, M., and Wakefield, L. Anthropometric measurements and dietary intakes of Cherokee Indian teenagers in North Carolina. *Journal of American Dietetic Association* 86 (1986): 1555–60.

Terry, R. and Bass, M. Obesity among Eastern Cherokee Indian women: Prevalence, self-perceptions, and experiences. *Ecology, Food, and Nutrition* 14 (1984): 117–27.

U.S. Congress, Office of Technology Assessment. *Current health status and population projections of Native Hawaiians living in Hawaii.* Washington, DC: Office of Technology and Assessment, 1987.

U.S. Department of Health and Human Services, Public Health Service. *The Surgeon General's report on nutrition and health.* Washington DC: DHHS publication (PHS) 88-50210, 1988.

Warner, J. *All the best Mexican meals.* New York: Hearst, 1992.

Warner, J. *All the best stir-fries.* New York: Hearst, 1993.

Whitney, E., and Rolfes, S. *Understanding nutrition.* Minneapolis, MN: West, 1993.

Williamson, D. F., Kahn, H. S., and Byers, T. The 10-year incidence of obesity and major weight gain in black and white U.S. women aged 30–55 years. *American Journal of Clinical Nutrition* 53 (1991): 151S–8S.

Wolfe, W. and Sanjur, D. Contemporary diet and body weight of Navajo women receiving food assistance: An ethnographic and nutritional investigation. *Journal of American Dietetic Association* 88 (1988): 822–27.

CHAPTER

7 Ethnic Minority Drug Use

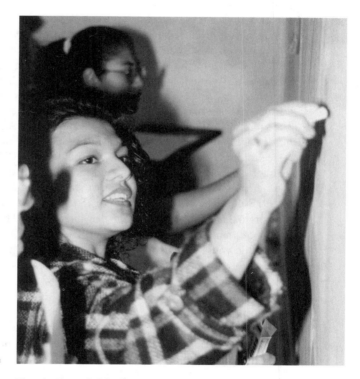

The power of people doing things for themselves is very strong medicine.
—Kate Lorig, Nurse

Photo by Everardo Martinez-Inzunza, published in *Cultures* magazine, volume 2, issue 2.

Few people would argue that the use of psychoactive drugs occurs in all 50 states. On closer examination, because of population demographics, Johnson and colleagues (1990) reported a higher level of drug use in areas with dense populations. Major metropolitan areas such as New York, Miami, Detroit, and Washington, DC, tend to show greater drug use patterns among minority Americans. This does not mean that minority Americans have a greater drug problem but rather that in these cities minority Americans collectively are in the majority.

The news media have contributed to the notion that ethnic minority Americans use more drugs by frequently reporting stories, along with photographs, of minority Americans being arrested for drug-related crimes. In addition, it is not unusual to see harrowing stories of drug use in public housing projects and poor neighborhoods. Very seldom is this vision countered by stories and photographs of drug use in affluent, nonminority communities and neighborhoods.

The use and abuse of licit and illicit drugs has been implicated as a reason for the relatively high number of arrests among black and Hispanic males, as a major factor in the health disparities between whites and America's black and Hispanic populations, and, of course, as a primary cause for the disproportionate share of black and Hispanic adults in drug and alcohol treatment (Secretary's Task Force on Black and Minority Health, 1995). In light of the media attention and the "drug-related" problems that African American and Hispanic Americans appear to have, a relatively high prevalence of drug use and abuse might be expected. This negative image of minority Americans, especially African Americans, has led many to believe that ethnic minorities and, in particular, African Americans are more likely to have drug problems than white Americans.

Despite this expectation, The National Institute on Drug Abuse (U.S. Department of Health and Human Services, 1991c; Trimble, et al. 1987) reports that drug use occurs among almost all races and that ethnic minorities and, in particular, African Americans and Hispanic Americans do not use more drugs more than whites. In fact, they generally use less. The 1991 National Household Survey (U.S. Department of Health and Human Services, 1991d) reported that a higher percentage of whites reported higher use of cigarettes, marijuana, and alcohol than African Americans and Hispanic Americans. One possible exception is that Hispanic youth in general, and Hispanic males in particular, report a higher prevalence of cocaine use than other groups. Table 7.1 represents the percent of people who reported use of selected drugs by race or ethnicity in 1988.

Has the drug scene changed since 1988? This is a difficult question to answer because of the scarcity of coordinated research on drug use and abuse of the many different subgroups within each of the major racial categories. The research on ethnic minority drug use is still very limited. Studies are sporadic and usually limited to certain geographical areas. Most of the drug research has come from national surveys that have often ignored the significant differences within minority groups. Because drug research is limited, information that is available on both minority groups and subgroups is speculative. Consequently, thoughtful reflection will be necessary as a substitute for firm data.

The most comprehensive study was the National Household Survey on Drug Abuse (NSHDA, 1991a), which compiled data from over 35,500 respondents in four regions of the United States. African Americans and Hispanic Americans were well represented in the survey but Asian Americans, Native Americans, and other ethnic minority groups were placed into one general category designated as "Other." The NHSDA report did not differentiate between cultures within each category. For example, there was no distinction between Mexican Americans, Cuban Americans, Puerto Ricans, and other cultures within the Hispanic American category. In addition, there was no distinction between foreign-born and American-born individuals, nor was there any distinction between traditional, bicultural, and acculturated individuals..

TABLE 7.1   Illicit Drug Use, by Substance

Substance	Total %					
	Ever Used			Used in Past Months		
	Hispanic	**White**	**Black**	**Hispanic**	**White**	**Black**
Marijuana	27.9	33.7	33.3	6.0	5.6	6.3
Cocaine (including crack)	11.0	10.8	9.3	2.6	1.3	2.0
Crack	2.2	1.0	2.4	0.5	0.2	0.8
Inhalants	5.8	6.0	3.6	0.4	0.7	0.3
Hallucinogens (including PCP)	6.1	8.1	2.9	0.3	0.5	—*
PCP	3.0	3.3	1.6	—	—	—
Stimulants	5.2	8.0	2.6	0.8	1.0	0.6
Sedatives	2.5	3.8	2.3	0.5	0.4	0.5
Tranquilizers	3.3	5.2	3.1	0.6	0.6	—
Analgesics	4.4	5.4	4.1	1.2	0.5	0.7
Heroin	1.1	0.8	2.3	—	—	—
Needle use	1.3	1.2	2.9	—	—	—

The percent of people surveyed who reported use of each drug is shown, by race/ethnicity, as of 1988.

*—insufficient data

Source: Adapted from Percent surveyed reporting drug use in 1988: U.S. civilian noninstitutionalized population, by sex and race, *Health status of minorities and low-income groups, 3rd ed.,* 1991, p. 267. Primary source: National Institute on Drug Abuse, *National Household Survey on Drug Abuse: Population Estimates 1988.* Department of Health and Human Services Pub. No (ADM)89–1636.

A Comparison of the 1990 and 1995 National Household Survey on Drug Abuse

This section compares the results of the 1990 National Household Survey on Drug Abuse (U.S. Department of Health and Human Services 1991a) and the 1995 National Household Survey (U.S. Department of Health and Human Services, 1995). The comparison is made to reflect the changing drug patterns among minority Americans.

The 1990 National Household Survey on Drug Abuse

The 1990 National Household Survey on Drug Abuse reported the following:

- A decrease in drug use among African Americans during their lifetime, from 37.1 percent to 35.9 percent;
- A significant decrease in drug use among African Americans in the past year from 21.8 percent to 14.9 percent;

B O X   **7.1**
Types of Drugs

A drug is any chemical substance, aside from food, that, on entering the body, alters the functioning of the body. A drug that alters sensory perceptions, mood, thought processes, or behavior is called as a *psychoactive* drug

Drugs are currently divided into seven basic categories based on their chemical properties and the effects that they cause.

Depressants include alcohol, tranquilizers, and sedatives.

Stimulants affect physical and/or mental processes and include amphetamines, cocaine, nicotine, and caffeine.

Narcotics include opiate derivatives such as morphine, heroin, and codeine, as well as synthetic drugs like methadone. These drugs were originally designed for pain relief.

Hallucinogens distort information and include LSD, mescaline, psilocybin, and PCP.

Marijuana and its derivatives are in a separate category due to their potential multiple effects.

Inhalants are the mind-altering vapors from a variety of sources including household solvents and aerosols.

Other drugs include designer (human-made) drugs and anabolic steroids.

Source: P. Reagan and J. Brookins-Fisher. *Community Health in the 21st Century,* Boston, MA: Allyn and Bacon, 1997, 381–382.

- A significant decrease in drug use among blacks in the past month, from 15.7 percent to 7.8 percent;
- Over one-third of African Americans between the ages of 18 and 19 have dropped out of high school, with drug use higher among them;
- African American students who stay in school are less likely than white students to use illicit drugs;
- Thirteen percent of white seniors reported using cocaine as compared to 6 percent by African American seniors;
- Fifty percent of white seniors reported using marijuana as compared to 37 percent by African American seniors.

The results of this survey suggest that the prevalence of drug use within the African American community is decreasing. However, a closer examination by the 1990 National Household Survey on Drug Abuse (NHSDA) revealed that a significant number of drug users are still using illicit drugs within the African American community. The NHSDA defined "illicit drug" use as any nonmedical use of marijuana or hashish, cocaine (including crack), inhalants, hallucinogens (including PCP), heroin, or psychotherapeutics (stimulants, tranquilizers, and sedatives). The survey revealed that:

- Thirty-six percent or 8 million African Americans have used illicit drugs at least once in their lifetimes;
- Three million African Americans have used illicit drugs in the past year;
- Almost 2 million African Americans have used illicit drugs in the past month;
- African Americans 35 years and older were more likely than whites or Hispanic Americans to have used an illicit drug in the past month;
- African Americans in the 18–34 age group had a 24 percent usage rate, the highest rate among all racial or ethnic groups;
- African American rates were lower than white rates for those 12–25 years old;
- African Americans were more likely than whites or Hispanic Americans to have used heroin once in their lifetime;
- African Americans were more likely than Hispanic Americans, but less likely than whites, to have smoked cigarettes;
- African American women were more likely than women in any other racial or ethnic group to have used crack cocaine.

The 1995 National Household Survey on Drug Abuse

The 1995 National Household Survey on Drug Abuse reported the following:

- An estimated 12.8 million Americans were current illicit drug users (used an illicit drug in the past month) and represent 6.1 percent of the population 12 years old and older;
- Marijuana continues to be the most commonly used illicit drug, used by 77 percent of current illicit drug users. Approximately 57 percent of current illicit drug users used marijuana exclusively, 20 percent used marijuana and another illicit drug, and the remaining 23 percent used an illicit drug other than marijuana in the past month;
- An estimated 5.6 million Americans (2.6 percent of the population) were current users of illicit drugs other than marijuana and hashish;
- The current illicit drug use (within the past month) for African Americans (7.9 percent) was somewhat higher than for white Americans (6.0 percent) and Hispanics (5.1 percent);
- Among youths, the rates of illicit drug use are about the same as those for the three groups. These numbers may reflect a change in the use of illicit drugs by different minority groups. Most current illicit drug users were white Americans;
- There were an estimated 9.6 million whites (75 percent of all users), 1.9 million African Americans (15 percent), and 1.0 million Hispanics (8 percent) that were current users in 1995;
- There was an increase in illicit drug use among white American, African American, and Hispanic American youths between 1992 and 1995.

The rate of current illicit drug use for youths in "other" race/ethnicity groups increased from 2.7 percent to 11.2 percent between 1994 and 1995. This result should be viewed with caution, however, as the NHSDA sample size is small for this group. This racial/ethnic group is comprised mainly of Asian Americans, Pacific Islanders, and Native Americans.

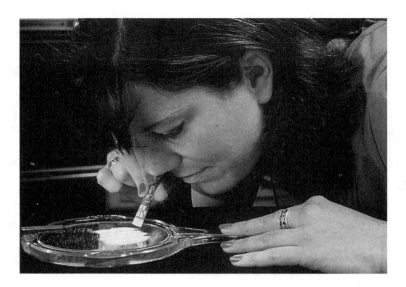

Photo by Will Hart.

Of all the tyrannies which have upsurped power over humanity, few have been able to enslave the mind and body as imperiously as drug addiction.
—Sisters in Crime, 1975

Drug Use by the "Other" Race

The following section discusses some independent drug research on Native Americans and Asian and Pacific Americans, the members who make up the "Other" category of the National Household Drug Abuse Survey. Unfortunately, published studies describing prevalence rates are few and limited in scope. Caution must be taken in interpreting them.

Native Americans

One of the few longitudinal studies on Indian drug use reported that, over a three-year period: (a) 80 percent of Indian youth reported using alcohol and 20 percent use alcohol every weekend, (b) 70 percent reported using marijuana, and 40 percent of those used it at least 10 times during the past month, and (c) 40 percent reported using other drugs at least three times in the past month (King et al., 1992).

Segal (1995) conducted a comprehensive survey of Alaska Natives and reported that Native youth showed higher drug and alcohol use than all other ethnic groups, including white Americans. Segal found that 71 percent of Alaska Natives and 66 percent of Indians had tried marijuana; 40 percent reported using stimulants; 33 percent used inhalants; 70 percent of the Alaska Natives and 53 percent of the Indians used chewing tobacco. Eighty-eight percent of the Indians and 75 percent of the Alaska Natives had tried alcohol. Table 7.2 reports the percentage of high school seniors who reported using selected drugs in the past year, 1985–1989.

TABLE 7.2   Percentage of High School Seniors Who Reported Using Selected Drugs in the Past Year, 1985–1989

Marijuana

Am. Indian		White		African Am.		Hispanic Am.		Asian Am.	
M	F	M	F	M	F	M	F	M	F
42	44	40.2	36	29.8	18.4	34.5	24	19.6	17.1

Cocaine

Am. Indian		White		African Am.		Hispanic Am.		Asian Am.	
M	F	M	F	M	F	M	F	M	F
14.2	15.5	11.9	9.3	6.1	2.6	15	7.6	5.8	5.7

Alcohol

Am. Indian		White		African Am.		Hispanic Am.		Asian Am.	
M	F	M	F	M	F	M	F	M	F
82	81.3	88.3	88.6	72.5	63.9	81	75	69.3	67.5

Inhalants

Am. Indian		White		African Am.		Hispanic Am.		Asian Am.	
M	F	M	F	M	F	M	F	M	F
5.2	0.9	3.4	2	1.4	1.4	2.1	1.5	1.3	0.8

LSD

Am. Indian		White		African Am.		Hispanic Am.		Asian Am.	
M	F	M	F	M	F	M	F	M	F
3.1	2.2	2.8	1.1	0.6	0.2	1.8	0.25	1.1	0.1

Cigarettes

Am. Indian		White		African Am.		Hispanic Am.		Asian Am.	
M	F	M	F	M	F	M	F	M	F
36.8	43.6	29.8	34	15.6	13.3	23	21	16.8	14.3

Data have been combined for 1985 to 1989.

Source: Adapted from U.S. Department of Education, National Center for Education Statistics, *The condition of education,* 1992, Washington, DC: 1992. Primary source: U.S. Department of Health and Human Services; Alcohol, Drug Abuse, Mental Health Administration; National Institute of Drug Abuse, *Drug use among high school students, college students, and other young adults,* 1991.

The average percentage of American Indian high school seniors (both male and female) who have used drugs in the past 12 months (1985–1989) was higher than other racial/ethnic groups (U.S. Department of Health and Human Services, 1991).

Asian Americans

There is a relatively small number of research papers devoted to the use of drugs among Asians and Pacific Americans. Most of the information pertaining to alcohol, tobacco, and other drug use among Asian Americans comes from isolated, nonrandom surveys. Unfortunately, the number of published articles describing prevalence rates among this ethnic groups is few and limited in scope. In general, the research reports that Asian and Pacific Americans use and abuse substances less frequently than do members of other racial and ethnic groups (McLaughlin et al., 1987; Trimble et al., 1987; Tucker, 1985). Flaskerud and Hu (1992) found lower rates of substance abuse among Asian Americans than among white Americans, African Americans, or Latino Americans. However, most samples are small and primarily drawn from West Coast cities like San Francisco and Los Angeles.

There are no prevalence data pertaining to the Asian American populations at the national level. Most of the available survey data are on the use of alcohol and tobacco. The three major surveys—the National Institute on Drug Abuse (NIDA) National Household Survey, the NIDA National Adolescent School Health Survey, and the National High school Seniors Survey—do not report data on Asian American groups. In addition, the majority of studies conducted primarily on Chinese and Japanese populations do not include recent immigrant and refugee groups. These later groups are at high risk for illegal drug use and are also the fastest growing populations among Asian Pacific groups.

Tobacco and Smokeless Tobacco

When a smoker puffs from a lit cigarette, he or she is inhaling more than 2000 different chemicals and chemical compounds, many of which are poisonous and cancer-causing agents. In general terms, the two major categories of components in tobacco smoke are the particulates or tar and the gas components. The particulates (tar) are the small particles that are suspended in the smoke, which includes water droplets, nicotine, and a host of other compounds, some of which are poisonous, carcinogenic, and co-carcinogenic. The other components are the gas compounds in the smoke, which includes carbon monoxide, ammonia, hydrogen cyanide, and acetone. Among these gases, carbon monoxide is extremely toxic.

The following discussion will focus on only three of the most important compounds in tobacco smoke: tar, nicotine, and carbon monoxide.

Tar

When an individual smokes a filtered cigarette, the filter will turn yellow. This discoloration is due to the accumulation of tar. In laboratory experiments in which special smoking machines are designed to collect the tars from cigarettes, the tar is collected in a flask. As the tar accumulates in the flask, it takes on a dark, sticky appearance not unlike the tar used to pave roads. The sticky characteristic allows the tar to adhere to the cells of the respiratory system (the lungs and air passages). The respiratory system has a specialized mechanism consisting of small hairlike projections, called *cilia,* that are capable of removing unwanted contaminants that impede the breathing process. Components in tar eventually affect the normal functioning of the cilia, allowing the sticky tar to remain in the lungs and other parts of the respiratory system. The carcinogenic and co-carcinogenic compounds eventually cause cellular changes in the lung tissue that may result in cancer.

Nicotine

Nicotine is the dependency-producing psychoactive drug that stimulates the central nervous system, giving the smoker a brief "kick." Nicotine increases blood pressure, heart rate, and vasoconstriction, inhibits the gastrointestinal system, decreases peripheral circulation and fibrinolytic activity, and increases the release of glycogen by the liver. Nicotine also increases blood-clotting potential. The dependency-producing effect is enhanced by: (1) the speed with which smoked nicotine reaches the brain, (2) the learned rewards received in the social environment, and (3) the sheer number of times a smoker experiences a dose of nicotine throughout the day.

Over time, tolerance increases in the nicotine receptors of the brain and the smoker increases the number of cigarettes needed to maintain his or her addiction. Common symptoms of physical withdrawal from tobacco will usually include headache, an inability to concentrate, irritability, drowsiness, fatigue, and sleep disturbances. Physical withdrawal from tobacco usually takes from seven to ten days. However, the most difficult aspect of withdrawal is the psychological craving for a cigarette. These cravings can take months to years before they completely diminish.

Carbon Monoxide

Carbon monoxide (CO) is an odorless, colorless, tasteless toxic gas that is formed when tobacco burns. The danger in carbon monoxide is that it has a 200 times greater affinity to hemoglobin than oxygen. Consequently, carbon monoxide easily attaches to hemoglobin and is transported through the bloodstream instead of oxygen. In addition, carbon monoxide is also more resistant to detaching itself from hemoglobin, resulting in an accumulation of carbon monoxide over time. Accumulation of carbon monoxide may contribute to coronary disease as well as deficiencies in physiological functioning and behavior.

Health Effects of Smoking

Smoking remains one of the most preventable causes of death, accounting for approximately 125,000 deaths per year or 30 percent of all deaths from cancer (American Cancer Society, 1989). Smoking also plays a major causative role in heart disease, stroke, hypertension, and respiratory disorders such as emphysema and bronchitis.

Cancer

As discussed earlier, the exposure to the carcinogens and co-carcinogens found in cigarette tar can lead to the development of cancer, in particular, lung cancer.

Cardiovasuclar Disease, Stroke, and Hypertension

Smoking is responsible for approximately 30 percent of all deaths due to cardiovascular disease and stroke. The two major factors that lead to these situations are the combination of nicotine and carbon monoxide. Nicotine increases blood pressure by increasing heart rate while, at the same time, causing vasoconstriction of the blood vessels. In conjunction, nicotine increases the potential of blood clots by increasing blood platelets' adhesiveness. Finally, nicotine increases the possibility of atherosclerosis in the coronary arteries and the arteries of the brain by increasing the body's serum cholesterol and fatty deposits. Combining these nicotine factors with carbon monoxide's ability to decrease oxygen in the blood is the perfect recipe for hypertension, heart attack, or stroke.

Respiratory Diseases

Chronic obstructive pulmonary disease (COPD) is a term that refers to a group of diseases characterized by impaired breathing due to abnormalities in the air passages. Smoking is the major cause of COPD. Two significant COPD diseases are emphysema and bronchitis. Emphysema is a condition in which the air sacs (alveoli) in the lungs become enlarged or rupture, resulting in extremely difficult breathing. These tiny air sacs are the center at which the oxygen and carbon dioxide exchange takes place. Massive destruction of these air sacs leads to a debilitating condition in which gasping and struggling to breathe utilizes almost 80 percent of the patient's daily physical energy. Ingredients in tobacco smoke cause an oversecretion of mucus in the air passages of the respiratory system that ultimately impairs the lungs, leading to emphysema. Chronic bronchitis is a condition in which the bronchial tissues become inflamed, leading to coughing and shortness of breath.

Cigarette Smoking

Smoking remains the single most preventable cause of death (U.S. Department of Health, Education, and Welfare, 1985), accounting for approximately 125,000 cancer deaths per year or 30 percent of all deaths from cancer (American Cancer Society, 1989). Cigarette smoke consists of more than 2000 different chemicals and chemical compounds, many of which are known to be carcinogenic (cancer-producing), co-carcinogenic, and poisonous to the body. As a result, smoking plays a major causative role in heart disease, stroke, hypertension, and respiratory disorders such as emphysema and bronchitis.

Cigarettes also contain nicotine, which is addictive and a stimulant to the central nervous system. Nicotine will increase blood-clotting potential, heart rate, blood pressure, and vasoconstriction, At the same time, nicotine will also decrease peripheral circulation and fibrinolytic activity.

The 1995 National Household Survey reported that an estimated 61 million Americans were current smokers in 1995. This represents a smoking rate of 29 percent for the population aged 12 and older. In addition, current smokers were more likely to be heavy drinkers and illicit drug users.

African Americans

Hildreth and Saunders (1992) reported that smoking-related diseases are more prevalent among African Americans than whites, and among African American women, in particular (Klonoff et al., 1995). One in five college-age African American males are current cigarette smokers, more than twice the number of female African Americans. For African American men, lung cancer is the leading cause of cancer deaths. Over twice as many African American males than females die from lung cancer. African American women smoke more than nonminority women, and this difference is partially responsible for mortality rates for lung cancer that are twice as high for African American women (National Cancer Institute, 1988).

Hispanic Americans

The 1985 National Health Interview Survey (Centers for Disease Control, 1987a) reported that 31 percent of Hispanic men and 32 percent of non-Hispanic whites smoke cigarettes. The corresponding figures for women were 21 percent among Hispanics and 28 percent for non-Hispanic whites. Further studies by Marin and his colleagues (1995) also reported differences in the number of cigarettes smoked per day. Non-Hispanic whites reported smoking more cigarettes (mean = 21.5) per day than Hispanics (mean = 12.0).

Latina females are much less likely than African Americans or Anglos to smoke and much less likely to use drugs (Marin et al., 1989). Latinas drink much less than Anglo and African American women. Indeed Latinas are the group most likely to be abstainers (Gilbert, 1987).

Asian and Pacific Islanders

Cigarette use among Asian immigrant or refugee groups is higher than in other ethnic groups in the United States. Among California immigrants, smoking rates among men are 72 percent to 92 percent for Latinos, 71 percent for Cambodians, and 65 percent for Vietnamese (U.S. Department of Health and Human Services, 1990), compared with 30 percent for the overall white American male population. Table 7.3 reports cigarette use from the data taken from 1991 National Household Survey on Drug Abuse, organized by race and age.

The results of the survey still reflect greater cigarette use by males when compared to females, and white Americans smoke more than minority Americans.

The 1995 National Household Survey summary was prepared by Joseph Gfroerer of the Substance Abuse and Mental Health Services Administration, Office of Applied Studies (SAMHS/OAS). The National Household Survey reported that:

> Among adults, men had somewhat higher rates of smoking than women, but rates of smoking were similar for males and females aged 12–17;
>
> Approximately 4.5 million youths aged 12–17 were current smokers in 1995. This rate is about 20 percent of all youths in this age category. The rate was 18.9 percent in 1994;
>
> Youths aged 12–17 who smoked were about eight times as likely to use illicit drugs and eleven times as likely to drink heavily as nonsmoking youths
>
> The level of educational attainment was correlated with tobacco use. Thirty-seven percent of adults who had not completed high school smoked cigarettes, while only 17 percent of college graduates smoked.

TABLE 7.3 Cigarette Use by Race, Sex, and Age. Estimates Are Shown for 1991

	Total	Hispanic	White	Black
Percent rate estimates				
Ever used				
Age				
12–17	37.9	31.9	41.7	25.6
18–25	71.2	58.0	76.5	57.0
26–34	76.4	69.2	78.4	74.0
35+	78.0	66.3	80.0	75.6
Sex				
Male	77.3	70.7	79.7	70.2
Female	72.7	60.6	75.8	65.4
Used in past year				
Age				
12–17	20.1	16.7	23.2	9.6
18–25	41.2	33.0	45.3	28.9
26–34	38.0	34.6	38.3	40.8
35+	30.0	31.1	29.2	35.7
Sex				
Male	34.7	35.8	34.3	36.3
Female	39.7	24.8	30.7	28.5
Used in past month				
Age				
12–17	10.8	8.7	12.7	4.3
18–25	32.2	24.7	35.7	22.0
26–34	32.9	28.6	33.2	36.8
35+	26.6	27.7	25.8	32.6
Sex				
Male	28.7	29.7	28.1	31.5
Female	25.5	19.7	26.5	24.8

Source: Adapted from *National Household Survey on Drug Abuse: Population Estimates, 1991.* U.S. Department of Health and Human Services; Alcohol, Drug Abuse, Mental Health Administration; pp. 91–93. National Institute of Drug Abuse, 1991 National Household Survey on Drug Abuse.

Teen Smoking on the Rise

A Washington (AP) newspaper article titled "Teen smoking on the rise" summarized a Centers for Disease Control and Prevention study on the current teenage tobacco (includes cigarettes, cigars, and chewing tobacco) trends by race and gender in 1997. Among the findings by the Centers for Disease Control and Prevention reported in the article were that:

48.2 percent of all teenage boys and 36.0 percent of all girls smoke either cigarettes, cigars, or tobacco,

Cigarette smoking jumped from 34.8 percent of high school students in 1995 to 36.4 percent in 1997,

Smoking has doubled among black teen males since 1991—27.2 percent of them smoked in 1997. Smoking increased by 54 percent among black females, to 17.4 percent in 1997,

Smoking increased from 25 percent in 1991 to nearly 35 percent in 1997 among Hispanic teenagers. Smoking among Hispanic females rose from 23.5 percent in 1991 to 32 percent in 1997, and

The smoking rate among whites rose from 31 percent in 1991 to 40 percent in 1997. The percent of white female and male smokers is nearly equal.

These findings indicate that black and Hispanic teens are taking up smoking at a faster rate than whites. Smoking by black students—once hailed as a success story for their continually low cigarette use—has almost doubled. This trend is a potentially tragic reversal for the health of U.S. minorities.

Smoking and Women

More than 22 percent of all American adult women smoke cigarettes, compared to 28 percent for men. The American Lung Association projects that the gap between the men and women smokers will close by the year 2000. The lung cancer incidence rate in women continues to increase and reached a high of 41 per 100,000 in 1990. Since 1987, lung cancer has surpassed breast cancer as the leading cause of cancer deaths among women in the United States. Smoking causes an estimated 87 percent of all lung cancers in the United States and continues to be the leading cause of cancer deaths in the United States, with over 153,000 victims a year (American Cancer Society, 1995).

Unfortunately, for lung cancer victims cures are rare. Eighty-seven percent of all people who develop lung cancer will be dead within five years of diagnosis. Twenty-five percent of those diagnosed with lung cancer will die within the first year. Current female smokers aged 35 or older are 12 times more likely to die prematurely from lung cancer than nonsmoking females.

In general, male and female smokers tend to report more chronic health conditions such as emphysema and chronic bronchitis. The American Lung Association (1996) reported that female smokers aged 35 or older are 10.5 times more likely to die from emphysema or chronic bronchitis than nonsmoking females.

Smoking men and women also have more problems with their reproductive systems. Men have a higher risk of developing erectile dysfunction. Nicotine narrows and blocks the flow of blood to the reproductive area and eventually damages the penile artery, leading to impotence or the inability to have erections or sustained erections. Women who smoke more than a pack a day increase their chances of having an ectopic pregnancy (Coste et al., 1991).

Smoking and Pregnancy

Babies born to women who smoke during pregnancy weigh an average of 200 grams less than babies born to comparable nonsmoking women. The smaller size is directly correlated to the amount a woman smokes during the pregnancy. Cigarette smoking also causes a variety of other serious health problems to an unborn child. Cigarette smoking prevents as much as 25 percent of oxygen from reaching the placenta. The risks of preterm deliveries and infant deaths all increase directly with increasing levels of maternal smoking during pregnancy. Smoking accounts for up to 14 percent of preterm deliveries and about 10 percent of all infant deaths.

In addition, an infant's risk of developing sudden infant death syndrome (SIDS) is increased by maternal smoking. Haglund and Cnattingius (1990) reported that the more the mother smokes while pregnant, the greater the likelihood the infant will experience a stoppage of breathing during sleep.

Other Significant Facts about Smoking

Smoking tends to reduce bone density and promotes osteoporosis;

There is an increased risk of heart attack, stroke, and other circulatory diseases among women who smoke and also use oral contraceptives;

The combination of alcohol consumption and cigarette smoking increases the risk of cancer of the upper digestive tract;

CHICK: *"They say each cig-*
arette is just a little stick of
cancer. A little death stick.

MEG: *"That's what I like*
about it, Chick—taking a drag
off a death. Mmm! Gives me a
sense of controlling my own
destiny. What power! What
exhilaration! Want a drag?"
        —Act. 1: *Crimes of the Heart*

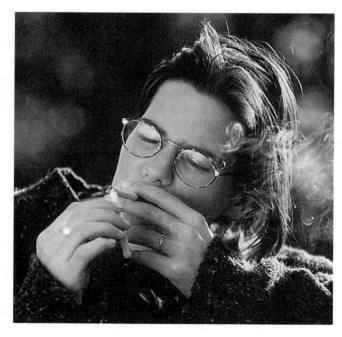

Photo by Will Hart.

Infants are more likely to develop colds, bronchitis, and other respiratory diseases if secondhand smoke is present in the home;

Women join smoking cessation groups more often than men, but are less successful than men in quitting smoking;

Kadunce and colleagues (1991) reported that cigarette smoking has been identified as an independent risk factor that causes skin wrinkling that could make smokers appear less attractive and prematurely old.

Smokeless Tobacco Use

Smokeless tobacco products include chewing tobacco and snuff. Chewing tobacco can be looseleaf, pressed into bricks or cakes (plugs), or twisted into ropelike strands. Snuff is made from powdered or finely cut tobacco leaves. Smokeless tobacco contains carcinogens, nicotine, and abrasives to the teeth and gums. Smokeless tobacco can cause halitosis, stained teeth, gingivitis (inflammation of the gums), ulcerations of the gums, leukoplakia (a precancerous condition), and cancer of the mouth, tongue, and palate. In addition, because of its nicotine content, smokeless tobacco has all the effects on the cardiovascular system attributed to nicotine.

Recently, the National Institute on Drug Abuse estimated that as many as 22 million Americans have used smokeless tobacco. Most users are male, but unfortunately, in some Native American tribes, smokeless tobacco use rates among adolescent females approach 45 percent. Table 7.4 reports the use of smokeless tobacco by race and age.

One out of every four males has used smokeless tobacco—eight times the number of females. More than one out of five college aged males uses smokeless tobacco (11 times the number of females). The 1995 National Household Survey on Drug Abuse found that an estimated 6.9 million Americans (3.3 percent of the population) were current users of

---

BOX **7.2**

Signs of Trouble from Smokeless Tobacco

- Lumps in the jaw or neck area
- Color changes or lumps inside the lips
- White, smooth, or scaly patches in the mouth, neck, lips, or tongue
- A red spot or sore on the lips or gums or inside the mouth that does not heal in two weeks
- Repeated bleeding in the mouth
- Difficulty or abnormality in speaking or swallowing

If you use smokeless tobacco, you are at risk for serious health problems. If you have any of the above symptoms, see your dentist or physician immediately.

Source: Payne, W. and Hahn, D. (1995). *Understanding your health.* St. Louis: Mosby, p. 232.

TABLE 7.4   Smokeless Tobacco Use by Race and Age. Estimates Are Shown for 1991.

	Total	Hispanic	White	Black
Percentage rate estimates				
Ever used				
Age				
12–17	11.8	4.2	14.9	4.0
18–25	21.8	9.2	26.4	7.6
26–34	16.4	8.9	19.2	7.5
35+	11.7	4.7	12.4	12.8
Used in past year				
12–17	6.1	2.0	7.9	1.2
18–25	8.7	2.7	11.0	2.0
26–34	5.0	2.0	5.9	2.3
35+	3.4	0.6	3.7	2.9
Used in past month				
12–17	3.0	1.1	3.8	0.8
18–25	5.8	1.7	7.5	1.2
26–34	3.5	0.8	4.3	1.5
35+	2.8	0.4	3.0	2.8

Source: Adapted from *National Household Survey on Drug Abuse: Population Estimates, 1991.* U.S. Department of Health and Human Services; Alcohol, Drug Abuse, Mental Health Administration; National Institute of Drug Abuse, 1991 National Household Survey on Drug Abuse.

smokeless tobacco. In addition, the rate of smokeless tobacco use continued to be significantly higher for men than for women in 1995 (6.2 percent versus 0.6 percent). Over 90 percent of smokeless tobacco users were men.

In 1995, the National Household Survey reported that smokeless tobacco use was more prevalent among whites (3.9 percent) than among blacks (1.3 percent) or Hispanics (1.2 percent).

Alcohol

Alcohol, a depressant drug, is one of the most widely used and abused drugs in the United States and throughout the world. Abusive alcohol consumption is related to a variety of health problems, such as destruction of brain cells, cirrhosis of the liver, cardiomyopathy, ulceration of the stomach lining, menstrual irregularities, and sexual impotency. However, the leading alcohol-related cause of death is injury due to drunk driving. Young drinkers are at highest risk of dying in an alcohol-related driving accident, while drinkers over 60 years face a higher risk of premature death from cirrhosis of the liver, hepatitis, and other alcohol-linked illnesses.

A misconception held by many people is that some alcoholic beverages are less dangerous than others (e.g., a belief that beer is safer than a mixed drink). This is not true. There is only one type of alcohol, ethyl alcohol, and it is found in all alcoholic drinks. However, different drinks contain different amounts of alcohol. One alcohol drink can be any one of the following:

- A 12-ounce container of beer, which contains 5 percent alcohol;
- A 4-ounce glass of wine, which contains 12 percent alcohol;
- A 2-1/2-ounce glass of fortified wine, which contains 20 percent alcohol;
- A one-ounce shot of distilled spirits in a mixed drink, which contains 50 percent alcohol.

All of the above drinks contain about the same amount of alcohol. Another danger of alcohol is mixing it with other drugs (either legal or illegal). Combining alcohol and other drugs produces a synergistic effect in which the effects increase dramatically. Synergism means that one plus one is no longer equal to two, but one plus one may be equal to five or ten. Because the effects of synergism are so great, combining alcohol with other drugs is the number one cause of drug-related death in the United States.

Alcohol can cause both psychological and physical dependency (addiction). Not all people who abuse alcohol become addicted, but those who do must have it daily to prevent symptoms of withdrawal. Symptoms of withdrawal include hyperarousal (e.g., the "shakes," insomnia, and irritability), hallucinations, convulsive seizures (loss of consciousness and severe muscle contractions), and delirium tremens or the DTs (a combination of hallucinations and shaking).

About 10 percent of people who drink alcohol will become alcoholics (National Institute on Alcohol Abuse and Alcoholism, 1987). Alcoholism is a disease in which the drinker loses control of his or her ability to drink alcohol in moderation. The cause of alcoholism is multifaceted and is a combination of genetic, psychological, and cultural factors. Genetic factors and psychological factors have been well established, but research is beginning to recognize the importance of cultural or social factors. Customs, attitudes, religious influences, and laws all influence drinking behaviors. For example, religious groups, such as Mormons, Muslims, and Seventh-Day Adventists, have a low rate of alcohol abuse within the group, whereas societies or social groups that promote drunkenness have a higher incidence of problem drinking and alcoholism.

Some Effects of Alcohol

Alcohol depresses an area of the brain that normally would inhibit certain behavior, resulting in the illusion of stimulation, impairment in judgment and thinking, and a loosening of social inhibitions.

When alcohol intake is increased, inhibitions may disappear and feelings of aggression or depression may be evident.

Concentration decreases, speech is slurred, and driving is extremely hazardous.

Excessive amounts of alcohol can severely depress the respiratory centers in the medulla, resulting in death by respiratory depression.

Alcohol irritates the stomach lining, which can result in vomiting.

Alcohol dilates the peripheral blood vessels, leading to a feeling of warmth and redness of the skin. This process leads to heat loss in the body.

Alcohol reduces REM (rapid eye movement) sleep, resulting in poor sleep.

Heavy consumption of alcohol can lead to some of the following hangover symptoms: headache, nausea, fatigue, thirst, the feeling of a furry tongue.

Alcohol has a synergistic effect when it interacts with other drugs, in particular with other depressant drugs (i.e., barbiturates and tranquilizers). This increased effect has contributed to many accidental overdose deaths.

Alcohol is high in calories but provides no nutritional value. Alcoholics often suffer from malnutrition.

If alcohol abuse continues, the body suffers great damage. The brain, liver, kidneys, pancreas, heart, and stomach will all be victimized. This further complicates health problems and can shorten the drinker's lifespan.

Alcohol is a major factor in problems of child abuse, broken marriages, and employment difficulties.

Pregnant women who consume alcohol can cause fetal alcohol syndrome in their newborns. It is discussed later in this chapter.

Alcohol and Multicultural Populations

Some results from the 1991 and 1995 National Household Surveys on drug abuse are discussed below. Although the data presented cannot be compared, the results do reflect the prevalence of alcohol use in the United States. The following table (7.5) reports the use of alcohol by race and age. The data were taken from the 1991 *National Household Survey on Drug Abuse.*

white Americans have the highest overall rate of alcohol use. Rates for Hispanics and African Americans were slightly lower. The survey also reported that 58.1 percent of men were had used in the past month, compared to 44.3 percent of women.

The following 1995 National Household Survey summary was prepared by Joseph Gfroerer of the Substance Abuse and Mental Health Services Administration, Office of Applied Studies (SAMHS/OAS). The 1995 *National Household Survey* defined the following three levels of alcohol use.

Current: At least one drink in the past month (includes bingeing and heavy use)

Binge use: Five or more drinks on the same occasion at least once in the past month (includes heavy use)

Heavy use: Five or more drinks on the same occasion on at least five different days in the past month.

TABLE 7.5   **Alcohol Use by Race and Age. Estimates Are Shown for 1991**

	Total	Hispanic	White	Black
Percent rate estimates				
Ever used				
Age				
12–17	46.4	45.9	48.2	40.3
18–25	90.2	82.2	93.2	82.5
26–34	92.4	85.7	94.4	88.6
35+	87.5	81.0	88.9	84.4
Sex				
Male	89.0	86.0	90.6	84.2
Female	80.7	68.9	83.3	74.7
Used in past year				
Age				
12–17	40.3	40.2	41.9	35.2
18–25	82.2	72.3	86.8	72.8
26–34	80.9	74.4	83.7	72.7
35+	65.1	64.4	66.4	56.6
Sex				
Male	72.7	75.0	73.6	66.1
Female	63.9	54.9	66.8	54.5
Used in past month				
Age				
12–17	20.3	22.5	20.4	20.1
18–25	63.6	52.8	67.2	56.0
26–34	61.7	57.2	63.8	57.1
35+	49.5	47.8	50.9	40.3
Sex				
Male	58.1	60.2	59.2	52.2
Female	44.3	34.9	46.6	36.5

Source: Adapted from *National Household Survey on Drug Abuse: Population Estimates, 1991.* U.S. Department of Health and Human Services; Alcohol, Drug Abuse, Mental Health Administration, pp. 85–87. National Instate of Drug Abuse, 1991 National Household Survey on Drug Abuse.

The 1995 *National Household Survey on Drug Abuse* reported that:

Approximately 111 million persons aged 12 and over were current alcohol users. About 32 million persons (15.8 percent) engaged in binge drinking, and about 11 million Americans (5.5 percent of the population) were heavy drinkers.

About 10 million of those drinkers were under the age of 21. Of these, 4.4 million were binge drinkers, including 1.7 million heavy drinkers.

The level of alcohol use continues to be strongly associated with illicit drug use in 1995. Of the 11.3 million heavy drinkers, 25 percent (2.8 million people) were current illicit drug users. Among binge (but not heavy) drinkers, 18 percent (3.8 million) were illicit drug users.

Education also plays an important role in patterns of alcohol use and abuse. The 1995 *National Household Survey* found that 68 percent of adults with college degrees were current drinkers, compared with only 42 percent of those having less than a high school education. However, the rate of heavy alcohol use was 3.7 percent among adults who had completed college and 7.1 percent among adults who had not completed high school. Binge drinking use rates were similar across all levels of education.

white Americans continue to have the highest rates of alcohol use at 56 percent. Rates for Hispanics were 54 percent and African Americans were at 41 percent. The rate of binge use was lower among blacks (11.2 percent) than among whites (16.6 percent) and Hispanics (17.2 percent). Heavy use showed no statistically significant differences by race/ethnicity (5.7 percent for whites, 6.3 percent for Hispanics, and 4.6 percent for blacks).

The survey also reported that 60 percent of men had used alcohol in the past month, compared to 45 percent of women, and that men were much more likely to be heavy binge drinkers (23.8 percent and 8.5 percent, respectively) and heavy drinkers (9.4 and 2.0 percent, respectively).

African Americans and Alcohol.   Herd (1988) reported that African American youth use alcohol less often than youth from other ethnic groups. However, Herd also reported that African American adult males consume more alcohol than white males on a per capita basis. Schinke et al. (1986) found that those African Americans who do drink, compared to white Americans and Hispanics, show higher polydrug use, such as alcohol and heroin, alcohol and PCP, and cocaine and heroin.

Another consistent finding is that alcohol-related problems were higher among African American men even though they did not have significantly higher rates of heavy drinking or drunkenness than white Americans (Herd, 1994). Malin et al. (1982) found that, for all ages, cirrhosis mortality rates among African Americans were nearly twice those for white Americans. They also found that the rate for those in the 25–34 years of age group was found to be as much as 10 times higher for African Americans than for white Americans.

Barnes and Welte (1986) report that African American youth have a lower rate of alcohol use and overall drug use (Skager, 1986; Hartford, 1985) than white youth. The proportion of abstainers is higher among African Americans than whites, mainly because of the high proportion of abstainers among African American women. Lillie-Blanton et al. (1991) reported that white women with 12 years of education or more were heavier drinkers than black women with similar educational backgrounds.

The homicide rate is much higher for African Americans compared to white Americans. In 1991, over 10,000 African Americans were victims of homicide (U.S. Bureau of the Census, 1994). If 50 percent of the homicides are attributable to alcohol, more than 5,000 African Americans lost their lives due to alcohol abuse.

Obot (1996) found that African American problem drinkers were more likely to have been diagnosed as having arthritis, ulcers, cancer, hypertension, liver problems, kidney problems, and "nervous condition" when compared to those without a drinking problem, and that there were significant problems of alcohol abusers with people, police, love, and health, as well as with being victims of crime.

Harper (1981) suggested that one of the major barriers to the treatment of alcoholism for African American males is that heavy drinking is considered the norm and is positively associated with manhood and camaraderie. Harper (1979) has suggested that African American men generally do not draw a clear distinction between alcohol use and abuse.

Asian Americans and Alcohol.   Asian Americans consume less alcohol and have fewer cases of alcoholism than White, Hispanic, African, and Native Americans. Comberg (1982) reported that this may be due to the genetic–racial differences in alcohol sensitivity and aversion and Asian American attitudes and values toward the use of alcohol. Within Asian American groups, only native Hawaiians drink alcohol at levels similar to those of white Americans (Murakami, 1989). Outside of Hawaii, there is considerable variation in drinking patterns among different Asian groups, although it is generally believed that Japanese Americans drink the most, followed by Korean Americans, and Chinese Americans (Chi, et al., 1989). When comparisons are made within various Asian and Pacific American cultures, a relatively high proportion of heavy drinkers exists among Japanese American and Filipino American males. Foreign-born Korean Americans and Japanese Americans drink quite heavily in business entertainment and after-work hours in drinking establishments such as bars and nightclubs. By contrast, Chinese American men and women tend to have significantly lower incidence of alcohol use and abuse.

About 50 percent of all people of Asian descent have a genetically imposed lower level of acetaldehyde dehydrogenase in the liver. Acetaldehyde is a by-product created when alcohol is broken down in the metabolic process. Acetaldehyde dehydrogenase is an enzyme that breaks down the acetaldehyde into acetic acid. As a result of lacking acetaldehyde dehydrogenase, acetaldehyde builds up, causing nausea, itching, facial flushing, and cardiac acceleration (Nakawatase and Sasao, 1993). This response is referred to as the "flushing reflex." This condition, of course, can make alcohol consumption very unpleasant but is not necessarily a genetic trait that leads to alcoholism. The results of research (see Table 7.6) comparing Asians and whites support the hypothesis of racial differences in toxic responses to alcohol.

Native Americans and Alcohol.   Alcoholism and alcohol abuse remain the number one health problem facing Indian people, although patterns vary from tribe to tribe and region to region. *The Report of the Secretary's Task Force on Black and Minority Health* (U.S. DHHS, 1981) found that five of the top 10 leading killers of American Indian people were directly related to alcoholism and alcohol abuse. Table 7.7 presents the alcoholism deaths and mortality rates for American Indians and Alaskan Natives from 1986–88.

The rate of Native Americans' deaths due to alcohol is extremely high in comparison to all other races in the United States. The ratio of deaths between Native Americans and

TABLE 7.6   Frequency of ALDH Isozyme I-Deficiency in Different Populations

Population	No.	ALDH-Deficiency in % of Population Sample
Europeans	224	0
Egyptians, Sudanese	160	0
Liberians	169	0
Chinese	196	35
Japanese	79	48
Indonesians, Koreans	35	40
Vietnamese	82	57
Thais (Northern Thailand)	110	8
Highland Indians (Equador)	33	39

Source: H. Werner Goedde et. al., The role of alcohol dehydrogenase and aldehyde dehydrogenase iso-enzymes in alcohol metabolism, alcohol sensitivity, and alcoholism. Isozymes: Current Topics in Biological and Medical Research, Liss, New York 8: 175–193 (1983). In T. Watts and R. Wright. Alcoholism in Minority Populations. Springfield, IL: Charles C. Thomas Publisher, 1989, P. 146.

all other U.S. races is 5.4, an increase over the two previous years. Table 7.8 reports the alcoholism mortality rates for Native Americans by age and sex.

The National Technical Information Service (1986) reported a high rate of deaths among Native American youths due to causes related to substance abuse, particularly alcohol. Weibel (1984) reported that American Indian youth also have been found to begin abusing various substances at a younger age compared to white Americans.

Indian deaths from alcohol occur at younger ages, usually violently, and are related to risk-taking behaviors. In fact, of all Indian deaths annually, over 35 percent happen to people

TABLE 7.7   Alcoholism Deaths and Mortality Rates for American Indians and Alaskan Natives, 1986–1988

Year	Indian and Alaskan Natives		U.S. All Races	
	Number	Rate	Number	Rate
1988	389	33.9	16,882	6.3
1987	288	25.9	15,513	6.0
1986	272	24.6	15,525	6.4

Age adjusted rates are shown, per 100,000 population, for American Indians, Alaskan Natives, and all U.S. all races.

Source: Adapted from *Trends in Indian Health, 1991,* U.S. Department of Health and Human Services, Public Health Service, Indian health Service, p. 49. Note: All deaths include deaths due to alcohol dependence syndrome, alcoholic psychosis, and chronic liver disease and cirrhosis, specified as alcoholic.

under the age of 44, compared with 11 percent for all U.S. races. The two leading causes of death for Indians between ages 15 and 44 are accidents and cirrhosis of the liver (U.S. Indian Health Services, 1993). Among Indian people, alcohol has also been found to be a contributor to 90 percent of all homicides and 80 percent of suicides (Gunther et al., 1985).

Earlier biomedical theories of Indian alcoholism that suggested a genetic predisposition and the inability to metabolize alcohol at a normal rate are no longer accepted (Rex et al., 1985; Schuckit, 1980; Bennion & Li, 1976; Farris and Jones, 1978). At present, there is no reason to believe that American Indians are different from other groups as far as the physiology of alcohol metabolism is concerned.

Ethnic Differences in Alcohol Consumption. A genetic trait or metabolism predisposing someone to alcohol abuse belongs to individuals and not races or ethnic backgrounds. A few random facts about alcohol consumption by different minority groups are listed below.

Overall, African and white American men have similar drinking patterns, although African American men have higher abstention rates than do white American males.

Hispanic American males generally tend to drink heavily and to have a disproportionate number of alcohol-related problems, including alcohol dependence, compared to African and white American males.

African American women have higher rates of medical and other alcohol-related problems than white American women.

Hispanic American females are at considerably lower risk for developing alcohol-related problems than are white American females.

TABLE 7.8   Alcoholism Mortality Rates for American Indians and Alaskan Natives, by Age and Sex

	Indian and Alaska Native			U.S. All Races			U.S. Other Than White		
Age Group	Both Sexes	Male	Female	Both Sexes	M	F	Both Sexes	M	F
15–24 years	1.0	0.8	1.2	0.1	0.1	0.1	0.3	0.2	0.4
25–34 years	19.3	21.8	16.8	2.3	1.4	1.4	5.7	7.9	3.7
35–44 years	50.1	65.5	35.1	8.5	12.9	4.2	22.1	34.2	11.9
45–54 years	76.5	96.8	57.3	15.8	24.4	7.6	32.6	53.1	15.4
55–64 years	72.0	95.4	50.2	20.5	33.1	9.4	33.0	55.4	14.7
65–74 years	47.3	79.5	20.1	16.0	27.0	7.3	19.8	34.8	8.4
75–84 years	36.0	58.1	18.7	8.9	17.5	3.8	12.1	24.8	4.08
85 years +	10.6	13.3	8.9	3.2	7.3	1.6	5.1	10.8	2.3

Rate per 100,000 population for American Indians, Alaskan Natives, all races, 1955–1988.

Source: Trends in Indian Health, 1991, U.S. Department of Health and Human Services, Public Health Service, Indian Health Service, p. 50.

Native American women drink much less than Native American men do.

Three times as many African American males as females use alcohol once a week or more.

The death rate for African American men is more than one and a half times that of white American men and almost two and a half times that of African American women.

The U.S. Department of Health and Human Services (1991) reported in the National Household Survey on Drug Abuse: 1990 that Hispanic American adolescents have a higher percentage of abstainers than the general student population.

Menon et al. (1990) showed that problems in school performance, school conduct, peer associations, and attitudes of the peer group were significantly related to adolescent Mexican American inhalant use. Students with better grades were also less likely to use inhalants regularly.

McRoy et al. (1985) reported that greater use of alcohol and other drugs by Mexican American youth is associated with lower grades, increased school dropout rates, and high unemployment in adulthood.

Latina females drink much less than Anglo and black women. Indeed, Latinas are the group most likely to be abstainers (Gilbert, 1987).

Latinas are much less likely than blacks or Anglos to smoke (Marin et al., 1989), and much less likely to use drugs.

Fetal Alcohol Syndrome and Fetal Alcohol Effects.   Alcohol is widely recognized as a powerful teratogen, a drug capable of interfering with the development of an embryo and fetus and responsible for one or more birth defects. Fetal alcohol syndrome (FAS) occurs in 1.9 per 1,000 live births (Abel & Sokol, 1986) and as high as 29 per 1,000 live births in alcoholic women (Rosett & Weiner, 1985). In general numbers, this means that nearly 5,000 infants—one in every 750—are born with FAS every year. The main features associated with fetal alcohol syndrome are grouped into three major categories: growth deficiencies before and after birth, abnormal features of the face and head, and central nervous system disorders.

Growth Deficiencies before and after Birth.   Infants are smaller in weight, length, and head circumference and FAS children do not "catch up" in growth, but remain small for their age and are likely to show continued mental retardation. Such children are often only about 65 percent of normal birth length and 38 percent of normal birth weight (Day, 1992). Pregnant women who consume between one and two drinks per day are twice as likely as nondrinking mothers to bear a growth retarded infant weighing under 2,500 grams, about 5.5 pounds. (Mills et al., 1984). Little and colleagues (1986) have also indicated that even modest levels of alcohol consumption (about one drink per week), just prior to realizing one is pregnant, is also associated with decreased birth weight.

Abnormal Features of the Face and Head.   The most frequently observed characteristics are shortness of the palpebral fissures (the slits between the opposed lids of the closed eyes), a short, upturned nose with an underdeveloped ridge between the nose and the upper lip, a sunken basal bridge, folds on the inner aspect of the eyelids, a thin upper lip, an underdeveloped midface, and growth retardation of the jaw (Day, 1992).

Central Nervous System Disorders.   Mental retardation is particularly prevalent. FAS children will have difficulty with learning, attention, memory, and problem-solving, along with lack of coordination, impulsive behavior, and speech and hearing disorders (Day, 1992). Most significantly, fetal alcohol syndrome is the leading cause of mental retardation in the United States (Abel and Sobol, 1986), surpassing Down syndrome and spina bifida.

Alcohol exposure can also have a direct effect on a pregnancy, causing high rates of morbidity and mortality for the mother and the baby. The risk of spontaneous abortions or miscarriages increases by a ratio of 3.53 for heavy drinkers (three or more drinks a day) compared to nondrinking women (Hill & Kleinberg, 1984). Rosett and Weiner (1985) reported that consumers of an average of two or more drinks per day have been found to triple the likelihood of a premature delivery compared to nondrinking mothers.

Fetal alcohol effects (FAE) is less severe than FAS and represents a milder expression of complications due to prenatal alcohol exposure. Rossett and Weiner (1985) reported that there are approximately 36,000 cases of FAE each year in the United States, and that FAE often includes some degree of growth retardation, but also manifests itself in overt behavioral problems in the child. Streissguth and colleagues (1985) also found that FAS children often have deficits in attention and short-term memory. FAE is undoubtedly more common than FAE and less easily identified.

Prevention of FAS and FAE.   Until the exact amount of alcohol that might be safe to drink during pregnancy is known, most medical authorities recommend complete abstinence from alcohol during pregnancy and breast-feeding.

The FAS risk for African American women is nearly seven times higher than for white American women. Although African American women drink less than white American women, the overall estimated rates of substance use during pregnancy are higher for them (National Institute on Drug Abuse, 1994). Caetano (1994) found that African American females consume a higher number of drinks each month and have longer histories of drinking when compared with white women. African American women also have higher rates of medical and other alcohol-related problems than do white women. The drinking consumption and patterns may explain why twice as many African American women report health problems due to drinking than do African American men (Wilsnack & Beckman, 1987).

The FAS statistics for Native American women are even more alarming. In some American Indian communities, the FAS rate is two to five times the general U.S. rate (Streissguth et al., 1991) and, in some southwest plains Native Americans, the prevalence of FAS is extremely high, one case for every 102 births. Flemming and Manson (1990) reported that the two fastest growing rates of alcoholism are among Indian women and adolescents. Flemming and Manson suggest that Indian women abuse alcohol and other drugs because of: (a) cultural disruption, (b) loss of social controls, (c) prejudice, (d) poverty, (e) role reversals, (f) peer group dynamics, (g) familial socialization, and (h) decreased self-worth and alienation.

Gender Differences in Alcohol Consumption

Women may develop cirrhosis of the liver at lower levels of alcohol consumption and after a shorter history of excessive drinking than do men.

All grades of liver damage seem to develop more rapidly in women (Saunders et al., 1981).

Schatzkin et al. (1987) found that consumption of any amount of alcohol conferred an increase in the risk for breast cancer of 40 percent to 50 percent among women who drank less than 5 grams of alcohol per day (equivalent to about three drinks per week). The greatest risk was seen among women who drank 5 grams of alcohol or more per day.

The association between drinking and breast cancer was stronger among younger women than older, leaner rather than heavier, and premenopausal rather than postmenopausal (Schatzkin et al., 1987).

Five times more males than females are heavy drinkers.

Nearly one third of the estimated 15 million alcohol-dependent Americans are women.

Alcohol is involved in nearly one-half of all male accidents, homicides, and suicides.

Only one in every 10 drivers arrested for drunk driving are female.

Three and half times more males than females die from "alcohol-induced causes," which does not include accidents and homicides.

The time period between onset of drinking-related problems and entry into treatment appears to be shorter for women than for men.

Adult females' role deprivation—loss of one's role as wife, mother, or worker—seems to increase a woman's risk for abusing alcohol.

Men's greater use of alcohol and tobacco is the main cause of their higher rates of cancer and heart disease.

When compared to males, females have less body fluid and a lower water content in which to dilute any alcohol consumed. Women, therefore, become more intoxicated than men after drinking the same amount of alcohol.

Women are more susceptible to alcohol's effect because, when compared to men, they have less of the enzyme alcohol dehydrogenase in their stomachs. This enzyme helps break down a portion of the alcohol before it enters the bloodstream.

Drugs and Women of Childbearing Age.

The *National Household Survey* summary was prepared by Joseph Gfroerer of the Substance Abuse and Mental Health Services Administration, Office of Applied Studies (SAMHS/OAS). The *National Household Survey on Drug Abuse* (1995) reported the following facts about women of childbearing age.

Overall, 7.3 percent (4.3 million) of women aged 15–44 in 1995 had used an illicit drug in the past month. The corresponding rate for men aged 15–44 was 11.6 percent.

Of the 4.3 million women aged 15–44 who were current illicit drug users, more than 1.6 million had children living with them. About 400,000 had at least one child under two years of age.

Among women aged 15–44 with no children who were not pregnant, 9.3 percent were illicit drug users. Only 2.3 percent of pregnant women were current drug users, which suggests that most women may reduce their drug use when they become pregnant. However, women who recently gave birth (have a child under two years old, and not pregnant) have a use rate of 5.5 percent, suggesting that many women resume their drug use after giving birth. Similar patterns are seen for alcohol and cigarette use.

Among pregnant women, rates of illicit drug use and cigarette use were highest among women in the first trimester and lowest among women in the third trimester.

Among pregnant women, rates of substance use generally varied as they do among nonpregnant women. Rates were higher among women 15–25 than among those 26–44, and they were higher among unmarried women than among married women. One exception to this pattern was evident in smoking rates by age. Nonpregnant women aged 15–25 and aged 26–44 had about the same rates of smoking. However, among pregnant women, those aged 26–44 had a significantly lower past month

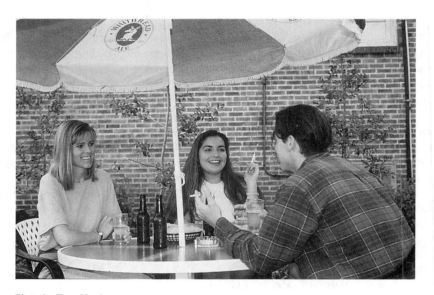

Photo by Tony Nesti.

In our society, we get to know one another over drinks, we associate feasts and celebrations with liquor. We think we have to drink, that it's a social necessity…It's romantic as long as you can handle it—for years I could and did—but it's misery when you become addicted.

—Betty Ford (*The Times of My Life,* 1979)

smoking rate than those aged 15–25, suggesting that older women smokers are more likely to reduce their smoking during pregnancy than are younger women smokers.

Peyotism: An American Indian Religion

Peyote is a small, spineless cactus having psychedelic properties that is used by American Indians for religious purposes. Peyote has a long history of medicinal use in Mexico, and mescaline, the active psychoactive ingredient in peyote, is used medicinally to treat angina pectoris and as a respiratory stimulant for pneumonia patients. The clustered tops of the cactus (called "buttons") are dried before eating and produce euphoria, relaxation, emotional calmness, timelessness, and a shift toward introspection and meditation, which is conducive to the all-night ceremony of the Native American Church.

The Native American Church of North America was organized in the early 1900s for the purpose of bringing together the religious beliefs of several tribes of Indians. At that time, state laws had little jurisdiction on Indian reservations, so peyotism continued to flourish and the Native American Church continued to grow. Even though there was opposition to the religious use of peyote, in 1978 the United States passed the American Indian Religious Freedom Act and allowed the practice of peyotism by American Indians. Peyote for recreational purposes is not legal and Indians must show that possession of peyote is for use in sacramental purposes. Peyote is still classified as a dangerous drug and forbidden under the Drug Abuse Control Act of 1965.

Peyotism is still practiced throughout the western United States with little interference. In 1990, by a vote of six to three, the U.S. Supreme Court ruled that each state may forbid peyote use, even for religious purposes. Because peyotism is not allowed in every state, Indians using peyote, even for religious purposes, in states where it is illegal, can be arrested or lose their jobs for drug use.

Although there are many variations of peyote ceremonies, they generally consist of an all-night meeting in which participants sit inside a tepee or other structure facing a fire in a crescent-shaped altar. The ceremony consists basically of four parts: praying, singing, eating peyote, and quietly contemplating (Anderson, 1996). The prayers, songs, and quiet contemplation, coupled with the effects of peyote, frequently lead to personal revelations. These are often in the form of visions and audible messages directly from Peyote or the Great Spirit. Peyote often "speaks" to the participants and promises them forgiveness of their sins; members are confident that Peyote will overcome both bodily and spiritual ills, for it is the "comfort, healer, and guide for many Indians" (Slotkin, 1956).

Drug Treatment Problems Associated with Race

Treatment is required when an individual's drug use has progressed to compulsive or addictive use. Once addiction has been established, its treatment requires specific interventions in order for successful recovery to occur. Abstaining from alcohol is the ultimate goal for the alcoholic, but there is no cure for alcoholism. Early treatment is a positive predictor for success. The longer the individual is addicted, the greater the physical, social, and emo-

TABLE 7.9   **Alcohol and Drug Abuse Treatment Programs**

	Hispanic	White	Black	Other	Unknown
Alcohol clients (n = 349,771)	9.3	67.4	14.6	3.0	5.7
Drug abuse clients (n = 253,748)	15.1	54.4	23.5	1.7	5.2
Total clients (n = 603,519)	11.8	62.0	18.3	2.5	5.5

Percent distribution of clients in alcohol and drug treatment units is shown in 1987.

Source: Adapted from *Health Status of Minorities and Low-Income Groups:* Third Edition, U.S. Department of Health and Human Services, Public Health Service, Health Resources and Services Administration, Government Printing Office, Washington, DC., p. 278. National Institute on Drug Abuse and National Institute on Alcohol abuse and Alcoholism, National Drug and Alcoholism Treatment Unit Survey, 1987 Final Report. Department of Health and Human Services Pub. No. (ADM) 89–1626.

tional damage, and there is less chance of successful treatment. Table 7.9 reports the percent of people in drug treatment programs by race.

The data report that, of the Americans who are getting treatment for alcohol and drug abuse problems, a large majority of them are white Americans. Two-thirds of all people who are in alcohol treatment centers are white Americans.

Recommendations for Prevention and Treatment of Drug Abuse

What is known is that community leaders, parents, educators, and youth from all over the United States are concerned, even angry, about drug use within and outside of their cultural groups. Opinions vary as to what is the best approach to solving this problem. Most researchers, however, would support the premise that the development of effective drug abuse prevention and intervention strategies for minority Americans has been seriously hampered by the absence of conceptual models about drug abuse and its etiology and functions (Becerra et al., 1982). If culturally appropriate prevention and treatment interventions are to be developed, they need to be culturally sensitive to basic issues in the problem of drug abuse (Becerra et al., 1982).

Given the fact that minority Americans tend to underutilize substance abuse treatment programs, various strategies and solutions need to be implemented to respond to the needs of the different populations. Certain features that may enhance cultural responsiveness have been identified by Murase (1977): (1) delivering services from community-based sites, (2) incorporating community input into service delivery decisions, (3) using bilingual and bicultural staff, (3) linking with indigenous formal and informal community care/support systems, and (4) developing intervention methods that address culturally salient aspects of the different minority American lifestyles and values.

In addition, in order for prevention and intervention programs to be more effective, researchers must continue to explore the many reasons for ethnic minority drug use and answer these two questions: (1) What are the specific cultural and ethnic activities that either enhance or discourage drug use? and (2) How can specific cultural activities be utilized to enhance positive influences on peer groups and their use of drugs? From a cultural perspective, the following two recommendations must also be researched: (1) Each ethnic group must be distinguished from others and studied separately; (2) It is important to research the differences among members of the same ethnic group. Presently, there are no large-scale longitudinal studies focusing on each of the specific cultural groups, studies that tell us something meaningful about each of the cultural groups.

It is also known that a variety of substance abuse prevention or treatment programs have been developed and the chance of success is increased when the right prevention or treatment program is matched to the needs of the client. No one program is right for every client. Therefore, it will require communities to develop consortiums of community-based agencies to develop coordinated programs that: (1) match different programs to the needs of the client: and (2) draw from a number of empirically validated prevention approaches, including individual and family counseling, parenting skills, education, social support systems, and social competence. The successful development of substance abuse programs will require communities to make modifications in order to make such programs effective and culturally responsive to the needs of community members.

REFERENCES

Abel, E., and Sokol, R. Fetal alcohol syndrome is now the leading cause of mental retardation (Letter to the editor). *Lancet* 2 (1986), 1222.

American Cancer Society. *Cancer facts and figures, 1989.* Atlanta, GA: Author, American Cancer Society, 1989.

American Cancer Society. *Cancer facts and figures, 1994.* Atlanta, GA: Author, American Cancer Society, 1995.

American Lung Association. *Lung cancer in diverse communities,* 1996. http://www.lungusa.org/noframes/learn/health/healungdes.html

Anderson, E. *Peyote: The divine cactus.* Tucson, AZ: University of Arizona Press, 1996.

Barnes, G., and Welte, J. Alcohol consumption of Black youth. *Journal of Studies on Alcohol* 47 (1986) 53–61.

Becerra, R., Karno, M., and Escobar, J. *Mental health and Hispanic Americans: Clinical perspectives.* New York: Grune & Stratton, 1982.

Bennion, L., and Li, T. Alcohol metabolism in American Indians and whites. *New England Journal of Medicine* 284 (1976), 9–13.

Caetano, R. Drinking and alcohol-related problems among minority women. *Alcohol, Health, and Research World* 18 (1994) 233–241.

Centers for Disease Control. *Surgeon General's report on smoking.* Washington, DC: Central Office for Health Promotion and Education on Smoking and Health, Government Printing Office, 1989.

Chi, I., Lubben, J. E., and Kitano, H. Differences in drinking behavior among three Asian-American groups. *Journal of Studies on Alcohol* 50 (1989), 15–23.

Comberg, S. Building on the strength of minority groups. *Practice Digest* 5 (1982), 6–7.

Coste, J., Job-Spira, N., and Fernandez, H. Increased risk of ectopic pregnancy with maternal cigarette smoking. *American Journal of Public Health* 81, 2 (February 1991): 199–201.

Day, N. "The effects of prenatal exposure to alcohol," *Alcohol Health and Research World* 16, 3 (1992) 238–44.

Farris, J., and Jones, B. Ethanol metabolism in male American Indians and whites. *Alcoholism: Clinical and Experimental Research* 2, 1 (1978) 77–81.

Flaskerud, J., and Hu, L. Relationship of ethnicity to psychiatric diagnosis. *Journal of Nervous and Mental Disease* 180, 5 (1992), 296–303.

Flemming, C., and Manson, S. Native American women. In R. C. Engs (Ed.), *Women: Alcohol and other drugs.* Dubuque, IA: Kendall Hunt, 1990, pp. 105–117.

Gfroerer, J. *Summary of the National Household Survey on Drug Abuse: Main Findings 1995.* National Clearinghouse for Alcohol and Drug Abuse (NCADI). Rockville, MD: United States Department of Health and Human Services, 1995. Http://www.health.org/pubs/95hhs/any.htm

Gilbert, M. Alcohol consumption patterns in immigrant and later generations. *Hispanic Journal of Behavioral Sciences* 9, 3 (1987)299–314.

Gunther, J. F., Jolly, E. J., Wedel, K. Alcoholism and the Indian people: Problem and promise. In E. M. Greeman (Ed.), *Social work practice with clients who have alcohol problems* (pp. 229–241). Springfield, IL: Charles C Thomas, 1985.

Haglund, B., and Cnattingus, S. Cigarette smoking as a risk factor for Sudden Infant Death Syndrome: A population-based study. *American Journal of Public Health* 80, 1 (January 1990) 29–32.

Harper, F. *Alcoholism treatment and Black Americans.* Rockville, MD: Department of Health, Education and Welfare, National Institute on Alcohol Abuse and Alcoholism, 1979.

Harper, F. Alcohol use and abuse. In L. E. Gary (Ed.), *Black Men.* Beverly Hills, CA: Sage, 1981, pp. 169–178.

Hartford, T. C. Drinking patterns among black and nonblack adolescents: Results of a national survey. In E. M. Greeman (Ed.), *Social work practice with clients who have alcohol problems* (pp. 229–241). Springfield, IL: Charles C. Thomas, 1985.

Herd, D. Drinking by black and white women: Results from a national survey. *Social Problems* 35 (1988) 493–505.

Herd, D. Predicting drinking problems among black and white men: Results from a national survey. *Journal of Studies of Alcohol* 55, 1 (1994) 61–71.

Hildreth, C., and Saunders, E. Heart disease, stroke, and hypertension in Blacks. In R. L. Braithwaite and S. E. Taylor (Eds.), *Health issues in the Black community* (pp. 90–105). San Francisco, CA: Jossey-Bass, 1992.

Hill, L. M., and Kleinberg, F. Effects of drugs and chemicals on the fetus and newborn (2). *Mayo Clinic Proceeding,* 59 (1984) 755–765.

Johnson, B., Williams, T., Dei, K., and Sanabria, H. Drug abuse in the inner city: Impact on hard-drug users and the community. In M. Tonry and J. Q. Wilson (Eds.), *Drugs and crime (Crime and justice: A review of research,* vol. 13). Chicago: University of Chicago Press, 1990, pp. 35–42.

Kadunce, D., Burr, R., Gress, R., Kanner, R., Lyon, J., and Zone, J. Cigarette smoking: Risk factor for premature facial wrinkling. *Annals of Internal Medicine,* 114, 1015 (May 1991) 840–44.

King, L., Beals, J., Manson, S., and Trimble, J. (1992). A structural evaluation model of factors related to substance abuse among American Indian adolescents. In J. Trimble, C. Block, and S. Niemcryk (Eds.), *Ethnic and multicultural drug abuse: Perspectives on current research.* Binghamton, NY: Haworth, 1992, pp. 72–93.

Klonoff, E. A., Landrine, H., and Scott, J. Double jeopardy: Ethnicity and gender in research. In H. Landrine (Ed.), *Bringing cultural diversity to feminist psychology: Theory, research, and practice* (pp. 335–380). Washington, DC: American Psychological Association, 1995.

Lillie-Blanton, M., Mackenzie, E., and Anthony, J. Black-white differences in alcohol use by women: Baltimore survey findings. *Public Health Reports* 106, 2 (1991) 124–133.

Little, R. E., Uhl, C. N., Labbe, R. F., Abkowitz, J. L., and Phillips, E. L. Agreement between laboratory test and self reports of alcohol, tobacco, caffeine, marijuana and other drug use in postpartum women. *Social Science and Medicine* 22 (1986) 91–98.

Malin, H., Coakley, J., Yaelber, C., Munch, N., and Holland, W. An epidemiologic perspective on alcohol use and abuse in the United States. In *Alcohol consumption and related problems: Alcohol and health,* monograph 1 (DHHS Publication No. ADM 82-1190, pp. 99–153). Washington, DC: Government Printing Office, 1982.

Marin, G., Perez-Stable, E. and Marin, B. Cigarette Smoking among San Francisco Hispanics: The role of acculturation and gender. *American Journal of Public Health* 79, 2 (1989) 196–198.

Marin, G., Marin, B., Perez-Stable, E., Sabogal, F., and Otero-Sabogal, R. Cultural differences in attitudes and expectancies between Hispanic and non-Hispanic White Smokers. In A. Padilla (Ed.), *Hispanic psychology: Critical issues in theory and research.* Thousand Oaks, CA: Sage Publications, 1995, pp. 275–298.

McLaughlin, P., Raymond, J., Murakami, S., and Gilbert, D. Drug use among Asian Americans in Hawaii. *Journal of Psychoactive Drugs* 19 (1987) 85–94.

McRoy, R. G., Shorkey, C. T., and Garcia, E. Alcohol use and abuse among Mexican-Americans. In E. M. Greeman (Ed.), *Social work practice with clients who have alcohol problems* (pp. 229–241). Springfield, IL: Charles C. Thomas, 1985.

Menon, R., Burrett, M., and Simpson, D. School, peer, and inhalant use among Mexican-American adolescents. *Hispanic Journal of Behavioral Sciences* 12 (1990) 408–421.

Mills, J. L., Graubard, B. I., Harley, E. E., Rhoads, G. G., and Berendes, H. W. Maternal alcohol consumption and birth weight: How much drinking during pregnancy is safe?" *Journal of the American Medical Association,* 252 (1984) 1875–1879.

Murakami, S. R. An epidemiological survey of alcohol, drug, and mental health problems in Hawaii. In D. Spiegler, D. Tate, S. Aitken, and C. Christian (Eds.), *Alcohol use among U.S. ethnic minorities* (NIAAA Research Monograph No. 18. pp. 343–353). Rockville, MD: National Institute on Alcohol Abuse and Alcoholism, 1989.

Murase, K. Delivery of social services to Asian Americans. In *National Association of Social Workers* (Ed.), *The encyclopedia of social work.* New York: National Association of Social Workers, 1977.

Nakawatase, J., and Sasao, T. The association between fast-flushing response and alcohol use among Japanese Americans. *Journal of Studies on Alcohol,* 54 (1993) 49–53.

National Cancer Institute. *Cancer in Hispanics.* Bethesada, MD: National Institutes of Health, 1988.

National Institute on Drug Abuse, Department of Health and Human Services, Health Status of Minorities and Low-Income Groups; the Drug Abuse Warning Network, Annual Data. Series 1, No. 8, Table 2.11, p. 35, 1988.

National Institute on Drug Abuse. *National household survey on drug abuse: population estimates, 1991* (ADM 92-1887). Rockville, MD: Division of Epidemiology and Prevention Research, National Institute of Drug Abuse, 1991c.

National Technical Information Service. *American Indian health.* Washington, DC: U.S. Department of Health, Education, and Welfare, 1986.

(NIAAA). National Institute on Alcohol Abuse and Alcoholism. *Sixth Special Report to the U.S. Congress on Alcohol and Health from the Secretary of Health and Human Services.* Rockville, MD: National Institute on Alcohol Abuse and Alcoholism. 1987.

Obot, I. Problem drinking, chronic disease, and recent life events. In H. Neighbors and J. Jackson, (Eds.), *Mental health in Black America.* Thousand Oaks, CA: Sage, 1996.

Payne, W., and Hahn, D. *Understanding Your Health.* St. Louis: Mosby, 1995, p. 232.

Reagan, P., and Brookins-Fisher, J. *Community Health in the 21st Century.* Boston, MA: Allyn and Bacon, 1997, pp. 381–382.

Rex, D., Boyron, W., Smialek, J., and Li, T. Alcohol and aldehyde dehydrogenase isoenzmes in North American Indians." *Alcoholism* 9, 2 (March–April 1985) 147–152.

Rosett, H., and Weiner, L. Alcohol and pregnancy: A clinical perspective. *Annual Review of Medicine* 36 (1985) 73–80.

Saunders, J. B., Davis, M., and Williams, R. Do women develop alcoholic liver disease more readily than men? *British Medical Journal* 282 (1981) 1141–1143.

Schatzkin, A., Jones, Y., Hoover, R., Taylor, P., Brinton, L., Ziegler, R., Harvey, E. Carter, C., Licitra, L., Dufour, M., and Larson, D. Alcohol consumption and breast cancer in the epidemiologic follow-up study of the first national health and nutrition examination survey. *New England Journal of Medicine* 316 (1987) 1169–1173.

Schinke, S., Botvin, G., Trimble, J., Orlandi, M., Gilchrist, L., and Locklear. "Preventing substance abuse among American Indian adolescents: A bicultural competence skills approach. *Journal of Counseling Psychology,* 35, 1 (1988) 87–90.

Schuckit, M. *Theory of alcohol and drug abuse: A genetic approach. Theories on drug abuse* (pp. 297–302). Washington, DC: Government Printing Office, 1980.

Secretary's Task Force on Black and Minority Health. (1986). Chemical dependency and diabetes, (vol. 7). Washington, DC: Government Printing Office. In G. J. Botvin, S. Schinke, and M. A. Orlani (Eds.), *Drug abuse prevention with multiethnic youth.* Thousand Oaks, CA: Sage, 1995, pp. 260–275.

Segal, B. Drug-taking behavior among school aged youth: The Alaska experience and comparisons with lower-48 states. *Drugs and Society* 4 (1992) 1–174. In R. Coombs and D. Ziedonis (Eds.), *Handbook on drug abuse prevention.* Boston: Allyn & Bacon, 1995.

Skager, R. *A statewide survey of drug and alcohol use among students.* Sacramento, CA: Office of the Attorney General, 1986.

Slotkin, J. *The peyote religion.* Glencoe, IL: Free Press, 1956.

Streissguth, A., Aase, J., Clarren, S., LaDue, R., Randals, S., and Smith, D. Fetal alcohol syndrome in adolescents and adults. *Journal of the American Medical Association* 265 (1991) 1961–1967.

Teen smoking on the rise, Washington (AP). (1998, April 17), San Louis Obispo Telegram-Tribune, page A-6.

Trimble, J., Padilla, A., and Bell, C. (Eds.). *Drug abuse among ethnic minorities* (DHHS Publication no. ADM 87-1474). Rockville, MD: National Institute on Drug Abuse, 1987.

Tucker, M. U.S. ethnic minorities and drug use: An assessment of the science and practices. *International Journal of Addictions* 20 (1985) 1021–1047.

Cigarette smoking among high school students. *USA Today* (July 15, 1992), p. 1-D.

U.S. Bureau of the Census. *Statistical abstracts of the United States: 1994* (114th ed.). Washington DC: Government Printing Office, 1994.

U.S. Department of Health and Human Services. *National household survey on drug abuse: Main findings 1990,* DHHS publication No. (ADM)91-1788. Rockville, MD: U.S. Department of Health and Human Services, 1991a.

U.S. Department of Health and Human Services. *National household survey on drug abuse: Highlights 1990,* DHHS publication No. (ADM)91-1789. Rockville, MD: U.S. Department of Health and Human Services, 1991b.

U.S. Department of Health and Human Services. *Overview of the National Household Survey on Drug Abuse: NIDA Capsules* NO. C-83-1(a). Rockville, MD: U.S. Department of Health and Human Services, 1991d.

U.S. Department of Health and Human Services. *Healthy people 2000: National health and promotion and disease prevention objectives* (Conference ed.). Washington, DC: Government Printing Office, 1990.

U.S. Department of Health and Human Services. *Report on the secretary's task force on black and minority health.* Washington, DC: Government Printing Office, 1981.

U.S. Department of Health and Human Services. *Drug use among high school students, college students, and other young adults.* Alcohol, Drug Abuse and Mental Health Administration, National Institute on Drug Abuse, 1991c.

U.S. Department of Health and Human Services. *Trends in Indian Health.* Washington, DC, Government Printing Office, 1991 (pp. 31, 49)

Watts, T. and Wright, R. *Alcoholism in minority populations.* Springfield, IL: Charles C. Thomas Publisher, 1989.

Weibel, O. Substance abuse among American Indian youth: A continuing crisis." *Journal of Drug Issues* 14 (1984) 313–335.

Wilsnack, S., and Beckman, L. *Alcohol problems in women.* New York: Guilford, 1987.

8 Cardiovascular Disease (CVD), Cancer, and Other Disorders in Minority Americans

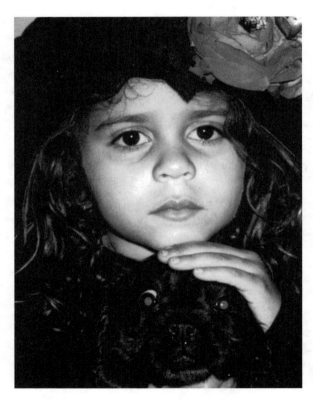

Health is a human right, not a privilege to be purchased.

—Shirley Chisholm, 1970

Photo by Elaine Walters, published in *Cultures* magazine, volume 3, issue 1.

Chronic diseases are the major killers in the United States today. Chronic conditions are those from which the patient does not expect to fully recover and are usually accompanied by some sort of residual disability. Chronic diseases get progressively worse over time and are often terminal. Many chronic diseases are related to lifestyle, habits, and behaviors, and are, therefore, preventable.

This chapter discusses some of the major chronic diseases among minority Americans: cardiovascular disease (atherosclerosis, hypertension, stroke), cancer, and diabetes. In addition, other conditions that affect minority Americans will be discussed: respiratory disorders (chronic obstructive pulmonary disease and asthma), lead poisoning, sickle-cell syndrome, and some genetic disorders.

Cardiovascular Disease

The leading cause of death for both men and women in the United States is cardiovascular disease (CVD). Nearly one million Americans will die each year from diseases of the heart and blood vessels and some 63 million Americans (one in four) suffer from some sort of cardiovascular disease. The good news for white Americans is that the death rate from heart disease has fallen 25 percent over the last decade and stroke fatalities have dropped by 40 percent. The bad news for African Americans is that their fatality rates from both heart disease and stroke continue to be dismal in comparison to White America. The three leading cardiovascular diseases are atherosclerosis or coronary artery disease, high blood pressure, and stroke. The patterns of mortality and morbidity from these diseases generally display strong associations with race, age, and gender.

Coronary artery disease is the most common CVD and a disease of the lining of the arteries (atherosclerosis). It is characterized by the accumulation of deposits of fat, fibrin (clotting materials), cholesterol, cellular debris, calcium, and other substances in the arteries, which narrows the artery channels. When the coronary arteries are narrowed and restricted because of this process, the risk of heart attack increases. When the arteries that supply the brain are narrowed and restricted, the risk of stroke increases.

Because of this process, the arteries begin to lose their ability to expand and contract. It becomes more difficult for the blood to flow freely through the narrowed arteries, making it easier for a blood clot (thrombus) to develop and block the artery. Such a blockage in an artery is called a *coronary thrombosis*. The blocked artery deprives the vital organs of blood. When this process blocks a coronary artery, a heart attack occurs. Atherosclerosis is the underlying cause of most heart attacks and strokes.

The medical name for a heart attack is *myocardial infarction* (MI). The muscle of the heart is called the *myocardium*. If its blood supply from the coronary arteries is blocked off due to the atherosclerosis process, the myocardial cells are deprived of sufficient oxygen and the portion of the myocardium deprived of its blood supply dies.

An alarming fact is that African Americans are far more likely to die of coronary heart disease than all other races. African Americans are also more likely to have heart attacks at an earlier age and more likely to die out of hospital or in emergency rooms than white Americans (Gillum, 1989). In addition, white Americans statistically have more reported cases of myocardial infarctions but African Americans' MI case fatality rate is higher (Roig et al., 1989). Table 8.1 provides the percentages of death by race for both male and females in 1992. The American Heart Association reported the following:

> In 1992, the death rates for cardiovascular disease were 335.6 per 100,000 people (46 percent higher than for white Americans) and 217.1 for African American females (69 percent higher than for white American females) (American Heart Association, 1996).

> One in five women has some form of cardiovascular disease.

> Since 1984 the number of cardiovascular disease deaths for women has exceeded those of men. The difference in deaths currently is over 35,000.

Epidemiologic patterns and trends in coronary heart disease risk factors have been extensively reviewed. The American Heart Association has identified four major risk factors associated with the development of CVD: tobacco use, high blood pressure, high cholesterol levels, and physical inactivity. Other risk factors, such as being overweight and diabetes, are also considered as important in the development of CVD. The higher prevalence of cigarette smoking as well as hypertension are continuing causes of concern, in particular, for African Americans. Further, knowledge about cardiovascular disease risk factors was lower in African Americans than white Americans, even after controlling age and education, in the United States (Ford & Jones, 1991). The four major risk factors associated with the development of CVD are discussed below in relation to the high rate of CVD death in African Americans.

Four Major CVD Risk Factors

Tobacco Use.   The risk of heart attack doubles if a person smokes cigarettes, and the more a person smokes the greater the risk. A smoker who has a heart attack also has less chance of surviving the heart attack than the nonsmoker. How smoking increases the risk of heart attack is not completely understood, but the nicotine may repeatedly overstimulate

TABLE 8.1   CVD, the Leading Cause of Death for African American, Hispanic American, Asian/Pacific Islander Americans, and Native American Males and Females, and the Percentages of Death in 1992

Race	Male/Percent of Deaths	Female/Percent of Deaths
African Am.	32.6%	42.5%
Asian/Pacific Am.	36.2%	39.7%
Hispanic Am.	25.7%	34.0%
Native Am.	27.7%	31.7%

Source: American Heart Association (1996)

the heart, the carbon monoxide in cigarette smoke may displace oxygen, which affects appropriate nourishment of the heart muscle, or the smoke may damage the inner lining (intima) of the coronary arteries, making it easier for atherosclerosis to develop. The latest estimates from the American Heart Association (1996) show that 33.2 percent of African American men and 19.8 percent of African American women are cigarette smokers.

High Blood Pressure (Hypertension).   Hypertension increases the work load of the heart, causing the heart to enlarge in an unhealthy manner and become less efficient over time, increasing the likelihood of stroke, heart attack, kidney failure, and congestive heart failure. Approximately 28 percent of African Americans suffer from hypertension (Saunders, 1985), well above the 15 percent prevalence rates among white Americans (Roberts & Rowland, 1981). (See the section on hypertension latter in this chapter for a more detailed discussion.)

Cholesterol Levels.   Cholesterol is a necessary and important part of the human body. It is an important part of cell membranes, sex hormones, and the protective layer that surrounds and protects nerve cells. Cholesterol is so important for body functioning that the liver manufactures it to insure appropriate amounts. However, we can also increase cholesterol levels in our blood through diet. In some individuals, excess cholesterol will contribute to the atherosclerosis process. Among non-Hispanic African Americans aged 20 and over, 47 percent of men and 51 percent of women had serum cholesterol levels over 200 mg/dl; 16 percent of men and 19 percent of women have 240 mg/dl or more. In 1993, over 500 million adult women had serum cholesterol levels of 200 mg or higher. Fifty-one percent of African American females are in this group (American Heart Association, 1996).

Inactivity.   Individuals who lead sedentary lives run a higher risk of heart attack than do those who exercise regularly. Nearly 68 percent of African American women and 62.8 percent of African American men have a sedentary lifestyle (American Heart Association, 1996).

In the past few years, a number of scientific findings have revealed that men and women have significantly different risk factors for heart disease. The death rate from coronaries is declining faster in men than women, and this may be due in part to a lack of recognition and treatment of these different risk factors. In addition to being tested for cholesterol levels, lipoprotein levels (HDL's and LDL's) and triglycerides, many women are now tested for lipoprotein(a), fibrinogen, homocysteine, and serum magnesium. Deter (1997) stated in a University of Texas-Houston Health Science Center report that high levels of lipoprotein(a), or LP(a)s, are more predictive of coronary disease in women than in men. Higher fibrinogen is more of a risk factor for women than men, and high levels are more prevalent in women. Finally, high levels of homocysteine (a metabolite of the amino acid) cause endothelial cells to decrease their production of clot-preventing and clot-dissolving substances and to increase their production of clot-promoting substances. Deter (1997) also reported that, over the past six years, 38 studies have documented that high homocysteine levels are independent predictors of heart attack, stroke, deep vein thrombosis, and peripheral arterial insufficiency.

Stroke

A *stroke* is the result of a lack of blood to brain cells. It is also known as a cerebrovascular accident (CVA) and occurs when the blood supply to the brain is blocked off. About 500,000 people suffer strokes each year, and stroke is the third leading cause of death in all Americans after heart disease and cancer. Strokes kill more than 150,000 people a year.

Strokes can also occur when a diseased artery bursts in the brain, which floods the surrounding tissue with blood (cerebral hemorrhage). A head injury or the bursting of an aneurysm (a weak spot) in the wall of an artery can cause hemorrhage (bleeding). Brain tissue deprived of oxygen may lead to a variety of effects, from slight to severe or temporary to permanent damage and/or death. Sadly, African Americans suffer disproportionately from stroke when compared to other races.

The 1992 death rates for stroke were 52.0 per 100,000 for African American males (97.7 percent higher than white American males) and 39.9 for African American females (77.3 percent higher than for white American females) (American Heart Association, 1996), Gillum (1988) reported that the prevalence, incidence, and hospitalization rates for stroke were higher in African Americans than white Americans and that the survival rate after acute stroke is poorer in African Americans.

Hypertension

Hypertension is both a risk factor and a disease. It forces the heart to work harder than normal and puts the arteries under greater strain. Over time, it can cause damage to major organs (kidneys, eyes, heart) and blood vessels. Hypertension is the leading cause of kidney failure and hypertension-related end-stage renal disease and is a major contributor to heart disease and stroke (U.S. Department of Health and Human Services, 1985).

Over 60 million people or about 20 percent of the adult population in the United States have hypertension in some form. Those at highest risk for hypertension are males, people over 55 years old, and people of color. Hypertension, or chronically elevated blood pressure, is generally recognized as a major health problem afflicting a large percentage of African Americans. Seven and one-half million African Americans have high blood pressure.

In the United States, the mortality rate for hypertensive heart disease is three times greater for African Americans compared to white Americans (Meyers, 1986; Cruickshank and Beevers, 1982). It is estimated that the rate of mortality from strokes among blacks is approximately 66 percent higher than among whites (Hypertension Detection and Follow-Up Program Cooperative Research Group, 1982). African Americans also develop high blood pressure at an earlier age and, at any age, hypertension is more severe in African Americans than in white Americans.

Equally alarming is the fact that the mortality rate for African Americans between the ages of 34 and 54 years is 6 to 10 times greater than that for whites (Hypertension Detection and Follow-Up Cooperative Research Group, 1982). Over half of African Americans over the age of 50 suffer from hypertension.

This condition can be caused by disorders such as atherosclerosis and kidney disease. However, in more than 85 percent of all causes of hypertension in African Ameri-

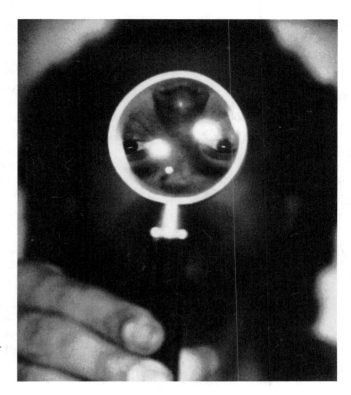

It is better to know the patient that has the disease than the disease that has the patient.
—William Osler

Photo by Evarardo Martinez-Inzunza

cans, the etiology is unknown; such cases are classified as "essential hypertension" (Cruickshank & Beevers, 1982). Studies have also indicated that essential hypertension may have its onset at earlier ages for African Americans than white Americans (Loggie, 1971; Londe & Goldring, 1976).

Even though it has been established that hypertension is more common in African Americans than among white Americans in the United States, little research has examined the proposed multiple factors that may account for the etiology of essential hypertension in African Americans. These include organic factors, high-salt diets, socioenvironmental factors, such as urban living and poverty, and psychological–emotional factors, such as stress and anger.

Cancer Morbidity and Mortality

Cancer accounts for one out of every five deaths in the United States. During the period between 1980–1990, trends in cancer incidence and mortality rates increased, with a more rapid increase for minority Americans than white Americans and a greater increase for men than women. For example, the five-year survival rate (1983–1988) for minority Americans was less than that of white Americans, about 38 percent compared with 54 percent for white Americans (National Cancer Institute, 1992). A major contributing factor related to this difference in survival is the late diagnosis that occurs more frequently in minority Americans.

African Africans (both men and women) have the highest age-adjusted cancer incidence and mortality rates of any population group in the United States, and the disparity in incidence, mortality, and survival point between African Americans and whites is increasing (Baquet et al., 1991). In 1995, African American men had a general cancer rate of 560 cases per 100,000 people and a cancer death rate of 319 per 100,000, the highest for any of the measured groups. Non-Hispanic males are second to African American males in incidence of disease. Cancer struck this group at the rate of 481 cases per 100,000. For cancer deaths, Hawaiian males were second to African American males, with a mortality rate of 230,000 per 100,000 (National Cancer Institute, 1996).

Among women in 1995, white non-Hispanics had the highest rates of all cancers, with 354 cases per 100,000. Alaskan native women were second, at 348 per 100,000. For cancer deaths, Alaskan native women had the highest rate at 179 per 100,000. African American and Hawaiian women were second, both with cancer death rates of 168 per 100,000 (National Cancer Institute, 1996).

The incidence of cervical cancer has dropped for both African American and white women in the past 14 years, but the incidence in African American women is still double that of white women (Avery, 1992). Although fewer African American women than white women get breast cancer, the survival rate is lower: 64 percent versus 76 percent. Avery suggested that early social, environmental, nutritional factors may weaken the immune system, making many African American women more vulnerable. Coates and colleagues (1992) suggested that African American women are more likely to be diagnosed at a later stage and, consequently, run a greater risk of death.

African American women who smoke have a mortality rate for lung cancer that is twice as high as that for white women (National Cancer Institute, 1989).

African Americans generally eat more nitrates and animal foods and lack adequate amounts of fiber, thiamin, riboflavin, vitamins A and C, and iron in their diets (Hargreaves et al., 1989). These poor dietary habits may be associated with African Americans' higher incidence of mortality from certain cancers, compared with whites.

Because certain chemicals and other agents in the environment are carcinogenic—solvents, dyes, heavy metals, pesticides, and herbicides—all of which can be found in the workplace, a new concern has arisen regarding employment of minority groups in less skilled jobs, in which exposures to hazardous substances tend to be greater (Baquet & Gibbs, 1992). Table 8.2 reports the distribution of cancer incidence by site for males in 1995.

The three leading cancers for all males are in order of incidence: prostate, lung, and colon and rectum cancer. However, lung cancer is the leading cause of cancer death, followed by prostate cancer. The number of males who develop lung cancer have a very low survival rate.

Table 8.3 reports the distribution of cancer incidence by site for females in 1995. The three leading sites for cancer in women are breast, lung, and colon and rectum. As with males, the leading cause of cancer death in women is lung cancer. Breast cancer was the number one cancer killer in women until the mid-1980s, when lung cancer became the

TABLE 8.2   Distribution of Cancer Incidence by Site and Gender (all races; 1995)

Male	Cancer Cases by Site	Cancer Deaths by Site
Prostate	244,000	40,400
Lung	96,000	95,400
Colon & rectum	70,700	27,200
Bladder	37,300	7,500
Lymphoma	34,000	12,820
Oral	18,800	*
Melanoma (skin)	18,700	*
Kidney	17,100	7,100
Leukemia	14,700	11,100
Stomach	14,000	8,800
Pancreas	13,200	11,000
Larynx	9,000	*
All sites	677,700	289,000**

*Cancer deaths by site not given for these cancers. In 1995, 7,300 males died of brain cancer, 8,200 males died of esophagus cancer, and 7,100 males died of kidney cancer. These cancers were not listed on cancer cases by site list but appeared on cancer deaths by site.

**This figure for all sites includes cancer deaths of the brain, esophagus, and kidney.

Source: Adapted from "Cancer Facts and Figures, 1995" American Cancer Society, Inc.

number one cancer killer. The gap between the two still continues to widen. Table 8.4 reports the distribution of cancer incidence by site for selected races in 1995.

When cancer deaths are broken down by race, similarities and differences are apparent. Lung cancer deaths and colon and rectum cancer deaths are high in all races. African Americans have an unusually high death rate from all cancers when compared to the other races. Native Americans have an unusually high death rate from stomach and esophagus cancer. Hispanic American and African American women have an unusually high death rate from breast cancer.

Risk Factors

Multiple risk factors contribute to cancer in minority Americans. The major risk factors include: (1) lifestyle, (2) occupational/environmental exposure, and (3) socioeconomic status. Familial predisposition and genetic factors are also known to contribute to cancer in all Americans.

Lifestyle Factors.   Lifestyle factors include smoking, alcohol consumption, and poor eating habits. Higher cancer rates in the lung, mouth, stomach, liver, and esophagus can be attributed to smoking and drinking. Other risk factors include diet and obesity.

TABLE 8.3 Distribution of Cancer Incidence by Site and Gender (all races; 1995)

Female	Cancer Cases by Site	Cancer Deaths by Site
Breast	182,000	46,000
Lung	73,900	62,000
Colon & rectum	67,500	28,100
Uterus	46,600	10,700
Ovary	26,600	14,500
Lymphoma	24,700	11,330
Melanoma (skin)	15,400	5,500
Bladder	13,200	*
Pancreas	13,000	13,800
Kidney	11,700	*
Leukemia	11,000	9,300
Oral	9,350	*
All sites	677,700	258,000**

*Cancer deaths by site for these cancers not given. In 1995, 6,000 females died of brain cancer, 6,500 died from liver cancer, and 5,900 died from stomach cancer. These cancers were not listed on cancer cases by site.

**This figure for all sites includes cancer deaths of the brain, liver, and stomach.

Source: Adapted from "Cancer Facts and Figures, 1995" American Cancer Society, Inc.

Smoking is a risk factor for cancer of the oral cavity, lung, esophagus, pancreas, larynx, bladder and, of course, the lungs. Alcohol has been associated with colon, breast, prostate, and esophageal cancers. The incidence of esophageal cancer in African Americans is almost four times higher than for white Americans. Mettlin (1980) reported that African American males drink heavier than do white American men of comparable age.

The estimated proportion of cancer deaths attributed to diet is 35 percent overall, with a range of 10 to 70 percent depending on the type of cancer (Surgeon General's Report on Nutrition and Health, 1988). African Americans consume higher levels of fats and fewer vegetables than white Americans (Mittlin, 1980). Numerous studies have shown daily consumption of vegetables and fruits is associated with a decreased risk of lung, prostate, bladder, esophagus, and stomach cancers. Diets high in fat and low in fiber are associated with various cancers—particularly colon, breast, and prostate cancers. Obesity is associated with cancers of the endometrium, breast, colon, and ovary (Hargreaves et al., 1989).

Occupational/Environmental Risk Factors. Various occupational hazards, such as ionizing radiation and chemicals like asbestos, benzene, chromium, lead, nickel, beta-naphthylamine, bioschloromethyl ether, and vinyl chloride, are known to cause cancer (Frumkin & Levy, 1983). Minority Americans are believed to be at higher risk because of their higher rate of placement in less skilled and more hazardous jobs.

TABLE 8.4   Some Cancer Deaths for Black, American Indian, Chinese, Japanese, and Hispanic Persons in the United States

Cancer Site	Black	American Indian	Chinese	Japanese	Hispanic*
All sites	57,921	1,454	1,632	1,099	14,689
Oral cavity	1,274	341	62	16	224
Esophagus	1,987	522	25	23	233
Stomach	2,383	916	102	110	824
Colon & rectum	6,020	143	184	156	1,399
Liver	1,405	81	206	67	860
Pancreas	2,933	77	94	79	810
Lung (male)	10,545	214	274	135	1,879
Lung (female)	4,656	130	145	82	848
Melanoma (skin)	119	8	4	1	89
Breast (female)	4,809	84	99	85	1,264
Cervix uteri	983	42	17	10	292
Other uterus	921	30	16	13	207
Ovary	1,067	34	29	41	369
Prostate	5,299	71	32	47	833
Bladder	840	22	17	12	221
Kidney	977	61	19	17	399
Brain & CNS**	681	26	23	15	429
Lymphoma	1,444	41	58	47	750
Leukemia	1,609	41	46	35	714
Multiple myeloma	1,580	26	20	7	314

*These numbers are believed to include over 90% of cancer deaths in Hispanics in 1991.

**CNS = Central nervous system

Source: Adapted from "Cancer Facts and Figures, 1995" American Cancer Society, Inc. reporting, however may be incomplete on death certificates in some states.

Socioeconomic Status (SES).   Low socioeconomic status is related to cancer incidence, survival, and mortality. Health habits among the poor are not as positive when compared to those who have a higher socioeconomic status, and the poor have less access to good health care. Both of these factors contribute to a higher incidence of cancer, (Bang et al., 1988) and a poorer survival rate (Smith et al., 1990).

Lung Cancer

Lung cancer is the leading cause of death from cancer in both men and women and responsible for more than 150,000 deaths each year in the United States. For example, in 1995, there were an estimated 170,000 new cases of lung cancer and 157,400 related deaths (American Cancer Society, 1995). Because few cases of lung cancer are cured, the number of cases today indicates probable lung cancer deaths in the years to come.

A major risk factor for lung cancer is smoking; it accounts for at least seven out of eight cases (American Lung Association, 1996). Various minority populations have high rates of smoking, and this has major implications for minority groups. Race has become an important factor in lung cancer deaths. Table 8.5 lists the lung cancer cases and deaths by gender and race in 1995.

African Americans. African American men have higher mortality rates from lung cancer than white Americans. Rates are comparable among women. The overall lung disease death rate for African Americans (85.9 per 100,000 population) is 19.6 percent higher than that for white Americans (71.8 per 100,000). based on 1992 data (American Lung Association, 1996). In addition, the age-adjusted lung cancer mortality rate per 100,000 persons is 67.5 for African Americans, versus 54 for white Americans.

Hispanic Americans. Earlier studies strongly suggested that Hispanics, especially women, were at reduced risk for lung cancer compared with other ethnic groups. However, as the tobacco industry continues to aggressively target Hispanics, along with other minority groups, the statistics are dramatically changing. For example, as reported by the American Lung Association (1996), the lung cancer mortality rate in 1982 was 28.8 per 100,000 for men and 11.2 per 100,000 for women. In 1990, the age-adjusted lung cancer mortality rates (per 100,000) for Hispanics was 35.6 overall and 56.8 for men and 20.1 for women.

Asian/Pacific Islanders. There is a great deal of variation among the different groups that make up this category. Lung cancer is the most common form of malignancy among Asians and Pacific Islanders, but the mortality rates are lower when compared to other ethnic groups. The American Lung Association (1996) reported that, in Asian/Pacific Islanders, the lung cancer death rates (per 100,00) were 39.3 for men and 16.7 for women (the overall rate was 26.8); the figures for white Americans were 80.8 and 34.7 (overall, 54.0), double the Asian/Pacific Islanders' rate.

TABLE 8.5   Lung Cancer Cases and Deaths by Gender and Race (1995)

	Male	**Female**
Number of cases (all races)	96,000	73,900
Number of deaths (all races)	95,400	62,000
Number of deaths by race		
African American	10,545	4,656
Native American	241	130
Chinese American	274	145
Japanese American	135	82
Hispanic American	1,879	848

Source: Adapted from "Cancer Facts and Figures, 1995" American Cancer Society, Inc.

American Indians/Alaskan Natives. Similar to Asian/Pacific Islanders, the lung cancer incidence rate among Native Americans is low compared with other populations in the United States. The National Center for Health Statistics for 1990, as reported by the American Lung Association (1996), shows an age-adjusted lung cancer mortality rate of 27.9 (per 100,000) for American Indians/Alaskan Natives, nearly half the white American rate of 54.

Breast Cancer

Breast cancer is the second leading cause of cancer death for women but the most frequently occurring cancer among women except Vietnamese Americans, who had more cervical cancer, and Alaskan Native women, who die more often of colon or rectum cancer (National Cancer Institute, 1996). Statistically, one out of every nine American women will develop breast cancer, and each year over 180,000 women are diagnosed with breast cancer, compared to approximately 1,000 new cases of breast cancer for men. Although statistically fewer in the number of cases of breast cancer, it is important for males to realize that breast cancer is not a female-specific disease.

There are an estimated 2.8 million women with breast cancer in the United States, and approximately 46,000 women will die from it each year. The risk factors for breast cancer include a woman's age (increases with age after 40), a personal or family history, early onset of menstruation, exposure to radiation, and late age at menopause. Alcohol consumption may also be linked to breast cancer in women.

Among women ages 35 to 55, breast cancer is the leading cause of death and accounts for nearly 30 percent of cancers in women. In 1995, there were an estimated 182,000 cases diagnosed and 46,000 women died from it. Breast cancer rates ranged from 28.5 per 100,000 for Korean American women to 115.7 per 100,000 among non-Hispanic white women (National Cancer Institute, 1996). Among women over 40, white Americans have higher rates than African Americans, whereas among women under 40, white Americans have lower rates than African Americans. Hispanic, Native, and Asian and Pacific Islander Americans have lower breast cancer rates than white Americans. Japanese Americans, in particular, have an extremely low risk of breast cancer. Table 8.6 reports breast cancer cases and death rates by race in 1995.

TABLE 8.6 Breast Cancer Cases and Death Rates by Race (1995)

Number of cases (all races)	182,000
Number of deaths (all races)	46,000
Number of deaths by race	
African American	4,809
Native American	84
Chinese American	99
Japanese American	85
Hispanic American	1,264

Source: Adapted from "Cancer Facts and Figures, 1995" American Cancer Society, Inc.

Although breast cancer incidence rates are 20 percent higher in white American women than in African American women, the five-year survival rate of African Americans is 17 percent lower than that of white Americans. The breast cancer mortality rate in 1989 was 27.5 per 100,000 for white American women and 30.4 for African American women (Miller et al., 1992).

Diagnosis.   Most deaths from breast cancer are unnecessary. Breast cancer can be survived if it is detected early by breast self-examination or mammography. If the breast cancer is detected before it has metastasized (spread) to other sites, the survival rate can be as high as 70 percent. In addition, the sooner it is detected the less extensive surgery will be required. To detect lumps or changes that could signal breast cancer, all women should perform monthly breast self-exams seven to ten days after their menstrual period. Symptoms of breast cancer include the appearance of a persistent lump or swelling of the breast, painful breast tissue, nipple tenderness, and the discharge of blood or other fluid from the nipple. The National Cancer Institute recommends that a woman should have a breast X-ray or mammogram every one to two years, for those between ages 40 and 49, and every year thereafter.

Mammography screening is an important tool in helping diagnose breast cancer. This process should, of course, be available to all women. Brown and colleagues (1990) reported that African Americans and Hispanic Americans were less likely than white Americans to undergo mammography. Low income and education and increasing age were also related to low use. They also reported that significant portions of the minority groups reported never having heard of the test.

If a lump is detected, ultrasound is used to determine whether the lump is benign or malignant, a fluid-filled cyst, or a solid one. A physician may also recommend a biopsy, or microscopic examination of breast tissue, if further diagnosis is necessary.

Treatment.   The surgical treatment of breast cancer is very controversial. The controversy surrounds the question of how much of the breast should be removed. A *lumpectomy* refers to removal of the lump and nearby tissue, and a *mastectomy* refers to removal of the breast itself (simple mastectomy) or the breast plus additional muscle and lymph nodes (radical mastectomy). In addition, most women receive one or more adjunct therapies such as radiation, chemicals, or hormones. The purpose of the additional therapy is to kill off any possible cancer that may have spread to distant sites. When mastectomy is necessary, breast reconstruction can be performed to help the patient start the emotional healing process.

Prostate Cancer

Prostate cancer is the most common cancer and the second leading cause of cancer death in men. Prostate cancer generally occurs in men over 65 and occurs frequently in African Americans. One in nine African American males will get prostate cancer. This is highest in the world and is 30 percent higher than for Anglo men (Floyd et al., 1995). A detailed discussion of prostate cancer is found in Chapter 10.

Colon and Rectal Cancer

Cancer of the colon and rectum (colorectal) is the third leading cancer for both men and women, and claims about 60,000 lives a year. Most of the patients are over the age of 50. There are three major risk factors associated with colorectal cancer: a family history of colon and rectal cancer, the growth of polyps in the colon or rectum, and ulcerative colitis. Diets high in fat and low in fiber have also been linked to increased risk. Regular exercise has been associated with lowering the risk of colon and rectal cancer in both men and women.

The symptoms associated with the development of colorectal cancer include bleeding from the rectum, blood in the stool (bowel movements), and changes in bowel habits, such as recurring constipation or diarrhea. Diagnoses for colorectal cancer include a digital rectal exam, a stool blood slide test that detects blood in feces, and proctosigmoidoscopy, which involves inserting a tube for a visual inspection of the colon and rectum. If there are any problems discovered, the physician can use more extensive diagnostic testing, such as a colonoscopy or a barium enema. Annual diagnosis for colorectal cancer should begin after the age of 40. The patient should discuss the frequency for each of the diagnostic procedures with his or her physician. Treatment includes surgery, radiation therapy, or chemotherapy.

Skin Cancer

Skin cancer is one of the most commonly diagnosed cancers. Every year, nearly one half million Americans are newly diagnosed with skin cancer (American Cancer Society, 1995). Skin cancer is most commonly found in people who are frequent exposed to the sun. Ultraviolet rays (UV rays) from the sun often are the cause. Repeated exposure to the sun's rays has cumulative effects.

The three main types of skin cancer are basal cell carcinoma, squamous cell carcinoma, and malignant melanoma. The first two are the most common and, fortunately, are not usually life-threatening. The much less common malignant melanoma can be very dangerous and life-threatening. Malignant melanoma accounts for the majority of skin cancer deaths.

Basal cell carcinoma, the most common of the three, starts with a small shiny bump on areas that are constantly exposed to the sun such as the head, neck, or hand. If left untreated, it may crust over and bleed. Squamous cell carcinoma begins as a knoblike bump, or as red blotches with a defined outline. They usually begin on the face and ear lobes but can spread internally to other body parts if left untreated.

Malignant melanoma starts in or near a mole and usually has a black and/or brown discoloration. It is not uncommon to also see blue and red areas in the melanoma. The borders of the melanoma are not defined, but ragged, and are not symmetrical as it continues to grow. A melanoma is different than a mole. A normal mole is less than 6 millimeters (about the size of a pencil eraser) and has well-defined borders. In addition, once developed, moles normally remain the same size. Almost everyone has moles, on the average about 25. A simple ABCD rule will help you remember the important signs of melanoma:

A. Asymmetry. One half does not match the other half.
B. Border Irregularity. The edges are ragged, notched, or blurred.

C. **Color.** The pigmentation is not uniform. Shades of tan, brown, and black are present. Red, white, and blue may add to the mottled appearance.

D. **Diameter Greater Than 6 Millimeters.** Any sudden or continuing increase in size should be of special concern.

If melanomas are detected early, they can normally be completely cured. Surgery is the recommended treatment. Later stages may require more extensive treatment. If not caught in time, a melanoma can spread to other parts of the body and cause death. If you have what appears to be a mole but it begins to grow and change in appearance, see a physician.

The individuals who are at greatest risk are people who sunburn easily, those with fair complexions and red or blonde hair, and those who have excessive exposure to the sun. Anyone, however, regardless of the darkness of skin pigmentation or coloration can develop skin cancer if exposed to prolonged and intense sunlight. It was once believed that dark brown or black skin was a guarantee against melanoma. We know now that African American people can develop this cancer, especially on the palms of the hand, the soles of the feet, and under the nails (American Cancer Society, 1995). In 1991, over 200 of the melanoma cancer deaths in the United States occurred in nonwhite populations (119 occurring in African Americans and 89 in Hispanic Americans) (American Cancer Society, 1995).

Other risk factors associated with melanoma are a family history of skin cancer and atypical moles. Individuals who live in year-round sunshine are also at greater risk. Some research has also shown that severe sunburn in childhood may increase risk later in life, so children should be protected.

Prevention is the best way to reduce the risk of skin cancer. By keeping your exposure to the sun at a minimum, wearing protective clothing, and wearing sun protection while in the sun you can reduce the risk of acquiring skin cancer. Use a 15 SPF (sun protection factor) or higher rated sunscreen, especially in the hottest and sunniest part of the day. Sunscreen should be reapplied after sweating or swimming.

Respiratory Disorders

Chronic Obstructive Pulmonary Disease (COPD): Emphysema and Chronic Bronchitis. The term *chronic obstructive pulmonary disease* (COPD) comprises emphysema and chronic bronchitis; together, they affect 15.4 million Americans (American Lung Association, 1996). In 1993 it was the fourth leading cause of death in the United States. Chronic bronchitis is a confusing condition because it is usually not a disease by itself, but rather a complication of some other preexisting condition, such as prolonged smoking and chronic heart disease. The vast majority (82 percent) of individuals who die from COPD are smokers, and smokers are ten times more likely than nonsmokers to die from COPD.

COPD is the only lung disease category, however, that disproportionately afflicts white Americans, and the only one for which the death rate for white Americans exceeds that for African Americans (American Lung Association, 1996).

Chronic bronchitis is the inflammation and swelling of the tiny air tubes (bronchioles) and the overproduction of mucus, which leads to shortness of breath. A prominent symptom of chronic bronchitis is the coughing up of the excess greenish-yellowish sputum that accumulates in the air passage. Over time, breathing becomes increasingly labored

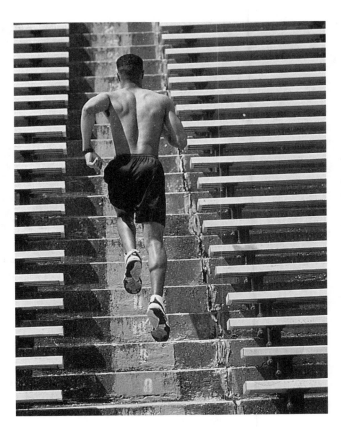

A man too busy to take care of his health is like a mechanic too busy to take care of his tools.
—Spanish proverb

Photo by Tony Nesti.

and oxygenation of the blood becomes more difficult. This condition places a severe burden on the heart and often leads to death by heart failure. Patients with chronic bronchitis must avoid cigarette smoke and environmental irritants, receive antibiotic treatment for any respiratory infections, and take prescribed medications of epinephrine or theophylline when recommended by a physician.

Emphysema is the breakdown or disintegration of the microscopic alveoli (air sacs) at the end of the bronchioles, producing a condition in which the disintegrating air sacs form one larger air sac. The larger air space remains filled with air but the lungs begin to lose their elasticity and the patient has difficulty removing the air on exhalation. The air cannot be adequately exhaled to allow oxygen to enter, creating a feeling of suffocation. Breathing becomes painful and distressful. As in chronic bronchitis, death often results from heart failure. Once the air sacs are destroyed, they cannot be restored. The patient can only try to stop the process and prevent it from becoming worse. Emphysema is treated in the same ways as chronic bronchitis.

Asthma.   Asthma is an inflammation of the airways resulting in wheezing and shortness of breath. An acute asthma attack is literally a struggle for breath, a battle that is sometimes lost. The death of Chicago's first African American mayor, Harold Washington, in 1987, following an asthma attack has been only one of the many thousands of fatalities (American Lung Association, 1996). There are an estimated 13.1 million Americans who suffer from asthma, 4.8 million under 18. (Contrary to popular belief, only about a quarter of afflicted children completely "outgrow" the condition.)

Bronchial asthma is caused by a hypersensitivity to various allergens in the environment. Air pollution, pollens, cat dander, cigarette smoke, animal hair, bacterial infections, drugs, exercise (especially in cold air), stress, and dust mites are common allergens that may precipitate an asthma attack. Asthmatic patients should consult a physician for appropriate treatment and medications, which may include inhaling bronchodilators.

In 1982, the prevalence rate among blacks (39.2 per thousand) exceeded that of whites (34.6) by 13.3 percent; by 1993, the rates were 61.4 and 50.2, respectively, per thousand: The figure for blacks was 22.3 percent higher (American Lung Association, 1996). Degree of severity also differs: In 1992, blacks were more than four times as likely as whites to be hospitalized for asthma. There were 4,964 deaths from asthma recorded in 1992. African Americans, who represent just 12.4 percent of the U.S. population, accounted for 1,032 (21 percent) of those deaths (American Lung Association, 1996). No one knows the reasons for the increase in prevalence, or for racial disparities. Unfortunately, there is little recent information available regarding other ethnic groups, but it appears that age-adjusted asthma prevalence among Asians/Pacific Islanders (2.8 percent) is substantially lower than that among whites (4.3); among Hispanics, slightly lower (4.1 percent); and among Native Americans, notably higher (5.3 percent) (American Lung Association, 1996).

Diabetes

The 1986 *Report of the Secretary's Task Force on Black and Minority Health* called attention to the alarming excess morbidity and mortality from noninsulin-dependent diabetes mellitus that exists in the United States. Diabetes is a disease that affects the body's ability to produce or respond to insulin. Insulin is the hormone made by the pancreas that enables blood sugar (glucose) to cross the bloodstream into the cells where it is used for energy. Without insulin, the glucose cannot enter most body cells. Inadequate insulin production by the pancreas will result in an excess glucose buildup that eventually spills into the urine. This process is caused by the inability of the kidney to process the excess glucose. Diabetes damages small blood vessels and can result in blindness, kidney failure, and amputations, and substantially increases the risk of heart attack and stroke.

Problems begin when the excess sugar spills into the urine. When sugar is excreted in the urine, urine volume rises because more water is needed to dissolve the abnormal sugar load. The first symptom to appear is increased urination followed by excessive thirst. A screening test for diabetes is a check for urine sugar. A color change on a dip-stick indicator pad reveals the presence of sugar. Sugar is not detectable in normal urine.

Two Types of Diabetes

Type 1, early onset insulin-dependent diabetes, occurs when the body doesn't produce any insulin, and generally strikes children and young adults. Type 1 is the more serious of the

BOX **8.1**

According to the National Diabetes Information Clearinghouse, a service of the National Diabetes and Digestive and Kidney Diseases, U.S. Public Health Service (Environmental Research Inc. [n.d.]):

Diabetes is the seventh leading cause of death in the United States.
169,000 people were diagnosed in 1992 with Type 1 diabetes.
127,000 children and teenagers aged 19 and younger have Type 1 diabetes.
An estimated 16 million people in the United States and Canada have Type 2 diabetes.
650,000 people were diagnosed in 1992 with Type 2 diabetes.
By age 70 1 person in 12 will have developed diabetes.
By age 80 1 in 4 will be diabetic.
Every year 30,000 Americans die from it.
300,000 more die from complications stemming from it.
Diabetes is the leading cause of blindness in adults.
Diabetes doubles the risk of heart attack or stroke.
Diabetes is associated with one third of all cases of kidney failure.

two because all patients must receive daily insulin shots in order to survive. Type 1 is far less common then Type 2 and accounts for only 5 to 10 percent of all cases of diabetes. Type 1 occurs equally among males and females, but is more common in whites than in nonwhites. The World Health Organization's Multinational Project for Childhood Diabetes Environmental Research, (n.d.) indicates that Type 1 is rare in most Asian, African, and Native American populations. Northern European countries, including Finland and Sweden, have the highest rates. Advances in both the control of insulin therapy and blood glucose control have allowed patients to live well into their sixties and seventies.

Type 2 diabetes is noninsulin-dependent and accounts for 90 to 95 percent of all cases of diabetes. It occurs when the body can't use the insulin it produces and usually doesn't develop until after age 40. An estimated 16 million people in the United States and Canada have Type 2 diabetes mellitus and half of these people don't know they have it.

The prevalence of Type 2 increases by age and occurs especially in older women who are obese. Type 2 patients have adequate or excessive amounts of insulin rather than a deficiency. However the insulin does not work properly and blood sugar rises. The result is the buildup of glucose in the blood and an inability of the body to make efficient use of its main source of fuel. The early symptoms of Type 2 develop slowly and are not very noticeable or dramatic. Symptoms include feeling tired or ill, frequent urination (especially at night), unusual thirst, weight loss, blurred vision, frequent skin and vaginal infections, extreme hunger, slow-healing wounds, and tingling or numbing sensations in the hands or feet. Doctors believe that one reason most people don't realize they have the disease is that the symptoms are mistakenly attributed to other medical problems or to the normal aging process. As a result, Type 2 diabetes often goes unnoticed in its early stages.

Risk Factors Associated with Type 2 Diabetes

Ancestry: Type 2 diabetes occurs more often among African Americans, Hispanics, and Native Americans. Compared with non-Hispanic whites, Type 2 diabetes rates are about 60 percent higher in African Americans and 110 to 120 percent higher in Mexican Americans and Puerto Ricans. Native Americans have the highest rates of Type 2 diabetes in the world. For example, half of the adult Pima Indians living in the United States have Type 2 diabetes (USDDHS, 1993).

Age: Type 2 diabetes is more common in older people.

Family History: Family history and genetics play a part in predicting diabetes. Persons with one diabetic parent are 2 to 3 times more likely to develop diabetes and 3 to 9 times more likely to develop diabetes if both parents were diabetic than individuals with no family history.

Obesity: One of the most significant risk factors, particularly for young adults, is obesity.

Treatment for Diabetes

Right now, there is no cure for diabetes, but, with proper care, it can be well managed. The goal of diabetes management is to keep blood glucose levels close to normal range. Individuals with Type 1 diabetes must take insulin every day to maintain a normal range. The first approach to controlling Type 2 diabetes is through proper diet, exercise, and weight control. In more advanced cases, medications and treatment of the medical complications are also required. The daily use of blood glucose monitors has helped diabetics keep tighter control of their blood glucose levels and has reduced their risk of medical complications.

Because the rise in blood sugar levels is similar whether a person eats simple sugars, such as candy and cakes, or complex carbohydrates, like rice, pasta, and potatoes, people with diabetes don't have to avoid sweets. Recommendations for those with diabetes are very similar to general dietary guidelines: control total caloric intake to prevent obesity or weight gain, limit fat to less than 30 percent of calories, limit foods that are high in calories that have little nutritional value, and eat carbohydrates (50 to 55 percent of your daily calories).

Diabetes among Minority Groups

African Americans.   Today, African Americans compose 12 percent of the United States population, more than 30 million people. Unfortunately, nearly 3 million African Americans (6 percent of African American men and 8 percent of African American women) have diabetes and are 1.6 times more likely to have diabetes than whites. In addition, African Americans experience higher rates of at least three of the serious complications of diabetes: blindness, amputation, and kidney failure.

African Americans and African immigrants show a basic predisposition to diabetes. A news release by Inter Press Services (1996) reported that Dr. Kwame Osei found that African Americans and African immigrants have a higher level of, and improper reactions to, insulin. In addition to possible insulin difficulties, Dr. Osei confirmed that obesity, in conjunction with genetic predisposition, significantly increases the chances of developing diabetes.

A Diabetes Association survey also reported that, unfortunately, 50 percent of African Americans believe that they themselves are not at risk and, if it should occur, there is nothing they could do to avoid it. The Diabetes Association also reported that the rate of diabetes among African Americans has tripled since the 1960s and now affects 1 in 4 African American women over the age of 55.

Hispanic Americans.   The growing rate of diabetes among Hispanic Americans has made this disease one of the major health problems among American Latinos.

Data from the Hispanic Health and Nutrition Examination Survey (HHANES) of 1982–1984 (U.S. Department of Health and Human Services, 1993) confirmed that 1.3 million Hispanics over 21 years of age have diabetes, almost 10 percent of the adult Hispanic population. Type 2 diabetes is the most common form among Hispanics. Compared with whites, rates of diabetes (diagnosed and undiagnosed) are 50 to 60 percent higher in Cubans and 110 to 120 percent higher in Mexican Americans and Puerto Ricans (USDDHS, 1993).

The HHANES also reported that severely overweight Hispanics are at higher risk, and, among Mexican Americans, 39 percent of the women and 30 percent of the men are overweight.

The Department of Health and Human Services (1993) also reported that Mexican Americans are six times more likely than non-Hispanics to develop end-stage renal disease, are more subject to severe hyperglycemia, and Mexican American women have high rates of gestational diabetes and resulting birth complications.

Native Americans.   Today, of the more than 2 million Native Americans in the United States, 47,000 of them have diabetes. The diabetes rate among the Native American population has reached epidemic proportions. Native Americans are more than 10 times more likely than white Americans to develop diabetes. Complications from diabetes are major causes of death and health problems in most Native American populations. Of major concern are the increasing rates of kidney failure, amputations, and blindness.

Type 2 diabetes has disproportionately disabled American Indian people, in particular, women, for whom amputation is a major complication. The majority of all amputations performed in Indian hospitals are related to complications of diabetes (Stemple, 1990). The incidence rate for Indian men peaks between the ages of 25 and 44; for Indian women the incidence peaks between 35 and 54.

Indian women are also at risk for developing gestational diabetes, which can cause significant health risks for the woman and the fetus and thus create increased risk for infant mortality and morbidity. Massion and colleagues (1987) found that gestational diabetes was present in 6.1 percent of all Navajo pregnancies, whereas nationally it appeared in only 1 percent to 3 percent of pregnancies for non-Indian populations.

One Native American tribe, the Pimas of Arizona, have the highest rate of diabetes in the world. About 50 percent of Pimas aged 35 years or older have diabetes, and more than 60 percent develop diabetes-related kidney disease.

Efforts to prevent and treat diabetes are hampered by the poverty that exists in Indian populations. Poverty diets of fast foods, U.S. government commodity food surplus, and fried foods make diet control difficult. Increased patient education that enlists the involvement of the entire family is needed.

Women.   Women are at higher risk for diabetes. Statistically, 55 to 60 percent of all people with diabetes are women. Each year, more than twice as many American women die from the disease than from breast cancer. Women with diabetes are also more prone to vaginitis, urinary tract infections, and endometrial cancer.

Another risk factor for Type 2 is giving birth to a baby weighing more than nine pounds, a sign that gestational diabetes (occurs in about 3 percent of pregnancies) may have been present. Older, heavier, and minority women are most at risk for gestational diabetes.

Women with insulin-dependent (Type 1) diabetes who have not gone through menopause have some trouble with vaginal lubrication or suffer more frequent yeast infections if their diabetes is poorly controlled. Women with noninsulin-dependent (Type 2) diabetes may be more likely to have sexual problems than women of the same age without diabetes. Changes in blood vessels and nerve damage caused by diabetes may play a role in these problems.

Lead Poisoning

Lead present in paint, soil, and household dust is possibly the most important toxic waste problem in the United States in terms of seriousness and extent of impact on human health. Lead poisoning is a more severe problem for young children than for adults. Lead poisoning causes impaired physical and mental development in infants and children, as well as acute illness in both children and adults.

Children come in contact with these sources of lead during normal indoor and outdoor play. A child can be poisoned from a single high dose of lead or from small amounts of lead ingested over time, or it can be breathed in. Lead can also be passed from a pregnant mother to the fetus, which can lead to low birth weight and slow, postnatal neurobehavioral development. Lead can cause damage to the brain, nervous system, and kidneys, as well as affect the development of red blood cells. Even at low levels, lead can result in problems with physical coordination, learning, and behavior. Excessive exposure may alter the number of organized connections between neurons, or the communication system between them, perhaps resulting in irreversible changes in structure and function. Lead is especially dangerous to children under six years of age because this is an important time in their growth and development.

Sources of lead are flaking paint from old houses, auto emissions, and industrial sources (airborne lead); old inner-city areas are the primary sites for lead poisoning. Within old buildings, lead dust originates from old, lead-based paint still clinging to the walls, affecting both those living in these deteriorating structures and those who might be renovating them. Soil lead derives from the deposition or "fallout" of airborne lead and, even more importantly, from the deterioration of exterior leaded paint that, in particular, has deteriorated into dust, weathered, or been scraped into soil. The dangers of such lead are increased by the small particle size, which enhances absorption. In particular, hand-to-mouth transfer of lead leads to the development and maintenance of subclinical chronic lead intoxication, which constitutes over 90 percent of all lead poisoning (Charney, 1982). It is a mistaken belief that children are at greatest risk from eating paint chips peeled off the walls of a deteriorated inner-city dwelling.

The Sickle Syndromes

The sickle syndromes are a group of genetic disorders that are hemoglobin-related. Hemoglobin is a protein that is carried in the red cells and is responsible for picking up the oxygen in the lungs and delivering it throughout the body. Hemoglobin is made up of two proteins that must be present to pick up and release the oxygen: one is called alpha, the other is beta. Alpha and beta proteins are genetically coded in DNA (the material that makes up genes). Occasionally, however, alterations in the code occur and an abnormal hemoglobin gene will be passed on to children. Although the changes that produce abnormal hemoglobin are rare, several hundred abnormal variants exist. Most variant hemoglobins function normally, but some can produce clinical disorders, such as sickle cell disease. Normal hemoglobin is referred to as hemoglobin A. Hemoglobin S is the hemoglobin produced by the "sickle gene" and is a mutation in the gene that produces normal hemoglobin A. Hemoglobin S is the hemoglobin found in patients with sickle cell disease.

Sickle Cell Disease

Sickle cell disease (formerly referred to as *sickle cell anemia*) is a blood disease that is inherited and is found most frequently in people of African ancestry, but is also seen in people of Mediterranean, Middle Eastern, and Indian backgrounds. The term *anemia* was changed to *disease* because it stressed anemia, which is the least important manifestation of this potentially devastating condition.

About 1 in 12 African Americans carries the gene for sickle cell trait (that is, they have the ability to produce children with sickle cell disease, but have no symptoms of the disease) (American Institute of Preventive Medicine, 1995). If both parents carry the trait, the chances of having a child with sickle cell disease is 1 out of 4, or 25 percent. The disease usually doesn't become apparent until the end of the child's first year. As many as 1 out of 4 children affected with sickle cell disease will die, usually before the age of five (American Institute of Preventive Medicine, 1995). For approximately 1.5 percent of African Americans, sickle cell disease is a painful, incapacitating, and life-shortening disease (Payne and Hahn, 1995). At any given time, over 50,000 Americans, including 1 in every 400 black Americans, have sickle cell anemia. Those afflicted have a less than 50 percent chance of living beyond their 20th birthday (Linde, 1972). Figure 8.1 displays how sickle cell trait is inherited.

		Father	
		S	s
Mother	S	SS	Ss
	s	sS	ss

SS	Sickle Cell Anemia 1 in 4 probability
sS/Ss	Sickle Cell Trait carrier (like parent) 2 in 4 probability
ss	Neither trait nor disease 1 in 4 probability

FIGURE 8.1 How Sickle Cell Trait Is Inherited

Sickle cell disease is a disorder that affects oxygen-carrying red blood cells. Red blood cells are normally round. In sickle cell anemia, the red blood cells are elongated, crescent-shaped (resembling a sickle), making the blood thicker, which affects the red blood cells' ability to carry oxygen to the body's tissues. Sickled cells are unable to pass through the body's minute capillaries. The disease can cause fatigue, pain, damage to vital organs, and death in early childhood. When blood vessels in the hands and feet get clogged, for instance, the hands and feet become painful and swollen. When blood flow is blocked to such vital organs as the kidneys, lungs, or brain, serious damage can occur.

Signs and symptoms of sickle cell disease include the following (American Institute of Preventive Medicine, 1995).

Pain, ranging from mild to severe, in the chest, joints, back, or abdomen;
Swollen hands and feet;
Jaundice;
Repeated infections, particularly pneumonia or meningitis;
Kidney failure;
Gallstones and gall bladder infection (at an early age);
Strokes (at an early age).

The severity of sickle cell disease varies tremendously from one person to another. Some patients have very few problems, while others are constantly troubled by complications of the condition, and in some cases become incapacitated. The most common problem experienced by patients is repeated attacks of pain, sometimes requiring over-the-counter medications, while others require narcotic pain relievers and others are hospitalized. In between bouts of pain, many patients carry on with their normal life activities. The level of activity is based on the individual patient's symptoms and level of tolerance. Other problems experienced by these patients include difficulties with bone, heart, lung, and kidneys. Youngsters sometimes develop severe and overwhelming infections (Bridges, 1996). It is also important to note that many people with sickle cell disease live long and productive lives.

Diagnosis and Treatment.   Diagnosis of sickle cell disease is a simple blood test that can identify the trait and/or disease. If an individual suspects or knows that he or she has a history of sickle cell, he or she should seek genetic counseling. At this time, no medicine exists to effectively treat sickle cell disease. The best approach is a prevention strategy in which individuals contemplating pregnancy voluntarily are tested to determine whether they carry the genes for the disease. The decision to have children and, perhaps, risk passing on the gene for defective hemoglobin to the next generation is a decision that must be carefully made (Payne and Hahn, 1995).

Because there is no known cure for sickle cell disease, it is imperative that counseling help patients understand the disease, and learn how to adjust their lifestyle to the disease and manage it. Schools are asked to shield sickle cell students from cold weather, competitive sports, long walks, and heavy stair climbing, all of which tend to bring on sickle cell crises.

The management of sickle cell disease includes education, counseling, prevention, social services, vocational guidance, and clinical support between periods of crisis as well as during crises.

Other Genetic Diseases

Thalassemia.   This is a group of disorders in which the normal hemoglobin protein is produced in lower amounts than usual. Thalassemia is difficult to explain because it is not a single disorder, but a group of defects that produce similar clinical effects. Thalassemia includes disorders affecting the alpha genes and the beta genes and the combination of beta and sickle genes. Thalassemia has been associated with patients of Mediterranean descent (Italian, Greek, Turkish) (Young, 1990). However, many are not aware of the high rate of thalassemia in South Asian and Chinese populations (Polednak, 1989). Presently, like sickle cell disease, there is no cure, and the same types of precautions must be taken.

Alpha Thalassemia.   Normally, there are four alpha chain genes found in DNA that makes up the normal alpha protein in hemoglobin. Alpha thalassemia involves a failure of function of one or more of the alpha chain genes. The loss of one gene diminishes the production of the alpha protein only slightly and has little effect on oxygen-carrying capacity. The loss of two genes (two-gene alpha thalassemia) produces small red cells and a mild form of anemia. The loss of three alpha genes (three-gene alpha thalassemia) produces serious hematological problems and patients often require blood transfusions to survive. The loss of four alpha genes usually results in death in utero or shortly after birth.

Beta Thalassemia.   Unlike alpha thalassemia, beta thalassemia rarely arises from the complete loss of a beta gene from the cell. More often, the gene is present, but its production of the beta protein is suppressed. The hemoglobin chain form is structurally normal, but the rate of synthesis is diminished, resulting in smaller than normal red cells, which can lead to anemia characterized by marked pallor and moderate spleenic enlargement. The growth of the child is retarded and mongoloid facial features and yellow skin may occur (Purtilo, 1978).

Sickle/Beta Thalassemia.   Sickle/beta thalassemia occurs when the patient has inherited a gene for hemoglobin S from one parent and a gene for beta-thalassemia from the other. The severity of the condition is determined to a large extent by the quality of normal hemoglobin produced by the beta-thalassemia gene. In some cases, this condition is almost indistinguishable from sickle cell disease. Sickle/beta thalassemia is the most common sickle syndrome seen in patients of Mediterranean descent because beta thalassemia is quite common and the sickle cell gene also occurs in some sections of these countries.

Tay–Sachs Disease.   Tay–Sachs disease is a genetically transmitted neurological disorder. It is characterized by a *deficiency* of the enzyme hexosaminidase A (Hex A), which is responsible for the breakdown of complex fat molecules called *gangliosides*. Without hex A, gangliosides accumulate in the brain and nerve cells, resulting in severe physical and mental problems as the entire central nervous system ceases to function. The symptoms of Tay–Sachs first appear at about three to six months of age, when an apparently normal healthy child gradually loses its ability to grasp or reach out, and eventually becomes deaf, blind, and paralyzed (NOAH, 1996). Seizures are also common. Death usually occurs by age five.

Tay–Sachs disease is extremely rare in the general population and is found mostly among descendants of Central and Eastern European (Ashkenazi) Jews. French Canadians in eastern Quebec, Cajun populations in Louisiana, Pennsylvania "Dutch" Germans, and certain isolated populations in Japan and Switzerland are also at similar risk (NOAH, 1996). About one out of every 30 American Jews carries the Tay–Sachs gene. This disease occurs in approximately 1 of every 3,600 Jewish infants.

Tay–Sachs disease is transmitted through heredity when two carriers of the gene become parents. Like sickle cell disease transmission, there is a 1-in-4 chance that any child they have will inherit a Tay–Sachs gene from each parent and have the disease. One-in-four children will be completely free of the disease and 2-in-4 will be carriers like their parents. A blood test can be taken to determine if a person is a carrier. Unfortunately, there is no treatment or cure for Tay–Sachs, but medications are available to help alleviate some of the many symptoms. It is recommended that couples seek genetic counseling if they are in a high-risk group for this disease, or if they have a family history of Tay–Sachs disease.

Although the infantile type of Tay–Sachs disease is the most common, there are other forms, including juvenile, chronic, and late-adult onset. These forms of Tay–Sachs have lower levels of hex A, which is missing entirely in infantile Tay–Sachs. This may help explain why symptoms begin later in life and are generally less severe than in the classical, infantile Tay–Sachs disease.

Cystic Fibrosis.   Cystic fibrosis (CF), also called *mucoviscidosis,* is an inherited metabolic disorder in which there is a production of a thick, sticky mucus that clogs the respiratory and gastrointestinal tracts. CF is a recessive gene disorder that causes a unique hypersecretion of sodium chloride in the perspiration and this, together with chronic respiratory infections and destruction of secretory glands (liver, pancreas), leads to chronic debilitation and early death if pulmonary therapy and antibiotics are not given (Purtilo, 1978).

The defective gene that causes cystic fibrosis causes the production of a protein that lacks the amino acid phenylalanine. This flawed protein distorts the movement of salt (sodium and chloride) and water across the membranes that line the lungs and digestive tract, resulting in dehydration of the mucus that normally coats these surfaces causing a thicker and stickier mucus that plugs the bronchial tubes and makes it difficult to breathe. Abnormal mucus also obstructs the pancreas, preventing enzymes from reaching the intestines to digest food. Other symptoms include very salty-tasting skin, persistent coughing, wheezing, or pneumonia, excessive appetite but poor weight gain, and bulky foul-smelling stools (Cystic Fibrosis Foundation, 1996). The abnormal mucus eventually clogs the lungs or leads to fatal infections.

Cystic fibrosis is the most common inherited fatal genetic disorder in the United States. CF is particularly concentrated in people of northwestern European descent. It is estimated to occur in 1 per 3,000 live births in these populations, is much less common among people of African ancestry, and is very rare in Asian populations (Cystic Fibrosis Foundation, 1996). Approximately 1,000 new cases are diagnosed annually in the United States, with a median survival rate of 30.1 years for these individuals.

The sweat test is currently the diagnostic test for cystic fibrosis, which identifies high salt content in perspiration. A high level of salt indicates the possibility of cystic fibrosis. The treatment for cystic fibrosis includes the intake of one or more of the following: pancreatic enzyme supplements, ibuprofen, vitamin supplements, a new drug, called Pulmozyme, which reduces respiratory infections and improves lung function, and a diet high in calories, protein, and fat. Antibiotics are also necessary when infection sets in. In conjunction with such treatments, vigorous physical therapy exercises are used to help loosen and drain the mucous secretions that accumulate in the lungs.

A child must inherit one defective copy of the CF gene from each parent in order to have cystic fibrosis. Each time two carriers conceive a child, there is a 25 percent chance that the child will have CF; a 50 percent chance that the child will be a carrier; and a 25 percent chance that the child will be a noncarrier. One in 29 Americans, more than 10 million, is an unknowing symptomless carrier of the defective gene.

REFERENCES

American Cancer Society. *Cancer facts & figures—1994.* Atlanta, GA: American Cancer Society, 1995.

American Diabetes Association. Diabetes. In Environmental Research, Inc., *Diabetes center—Type II or late onset diabetes.* (n.d.). http://www.nutranmed.com/zeno/Diabetes.htm

American Heart Association. *Biostatistical fact sheet—population.* 1996. http://amhrt.org/ha96/

American Institute of Preventive Medicine. 1995. *Sicklecell anemia.* http://healthy.net.80/LIBRARY/Books/Healthyself/sicklecell.htm

American Lung Association. 1996. *Lung Cancer in Diverse Communities.* http://www.lungusa.org/noframes/learn/health/healungdes.html

Avery, B. The health status of black women. In R. L. Braithwaite and S. E. Taylor (Eds.). *Health issues in the black community* (pp. 20–34). San Francisco: Jossey-Bass, 1992.

Bang, K., White, J., Gause, B., and Leffall, L. Evaluation of recent trends in cancer mortality and incidence among Blacks. *Cancer* 61 (1988) 1244–1261.

Baquet, C., and Gibbs, T. Cancer and black Americans. In R. L. Braithwaite and S. E. Taylor (Eds.). *Health issues in the black community* (pp. 20–34). San Francisco: Jossey-Bass, 1992.

Baquet, C., Harm, J., Gibbs, T., and Greenwald, P. Socioeconomic factors and cancer incidence among blacks and whites. *Journal of the National Cancer Institute* 83, 8 (1991), 551–557.

Bridges, R. *Sickle Cell Anemia.* Joint Center for Sickle Cell and Thalassemia Disorders, 1996. http://cancer.mgh.harvard.edu/medOnc/sickle.htm

Brown, M., Kessler, L., and Reuter, F. Is the supply of mammography machines outstripping need and demand? An economic analysis." *Annals of Internal Medicine* 113 (1990):547–552.

Charney, E. Lead poisoning in children: The case against household lead dust. In J. Chilson and D. O'Hara (Eds.). *Lead absorption in children.* Baltimore: Urban and Schwarzenberg, 1982.

Coates, R., Bransfield, D., and Wesley, M. Differences between black and white women with breast cancer in time from symptom recognition to medical consultation. *Journal of the National Cancer Institute* 84, 12 (June 1992), 938–950.

Cruickshank, J. K., and Beevers, D. G. Epidemiology of hyptension: Blood pressure in blacks and whites. *Clinical Science* 62, 1 (1982), 1–6.

Cystic Fibrosis Foundation. *Facts about cystic fibrosis.* Cystic fibrosis homepage, 1996. http://www.cff.org/factsabo.htm

Deter, P. *Gender-based screening for heart disease starts at UT-Houston.* News from the University of Texas-Houston Health Center, 1997. http://oac.hsc.uth.tmc.e…s/releases/protocol.html

Floyd, P., Mimms, S., and Yelding-Howard, C. *Personal health: A multicultural approach.* Englewood, CO: Morton Publishing, 1995.

Ford, E., and Jones, D. Cardiovascular health knowledge in the United States: Findings from the National Health Interview Study, 1985. *Preventive Medicine* 20 (1985), 725–736.

Frumkin, H. and Levy, B. Carcinogens. In B. S. Levy and D. H. Wegman (Eds.). *Occupational health* (pp. 145–175). Boston: Little Brown, 1983.

Gillum, R. F. The epidemiology of cardiomyopathy in the United States. *Progress in Cardiology* 2 (1989), 11–21.

Gillum, R. F. Strokes in Blacks. *Stroke* 19 (1988), 1–9.

Hargreaves, M., Baquet, C., and Gamshadzahi, A. Diet, nutritional status, and cancer risks in American blacks. *Nutrition and Cancer* 12, 1 (1989), 11–28.

Hypertension, Detection and Follow-Up Program Cooperative Research Group. Reduction in stroke incidence among persons with high blood pressure: Five-year findings of the Hypertension Detection and Follow-Up Program III. *Journal of the American Medical Association* 247, 5 (1982), 633–638.

Inter Press Services (IPS). *Blacks urged to take control of diabetes.* Inter Press Service (1996). http://www.lead.org/ips/demo/archieve/html

Linde, S. M. *Sickle cell: A complete guide to prevention and treatment.* New York: Pavillion, 1972.

Loggie, J. Systemic hypertension in children and adolescents. *Pediatric Clinics of North America* 18, 4 (1971), 1273–1310.

Londe, S., and Goldring, D. High blood pressure in children: Problems and guidelines for evaluation and treatment. *American Journal of Cardiology* 37, 4 (1976), 650–657.

Massion, C., O'Connor, P., Gorab, R., Crabtree, B., Nakamura, R., and Coulehan, J. Screening for gestational diabetes in a high-risk population. *Journal of Family Practice* 25, 6 (1987), 569–576.

Meyers, H. F. Coronary heart disease in black populations: Current research, treatment and prevention needs. In Health and human services secretary's task force report on black and minority health: vol. IV: *Cardiovascular and cerebrovascular diseases* (pp. 302–344). Washington, DC: Government Printing Office, 1986.

Miller, B., Ries, L., Hankey, F., Kosary, C., and Edwards, B. (Eds.). *Cancer statistics review: 1973–1989.* Bethesda, MD: National Cancer Institute; DHHS publication NIH 92-2789, 1992.

Mittlin, C. Nutritional habits of Blacks and Whites. *Preventive Medicine* 9 (1980), 601–606.

National Cancer Institute. Black men most likely to die of cancer, study says. Associated Press. StarText.NET: Fort Worth *Star-Telegram*, 1996. http://www.startext.net…71A/1:MED71A042796.html

National Cancer Institute (NCI). *Cancer statistics review 1973–1989.* NIH Publication Number 92-2789, 1992. Bethesda, MD:

National Cancer Institute. *1991 budget estimate.* Bethesda, MD: U.S. Public Health Service, 1989.

NOAH *Tay–Sachs Disease: Public Health Information Sheet.* Microsoft Corporation, 1996. http://www.noah.cuny.edu…s.html#Tay-Sachs Disase

Payne, W., and Hahn, D. *Understanding your health* (4th ed.). New York: Mosby, 1995.

Polednak, A. P. *Racial and ethnic differences in disease.* New York: Oxford University Press, 1989.

Purtilo, D. *A survey of human diseases.* Menlo Park, CA: Addison Wesley, 1978.

Report of the Secretary's Task Force on Black and Minority Health (1985), vol. 1: *Executive summary.* DHHS Publication No. 017-090-00078. Washington, DC: Government Printing Office, 1986.

Roberts, J., and Rowland, M. *Vital and health statistics (Series 11. No. 221), hypertension in adults 25–74 years of age: United States, 1971–75* (DHEW Publication No. PHS811671). Washington, DC: Government Printing Office, 1981.

Roig, E., Castaner, A., Simmons, B., Patel, R., Ford, E., and Cooper, R. In-hospital mortality rates from acute myocardial infarction by race in U.S. hospitals: Findings from the National Hospital Discharge Survey. *Circulation* 76 (1987), 280–288.

Saunders, E. Special techniques for management of hypertension in blacks. In W. D. Hall, E. Saunders, and N. Shulman (Eds.), *Hypertension in blacks: Epidemiology, pathophysiology, and treatment* (pp. 209–236). Chicago: Year Book, 1985.

Smith, C., Shipley, M., and Rose, G. Magnitude and cause of socioeconomic differentials in mortality: Future evidence from the Whitehall study. *Journal of Epidemiology and Community Health* 44 (1990), 265–270.

Stemple, T. Lower extremity amputations at the Phoenix Indian Medical Center. *IHS Provider* (December 1990), 165–167.

U.S. Department of Health and Human Services. *Diabetes in Hispanics: a growing public health concern.* Feb. 1993. Washington, DC: Government Printing Office, 1993. Http://www.iacnet.com/health/15032154.htm.

U.S. Department of Health and Human Services. *Surgeon General's report on nutrition and health.* Publication No (PHS) 88-50210, Washington, DC: Government Printing Office, 1988.

U.S. Department of Health and Human Services (U.S. DHHS). *Report of the Secretary's task force on black and minority health.* Washington, DC: Government Printing Office, 1985.

Young, I. Hereditary disorders. In B. R. McAvoy and L. J. Donaldson (Eds.). *Health care for Asians* (pp. 193–209). New York: Oxford University Press, 1990.

Infectious Diseases

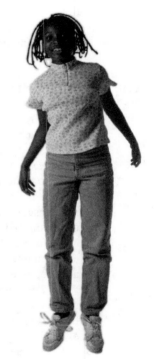

Every human being is intended to have a character of his own; to be what no other is, and to do what no other can do.

—Channing

Photo by Tess Camargo and Tessa Lee, published in *Cultures* magaine, volume 3, issue 1.

Infectious diseases are caused by a specific agent or its toxic products that arises through transmission of that agent or its products from reservoir to susceptible host, either directly, from an infected person or animal, or indirectly, through the agency of an intermediate plant or animal host, a vector, or the inanimate environment (American Academy of Pediatrics, 1977).

Infectious diseases are also known as communicable or contagious diseases. Throughout the history of human life, infectious diseases have had, and still have, significant impact on civilization. Diseases such as the plague, smallpox, polio, leprosy, and AIDS have altered the history of populations. Many life-threatening infections have been eradicated or greatly diminished in numbers through better public sanitation, antibiotics, and vaccinations. However, we have been recently reminded of their devastation through outbreaks of AIDS, tuberculosis, ebola virus, hepatitis, *E. Coli,* Hantavirus, and the Flesh-Eating Strep.

This first section of this chapter focuses on the infectious process and our body's defense system, followed by a discussion of the most prevalent sexually transmitted infections (syphilis, gonorrhea, chlamydia, hepatitis B, genital warts, herpes, and AIDS), tuberculosis, and parasitic infections. Concluding this chapter is a discussion of childhood diseases and immunizations.

The Infectious Process

Infectious diseases are still among the most frequent causes of absence from school and work. Each infectious disease is the result of a successive chain of events, the infectious process. An infectious disease is caused by a specific agent or microorganism, called a *pathogen.* For example, measles is caused by a special virus and gonorrhea is caused by a specific bacteria. When a person has an infectious disease such as the flu, his or her body will visibly react to the invading pathogen with signs and symptoms such as fever, a running nose, watery eyes, aches and pains, and a sore throat. Once in the body, these various organisms irritate and injure tissue by the poisons and toxins they induce.

In order for the infectious disease to develop, the following chain of events must exist: an infectious agent, a reservoir, a means of transmission for the infectious agent, and a susceptible host. If this chain is broken, the infection will not take place.

The infectious agent (causative or etiological agent) is a small living organism called a *pathogen.* There are a variety of different categories of pathogens but most infectious diseases are caused by viruses and bacteria. Bacteria are single-celled organisms that exist virtually everywhere, most of which are harmless. Only certain forms of bacteria can induce illness. Examples of bacterial infections include syphilis, conjunctivitis, strep throat, and chlamydia. Viruses are only a fraction of the size of a bacterium and can only survive in body cells that they infect. Examples of viral infections include the common cold, influenza, infectious hepatitis, measles, HIV/AIDS, and genital and oral herpes. Each infectious agent is specific for each disease. Other pathogens include fungi, protozoa, rickettsia, and parasitic worms.

Fungi are plant organisms and are responsible for such problems as athlete's foot and thrush. Protozoa are larger than bacteria but still require a microscope to see them. Most are also harmless but certain types can cause debilitating diseases such as malaria and amebic dysentery. Worms are parasites that can grow five or more yards in length within the intestinal tract. Parasitic worms can lead to intestinal obstruction and anemia.

The reservoir is the place where the pathogen resides and from which it can escape and be transmitted to the susceptible person or host. If the reservoir is a person, the infectious process can be controlled by keeping that person at home so that he or she cannot spread the disease to other people. Pathogens can reside in other places such as soil (tetanus) and animals (salmonellasis).

Transmission of the pathogen refers to the mechanism by which the pathogen is transmitted from the reservoir to the susceptible host. Pathogens can enter the host's body through several channels: direct contact, such as kissing, sexual intercourse, and touching; or indirectly by touching something with which an infected person has had contact. For example, the common cold is often transmitted from contaminated objects such as a telephone or escalator railing that has been touched by an infected person who covered his or her mouth with his or her hands while coughing. Cold viruses have the ability to live a few hours outside of the human body. Other means of transfer can occur through spreading airborne droplets (sneezing, coughing, or talking), vehicle spread (water, food, blood transfusion, etc.), vector spread (insects, invertebrates, or arthropods), and zoonosis (vertebrate animals).

The susceptible host refers to the person's susceptibility or resistance to the pathogen. No one really understands all the reasons why, at times, a disease develops after exposure, yet at other times it does not. Some of the factors involved include the amount of infectious agent received by the person on exposure, how long he or she was exposed to the infectious agent, the person's age, health history (malnutrition, presence of a chronic disease, fitness level, amount of stress in lifestyle, fatigue, etc.), and the specific immunity (antibodies that are present and prevent the development of the disease).

If a person becomes infected, he or she will go through the following course of infection: incubation period, prodrome period, acute stage, defervescent or decline stage, the recovery period, and defection.

The *incubation period* begins with the invasion of the pathogen in the susceptible host. The pathogens begin to multiply in the host, producing large numbers. During this time there are no symptoms of illness and the incubation period varies from one disease to another and from one person to another for the same disease.

The *prodrome period* begins when the body starts to react to the increased number of pathogens. It is a short interval characterized by the appearance of general symptoms such as headache, fever, nasal discharge, malaise, irritability, and/or discomfort. Specific symptoms of the illness are very difficult to diagnose at this time because they resemble those of other diseases, but the disease is highly communicable during the prodromal period.

The *acute stage* or *clinical disease* occurs when the illness is at its peak. The pathogens have reproduced in sufficient quantity to clearly diagnose the specific illness. For example, the specific symptoms of chicken pox or syphilis begin to appear during this time and can be easily identified by observation.

The *defervescent* or *decline stage* is marked by subsiding symptoms. The body is in the process of defending itself against the pathogens and the patient may feel well enough to become active before he or she is fully recovered. A patient must be careful during this time because too much activity may increase her or his chances of a relapse.

Convalescence is the period of recovery. During this time the body and mind begin to regain energy. However, pathogens are still present and certain diseases may still be communicable.

During *the defection period* the disease is eliminated and the illness has disappeared. Strength and vigor are fully recovered and the individual is prepared for the next assault.

Our Body's Defense System
against Infectious Diseases

When you are exposed to pathogens, your body has both an external (mechanical) and internal (cellular) defense mechanism that help your body defend against the invading pathogen. The external defense system consists primarily of the skin, the lungs, and the alimentary canal. The skin consists of a tough waterproof membrane that is slightly acidic in nature. The skin provides a cool hostile barrier to invading microorganisms. Sweat provides an inhospitable pH level for pathogen survival, helps control temperature, and contains an enzyme that breaks up bacteria and other organisms. Special areas of skin, such as around the eye and the vaginal lining, have special secretions that help protect against infection. The eyes have tear ducts, which contain a chemical, lysozyme, that effectively destroys bacteria. The lining of the vagina provides acidic secretions that help keep other organisms under control.

The respiratory tract is protected primarily by the nose, which acts as an efficient filter and air conditioner. The hairs in the nose keep larger particles out while smaller cilia (hairlike projections in lungs and respiratory tract), in conjunction with mucus, act as a sweep to move larger particles upwards into the throat for swallowing. The respiratory system is also protected by macrophage and lymphocyte cells, which wander over the surface of the mucous membrane and ingest foreign particles.

The digestive system is the most hostile port of entry; stomach acidity destroys most of the invading pathogens and digestive enzymes destroy many of those that penetrate deep into the intestines. If the pathogen eventually breaches any of the initial external barriers, it faces a formidable specialized network of defenses thrown up by the immune system.

The immune system is the internal defense system that counteracts the invading bacteria or virus by triggering an immune response. The activators of the immune system are known as *antigens*. When the body is bombarded by the pathogen, the immune system senses the invader's presence and produces a substance called *antibodies* that converge on infected areas to neutralize or destroy the antigens and assist in the repair of damaged cells.

When viruses attack the body cells, the cells release a substance called *interferon* that helps protect neighboring cells. Lymphocytes (specialized white blood cells) are stimulated to produce antibodies expert in combating virus infection. Macrophages (specialized scavenger cells) ingest the invading virus and produce a special protein called *interleukin*. Interleukin signals other immune system cells to produce specialized cells called T cells. There are three types of T cells. Helper T cells multiply and stimulate the production of specialized cells called B cells. B cells mature into plasma cells, which produce antibodies that are directed against the specific antigen. Killer T cells recognize and destroy the virus-infected cells. Once the cell is dead the virus dies with it. Finally, suppresser T cells send out signals to slow or stop the immune response after the antigen has been defeated.

Anyone who has suffered from viral infections acquires an immunity or resistance to the specific virus that has invaded the body. Special memory cells circulate through the body after infection, ready to respond to another invasion of the virus. Memory cells are the first line of defense against repeat invaders. In some diseases, such as measles and smallpox, immunity is lifelong while others last for weeks or months.

When bacteria invade tissues, they trigger an inflammatory response, the result of damaged cells and tissue and the bacteria's toxins. Proteins in the blood help to incapacitate the bacteria and neutralize their poisons. Lymphocytes and other cells are mobilized to produce antibodies, which act specifically against the antigens to destroy them or neutralize the toxins they produce. Antibodies can cause some bacteria to clump together, hindering their spread while others make the bacteria more susceptible to ingestion by phagocytes (specialized cells that engulf the bacteria).

The body's defense systems are formidable mechanisms that help us to remain free from harmful, infecting organisms. If we can combine these mechanisms with a general state of good health, we can remain free from harmful infections for most of our lives.

Sexually Transmitted Infections (STIs)

Sexually transmitted infections (STIs) are infections you catch through some form of sexual contact. The infectious agents that cause these infections prefer a dark, warm, and moist environment. The human body has perfect environments for these agents to thrive, particularly the mucous membranes that line the reproductive organs.

More Americans are infected with STIs now than at any other time in history. The most common sexually transmitted infections include chlamydia, genital herpes, genital warts, gonorrhea, syphilis, and HIV/AIDS. These diseases are caused and spread by identifiable pathogens, have definite courses of development, and can be treated. Because each is a separate disease, caused by separate pathogens, a patient can have more than one STI at a time. The bacterial pathogens that cause chlamydia, gonorrhea, and syphilis can be cured. The viral diseases, genital herpes and HIV, can be treated, but no cure is available. Genital warts, caused by a virus, can be treated by freezing, cauterization, chemicals, or surgical removal, but recurrences are common.

No one is immune to STIs. Everyone who is sexually active can get or transmit an STI. Race, religion, sexual preference, and socioeconomic status are not protective barriers to any of the sexually transmitted infections. "Nice" people get syphilis; heterosexuals get AIDS. STIs are equal opportunity diseases. However, the Division of Sexually Transmitted Disease prevention of the Centers for Disease Control (1995) reported that surveillance data show high rates of STIs for some minority racial/ethnic groups when compared with rates for white Americans.

There are no known biologic reasons to explain why racial or ethnic factors alone should alter risk for STIs. Rather, race and ethnicity in the United States are risk markers that correlate with other more fundamental determinants of health status, such as poverty, access to quality health care, health care seeking behavior, illicit drug use, and living in communities with a high rate of STIs. Acknowledging the disparity in STI rates by race–ethnicity is one of the first steps in empowering affected communities to organize and focus on this problem.

The incidence of sexually transmitted diseases in the black community is very high. While overall rates of gonorrhea and syphilis have decreased in the United States, one discouraging note is the extraordinarily rapid increase of infections, primary and secondary syphilis, among black men and women since 1985 (U.S. Department of Health and Human

Services, 1995). This increase in syphilis has predominantly occurred in heterosexual black men and women, at the same time, major declines in gay white men. The increase in the number of women with syphilis has led to a large increase in congenital syphilis, which is fatal to newborns.

HIV/AIDS

The human immunodeficiency virus (HIV) that causes the acquired immunodeficiency syndrome (AIDS) can be transmitted through blood, semen, or vaginal and cervical secretions. HIV is commonly transmitted through different types of sexual contact and by sharing intravenous needles, for any purpose. On rare occasions a person can become infected through blood transfusions or exposure to the blood of an infected person. Once infected, a pregnant woman can also transmit the virus to her unborn child. HIV-infected pregnant women have a 30 to 50 percent chance that their baby will be infected during pregnancy or delivery.

Individuals can protect themselves from acquiring HIV by abstaining from sexual intercourse (abstinence), using latex barriers (e.g., condoms) during intercourse, and not sharing intravenous needles.

People who carry the virus generally do not have symptoms and do not even know they are infected. However, HIV-infected individuals without symptoms may transmit the virus even if they do not realize they are infected. The symptoms of HIV infection move slowly or quickly along a continuum from less to more severe medical conditions. It can take years before the virus weakens the immune system so that the body can no longer fight off infections and disease. The most serious manifestation of HIV infections is AIDS, which is characterized by life-threatening opportunistic conditions, such as a number of protozoal, bacterial, viral, and fungal infections, rare forms of cancer, and neurological problems.

The common clinical manifestations in African Americans and others are generally similar (Greaves, 1987). However, opportunistic infections occur more frequently in African Americans, and HIV-renal disease is more severe (Cantor et al., 1991). Opportunistic infections are also common in IV drug users, which may account for the higher proportion of African American patients who develop these infections. In contrast, there is a relatively lower incidence of Kaposi's sarcoma among African American patients with AIDS.

The course of HIV disease appears to be more rapid in African American patients. This may reflect the underlying nutritional or other health status of these individuals, or presentation at a later stage of illness and destruction of the immune system. Prior to the availability of AZT, the median survival for African patients, that is from an AIDS-defining diagnosis to death, was approximately seven months in contrast to one year for white American patients (Greaves, 1987).

Diagnosis and Treatment

The AIDS test is not a test for AIDS but a test for the antibodies that are produced in response to the HIV infection. Testing for the HIV antibodies actually requires two tests.

The first screen is called the ELISA (enzyme-linked immunosorbent assay) test. If positive, a second test (IFA or immunoflourescent assay) is used to confirm the first test. There is no cure for HIV or AIDS, but a few drugs are available that help prolong survival. Zidovudine (trade name Retrovir), commonly known as AZT, has not only prolonged life but has improved the quality of life for those who are infected with HIV. However, like any other drug, there are negative side effects to AZT, including anemia and bone marrow damage. Newer drugs, such as DDI (didanosine or dideoxyinosine) and DDC (dideoxycytidine), are also helpful. Researchers have also been using different combinations of these drugs to make them more effective. The search for new and better treatments continues.

African Americans and Hispanic Americans.   There was a time when the media led the African American and Hispanic American communities to believe that AIDS was a disease of white gay men, while social scientists and epidemiologists ignored the racial aspects of the AIDS epidemic. The color and face of the epidemic have now changed as well as the attitude of society to the epidemic. From the start, AIDS has had devastating effects on African and Hispanic Americans who represent, respectively, 12.4 percent and 9.5 percent of the U.S. population. In 1981 African Americans accounted for 27 percent and Hispanic Americans for 15 percent of the first 100,000 reported AIDS cases. In August 1987, the CDC sponsored the first national conference on AIDS in minority communities and acknowledged that the HIV epidemic disproportionately affected African Americans.

Throughout the first half of the 1990s, there was a great increase in the number of cases in African Americans and a substantial one among Hispanic Americans. In July 1991, there were 182,834 cases of AIDS reported in the United States. 28.6 percent of these cases were among blacks. African Americans were 3.5 times more likely to contract AIDS than whites. Of all AIDS cases among blacks, 78 percent have been in adult men, 19 percent in adult women, and 3 percent in children younger than 13 years (National Commission on AIDS, 1993). Black children are 12.8 times more likely to contract AIDS than white children.

In 1994, the same upward trend for African Americans and Hispanic Americans continued. In 1994, a cumulative 441,528 U.S. cases had been reported. Hispanics accounted for 18.7 percent of the cases and African Americans 39 percent, or 3 of every 8 cases. Of the people who died from AIDS through 1992, 31 percent were African American and 14 percent Hispanic (American Lung Association, 1996).

There is no evidence to suggest that African or Hispanic Americans are biologically more susceptible to AIDS than white Americans. Differences in the distribution of risk behaviors, the existence of co-conditions (such as genital ulcer disease), and the lack of access to early diagnosis and treatment are major risk factors. Risk behaviors account for transmission of HIV infections, not membership in any particular ethnic group. However, some ethnic groups have a greater proportion of people exhibiting certain risk behaviors. White males account for 77 percent of AIDS cases in homosexual men (Mays, 1989). In 1989, among black males, 35.4 percent reported exposure to the disease through homosexual risk behaviors and 39.4 percent through intravenous drug use (National Center for Health Statistics, 1990).

Of all AIDS cases two years later, African Americans accounted for 13 percent of cases related to homosexual behavior and 28 percent of bisexual cases (Chu et al., 1992). Trends for African American homosexual men did not change significantly.

African Americans are somewhat more likely than any other group to use drugs intravenously. In 1991, twice as many African Americans as white Americans (2.4 percent versus 1.7 percent) reported lifetime needle use of cocaine, heroin, or amphetamines (National Institute on Drug Abuse, 1992). The incidence of IV drug abuse–related AIDS was 19.7 per million among white Americans and 188.9 per million among African Americans in 1987.

Among black men, who account for 26 percent of all AIDS cases in adult men, homosexual contact accounts for 43 percent of the cases and IV drug use accounts for 36 percent; homosexual men who inject drugs account for another 7 percent of cases (National Commission on AIDS, 1993). The greater proportion who use IV drugs in the black community accounts for many of the differences in the distribution of AIDS cases by race and the higher rate of disease among African Americans, particularly women and children.

Women.   The new cases of AIDS reported to the Centers for Disease Control and Prevention in 1992 showed a 9.8 percent increase for women, compared with a 2.5 percent increase for men; also, for the first time, more women were infected through heterosexual contact with HIV-infected men than were infected through IV drug use (Kelly & Holman, 1993). The most disturbing aspect of this new wave of cases in the United states is the disproportionate explosion of the virus among black (52%) and Latina (20%) women (World Health Organization, 1993).

Women represent the fastest growing group of HIV-infected people in the United States and abroad. Cases in women are increasing faster than they are in men. In 1991, the proportional increase in AIDS cases among women was 33 percent (Centers for Disease Control, 1991). African American and Latinas are the fastest growing group at risk of HIV infection; 52 percent of female AIDS patients are listed as black, non-Hispanic; 20.5 percent are Hispanic; and 26.5 percent are white, non-Hispanic (CDC, 1990), although black and Latina women make up only 19 percent of all U.S. women.

The trend for African American women continues. African American women are 13.8 times more likely to contract AIDS than white women. In 1994, of the number of women who were diagnosed with AIDS, nearly 75 percent were African American or Hispanic American (American Lung Association, 1996).

The majority of women acquire AIDS heterosexually, through IV drug use, or by being a sexual partner of an IV drug user. African American women are approximately 13.2 times more likely to contract AIDS than are white women and account for approximately 52 percent of all cases of AIDS among women (National Commission on AIDS, 1992). As of October 31, 1994, 53,978 (13% of all AIDS cases) women in the United States were reported to have AIDS (Rural Center for the Study and Promotion of HIV/STD Prevention, n.d.).

The increasing numbers of cases of AIDS among African American women is of concern because of the impact on pediatric cases of AIDS. Currently, 58 percent of all pediatric AIDS cases are African American children (CDC, 1992). AIDS among children is the result of infection in their mothers, and a significant number of cases are reported annually among African American newborns and children. The number of cases among African American women is growing rapidly, and faster than any major race or gender group. AIDS is the leading cause of death among women aged 15–44, and half of these women are African American.

In the United States, women infected with HIV have a 25–35 percent chance of passing the infection on to their children. Even women with relatively mild disease are more likely to transmit the virus. Women, of course, with advanced disease are more likely to transmit HIV to their babies (Rural Center for the Study and Promotion of HIV/STD Prevention, n.d.).

The number of AIDS cases is expected to increase rapidly among Hispanic women because of the high rate of positive HIV in this group. This trend is reflected in the following studies:

1. The CDC in 1990 reported a high rate of HIV among Hispanics (both sexes) applying for military service.
2. Stricof et al. (1991) reported a high rate of HIV-positive results in Hispanic runaways and homeless adolescents in New York City.
3. Novic et al. (1991) reported an increase of Hispanic HIV-positive newborns in New York City.
4. Stricof et al. (1991) reported an increase of HIV-positive Latina women of childbearing years at a New York City family-planning clinic.
5. Smith et al. (1991) reported the highest rate of HIV-positive rates among Latinas entering the New York State prisons (29%), compared with African American women (14%), and white women (7%).

Latinas are more vulnerable than white women to heterosexual transmission of HIV/AIDS through sex with bisexual men. This is particularly related to the fact that 20 percent of Hispanic gay men report having sex with both men and women, compared with 13 percent for white gay men.

Native Americans and Asian/Pacific Americans.   The research on Native Americans and AIDS is limited, but, according to the CDC (1994), the number of American Indians with AIDS as of September 1993 was 731. The data indicate 103 females afflicted with AIDS and 14 pediatric AIDS cases out of the 731 cases reported. It should be noted that improper ethnic identification has contributed to the omission of Native Americans in the AIDS reporting by states and the CDC.

Although the reported number of diagnosed AIDS/HIV cases is still low for Asian/Pacific American women, the AIDS/HIV problem should still be a major cause for concern. It is important that the disease does not spread among them and parallel the general U.S. trend of increased rates for women, particularly minority women.

The knowledge of Asian/Pacific American women, especially foreign-born women, is extremely limited. Wilkinson (1992) reported that, even if they understand the salient features of AIDS/HIV transmission, many have difficulty putting their knowledge of safe sex into practice because of their cultural background, which taught them to put their own needs last and to defer to the wishes of men.

Gonorrhea (commonly called *clap, the drip,* or *a dose*)

Nearly 1 million cases of gonorrhea are reported annually in the United States. The gonorrhea bacterium (*Neisseria gonorrhea* or *gonococcus*) is spread through genital, oral–genital, or genital–anal contact. Untreated gonorrhea can lead to serious consequences. Gonorrhea is a primary cause of pelvic inflammatory disease (PID), ectopic pregnancy, blocked fallopian tubes in women, and urethritis among men. PID is a major concern for women because of its link to infertility. Over time, untreated gonorrhea can also cause numerous other problems, such as inflammation of the scrotal skin, testicular swelling, heart problems, arthritis, reproductive problems, skin problems, and a variety of inflammations such as encephalitis and spinal meningitis. Gonorrhea can also be transmitted to infants as they pass through the birth canal. If the infant is exposed, the gonorrhea germ can infect the infant's eyes and, if left untreated, cause blindness. The newborn's eyes are treated with a solution (silver nitrate) to stop the infection.

Symptoms.   Gonorrhea is generally asymptomatic in women, who must, therefore, depend on the infected partner to notify them of the disease. Men, however, usually have very distinct symptoms, consisting of a purulent (pus) discharge from the penis and painful (burning sensation) urination. Some men, however, have no symptoms. Whether an infected person has symptoms or not, she or he can still transmit gonorrhea to her or his partner.

Diagnosis and Treatment.   Both are relatively simple: a culture test of the discharge from the penis or secretions from the cervix and, if positive, a treatment of penicillin or other antibiotic.

Gonorrhea has had a devastating impact on African Americans and Hispanic Americans who represent, respectively, 12.4 percent and 9.5 percent of the U.S. population. In 1994, the Division of Sexually Transmitted Diseases (DHHS) reported that African Americans accounted for about 81 percent of all reported cases of gonorrhea. The overall gonorrhea rates in 1994 were 1,219.3 cases per 100,000 for African Americans and 84.5 cases per 100,000 for Hispanics compared with 30.1 for non-Hispanic whites (Table 9.1).

Age-specific rates are very high for African American adolescents and young adults. In 1994, the Division of Sexually Transmitted Diseases of the Department of Health and Human Services (1995) reported that African American 15- to 19-year-old women had a gonorrhea rate of 4,911.9 cases per 100,000 population. African American men in this age group had a gonorrhea rate of 4,007.5. These rates were, on average, more than 28-fold higher than those in white American adolescents 15- to 19-years-old. Among 20- to 24-years-olds in 1994, the gonorrhea rate among blacks was 38 times greater than that of whites (4,479.3 versus 116.3, respectively).

Gonorrhea rates are rising in various Native American populations. Native American women, in particular, have a prevalence rate much higher than any other group of women in the United States. In 1992 the gonorrhea rate for Native American women was nearly 1200 per 100,000 population compared to less than 200 per 100,000 in all other female populations (CDC, 1993).

TABLE 9.1   **Gonorrhea: Reported Cases by Age, Gender, and Race/Ethnicity: United States, 1994**

	Total	Male	Female
All groups	380,381	207,581	172,800
white Americans	49,842	18,483	31,259
African Americans	300,997	170,016	130,981
Hispanic Americans	17,331	8,957	8,374
Asian/Pacific Americans	1,682	676	1,006
Native Americans	2,150	905	1,245

Source: Adapted from Division of STD Prevention. Sexually Transmitted Disease Surveillance, 1994. U.S. Department of Health and Human Services, Public Health Service. Atlanta: Centers for Disease Control and Prevention, September 1955.

Syphilis (commonly called *syph, pox,* or *lues*)

Syphilis is caused by a bacterium called *Treponema Pallidum,* commonly referred to as the spirochete. Each year, approximately 25,000 Americans contract syphilis. Most people think of syphilis only as a disease of the reproductive area, but it is more than that because the spirochete quickly enters the bloodstream after a person is infected. Syphilis quickly becomes a systemic disease. Syphilis is most often sexually transmitted, but kissing and other skin-to-skin contact with lesions can pass the spirochete from one person to another.

Once the person is infected, syphilis progresses through four stages. The first sign of syphilis is a *chancre,* a hard, red-rimmed, painless sore at the site of sexual contact. The chancre generally appears at the exact spot where the spirochetes invaded the body. Therefore, the sore can appear in other places besides the sex organs, such as the lip, tongue, or any other part of the body. If untreated, syphilis moves to a second stage often accompanied by the appearance of a rash, especially on the palms of the hand and soles of the feet. The rash does not itch and is variable in appearance and location. Other symptoms during the secondary stage can include large, moist lesions, low-grade fever, fatigue, alopecia (loss of hair), and pain in the joints.

Untreated syphilis progresses into latent syphilis, which generally does not have any external symptoms. During this stage, syphilis is not contagious. The latent stage can last from a few months to a lifetime. Internally, the body is trying to fight off this infection and some people will self-cure through their own natural body defenses. For those unfortunate individuals who do not recover, the disease will continue. The spirochetes will begin to invade the organs of the body—the brain, heart, skin, and other body parts. Progressive degeneration of these organs occurs, but goes unnoticed by the patient. Eventually, as destruction continues, symptoms become evident to the individual and this marks the beginning of the fourth or late stage of syphilis.

The late stage of syphilis often appears years later as the syphilis germs invade the internal tissues and organs. The complications of this stage lead to permanent damage to the body and can be fatal. Aneurysms in the arteries that rupture and permanent destruction of the cells of the brain and spine are common patterns in the late stage of syphilis. Treatment during the latent and late stage can stop the disease process, but any damage to the organs remains permanent.

Congenital syphilis results when the spirochete is transferred from an infected pregnant woman to her fetus. The baby, if it survives, usually has significant damage to the nervous system (both brain and spinal cord) that results in significant internal and external damage. Treatment in the first few months of pregnancy will prevent fetal infection.

Diagnosis and treatment are relatively simple. The two available diagnostic tests are the VDRL (Venereal Disease Research Laboratory test), which identifies the appearance of certain antibodies and confirms the disease, and the RPR (rapid plasma reagent). Syphilis can be treated with penicillin or other antibiotics.

The most recent epidemic of syphilis was largely an epidemic in heterosexual minority populations (R. T. Rolfs & A. K. Nakashima, 1990). Since 1990, the rates of primary and secondary (P&S) syphilis have declined among all racial and ethnic groups. However, rates among African Americans and Hispanics continue to be higher than for non-Hispanic whites. In 1994, African Americans accounted for about 87 percent of all reported cases of P&S syphilis. Table 9.2 reports the cases of primary and secondary syphilis.

In 1994, the Division of Sexually Transmitted Diseases reported the rate of congenital syphilis in African Americans was 202.1 per 100,000 live births and 66.9 in Hispanics, compared with 4.2 in white Americans.

Declining Syphilis Rates in the United States: 1998. An Atlanta (AP) article titled "Syphilis rate at an all-time U.S. low" (1998) summarized a Centers for Disease Control and Prevention study which reported that the syphilis rate in the United States has plummeted 84 percent this decade to its lowest level on record. For every 100,000 people, 3.2 contracted syphilis in 1997—the lowest rate since health officials started tracking the disease in 1941. The disease, however, still has a racial component. Twenty-two out of every 100,000 blacks contracted syphilis, compared with 0.5 of every 100,000 whites and 1.6 per 100,000 Hispanics.

TABLE 9.2   Primary and Secondary Syphilis: Reported Cases by Age, Gender, and Race/Ethnicity, 1994

	Total	Male	Female
All groups	26,352	13,942	12,410
white Americans	2,266	1,227	1,039
African Am.	22,605	11,724	8,724
Hispanic Am.	804	524	280
Asian/Pacific Am.	73	48	25
Native Am.	42	18	24

Source: Adapted from Division of STD Prevention. Sexually Transmitted Disease Surveillance, 1994. U.S. Department of Health and Human Services, Public Health Service. Atlanta: Centers for Disease Control and Prevention, September 1995.

Chlamydia (chlamydia trachomatis)

Nonspecific bacterial infections and chlamydia infections are the most common of all sexually transmitted diseases. They may affect as many as 45 percent of sexually active United States teens and college students (3 to 4 million a year) (Reagen & Brookins-Fisher, 1997). The CDC (1993) estimated that over 10 percent of sexually active young females and over 5 percent of sexually active young males have genital chlamydia.

Chlamydia is transmitted through sexual intercourse and is often asymptomatic. The bacteria infects a man's or woman's urethra (urinary tract) or a woman's vagina or other reproductive organs. When symptoms do appear, they include a burning sensation during urination and a urethral discharge in the male. Females may have a vaginal discharge, painful urination, abdominal pain, and bleeding between menstrual periods. If an infected person is asymptomatic, he or she can still transmit chlamydia to his or her partner.

If left untreated, chlamydia is associated with pelvic inflammatory disease, ectopic pregnancy, blocked fallopian tubes, and infertility in women and men.

Diagnosis and Treatment.   A culture test can identify the infection, and a treatment of antibiotics can cure the patient. It is strongly recommended that both sexual partners be treated simultaneously.

The Division of Sexually Transmitted Diseases (1995) reported that chlamydia is a widely distributed STI among all racial and ethnic groups but trends in positively tested women show consistently higher rates among minorities. Chlamydia is reported to occur more frequently among American Indian women, compared with other races. Alaskan Native Indian women have a higher rate of asymptomatic chlamydia compared with other races. Toomey (1989) found that 114 (23%) of the 493 Alaskan Native women studied had chlamydial infections; 39 (49%) of 80 teenagers had chlamydial infections, with rates declining to less than 6 percent among women over age 35.

Genital Herpes

Herpes is a family name of over 50 different viruses. Genital herpes or herpes simplex virus 2 (HSV-2) is just one of five herpes viruses that infect humans. Other herpes viruses can cause chicken pox, shingles, mononucleosis, and cold sores or fever blisters. Herpes simplex virus 1 (HSV-1) is responsible for the common cold sore. HSV-2 is similar to HSV-1 and causes similar lesions or blisters in the genital region. HSV-2 may also rival chlamydia in terms of prevalency. Some studies have shown that 15 percent of the adult population are infected with genital herpes virus.

If a person is infected with the genital herpes virus, a single sore or a small cluster of blisterlike sores will appear in the genital region, on the penis, inside the vagina, on the cervix, in the pubic region, on the buttocks, or on the thighs. The blisters are usually quite painful, and fever, sore muscles, and a feeling of general weakness are also present. The lesions may last from a few days to a few weeks. While the blisters are present, the disease is very contagious. Eventually the blisters begin to heal and both symptoms and the blister(s) disappear. However, the virus never entirely goes away. It retreats to a patch of nerves in the lower spinal cord called the *sacral ganglia.* There it remains dormant until a "trigger" such as stress, sudden changes in body temperature, a cold, or menstrual flow cause a recurrent attack. The infected individual is not infectious when the virus is in the dormant stage. During an active outbreak of genital herpes, some people are asymptomatic but are still infected and contagious. Fortunately, the attacks usually diminish in frequency and severity over time. Some infected individuals are very fortunate in that their defense mechanisms are able to keep the virus dormant and they do not suffer recurrent attacks.

If the virus crosses the placental barrier during pregnancy, it can lead to serious fetal damage or miscarriage. If a newborn infant is exposed to the virus at the time of delivery, there is a good chance that the baby will contract the virus, which then may spread throughout his or her body causing encephalitis (brain infection) and possible death.

There is no cure for genital herpes but there are medications that are effective in treating and controlling it. A prescription medication, Acyclovir, can reduce recurrences by about 75 percent. Symptoms can be relieved but the virus is not killed.

Genital Warts

Med Help International (no date) reported that an American College Health Association study found that 1 in 10 college women is infected with HPV, the human papilloma virus, one of the fastest growing sexually transmitted diseases (STDs). It is best known as genital warts. Some cause warts on the hand and face, while others cause visible genital warts. Some HPV infections cause no warts or warts that are microscopic in size, and the patient appears asymptomatic, even though infectious. When warts do appear, they may be raised or flat, single or multiple, and varied in size. Some appear as a cauliflower like lesion.

The sexually transmitted virus is responsible for the vast majority of the nearly 16,000 new cases of cervical cancer diagnosed in the United States. Several of the HPV's

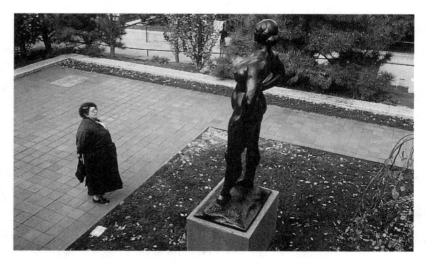

Photo by Robert Harbison.

You are the architect who ultimately designs the foundation for a healthy life.

—Mitsuru

many different strains cause genital warts or lesions that have been linked to both dysplasia and cancer. There are over 60 types of HPV that have been identified. Types 6 and 11 can cause warts on men's and women's bottoms (genital warts) and types 16, 18, 31, 33, and 35 may not cause warts but can cause changes to the cells of the vagina or cervix, such as dysplasia. The virus can lie dormant on the cervix for 20 years before it causes warts or changes to the cells (Midland Family Physicians, 1996).

Only one person in 100 with HPV will exhibit any warts. The PAP smear often detects HPV. At one time or another, about 5 percent of women will have a Pap smear indicating dysplasia. Even if HPV is not noted on the PAP smear, it is 80 percent to 90 percent certain that you have the virus if you have been diagnosed with any type of cervical dysplasia (Midland Family Physicians, 1996). Because most infected people carry HPV without knowing it, it is usually left untreated. It makes sense for sexually active women to minimize their risk of getting HPV by practicing safe sex (condoms and spermicide). Treatments for genital warts include topical preparations, freezing, laser surgery, and traditional surgery. Locally applied podophyllum resin is about 60 percent effective.

Risk Factors.   Having sex before age 18 or having more than three sexual partners in a lifetime increases a woman's likelihood of contracting HPV and cervical cancer. The combination of HPV and low folic acid (B vitamin) level may also increase a woman's risk of cervical cancer. Smoking has also been linked to increased risk for cervical cancer (Midland Family Physicians, 1996).

Hepatitis B

Hepatitis B, or serum hepatitis, is caused by a virus that lives in the bloodstream but is also found in semen and vaginal secretions. Of the five hepatitis viruses, hepatitis B virus (HBV) is the only DNA virus; the rest are RNA viruses. Hepatitis A and E appear in epidemic form and spread mainly through fecal–oral routes (Ramalingaswami and Purcell, 1988). Hepatitis B, C, and D appear to be sporadic or endemic in form and are transmitted mainly via blood, semen, or vaginal secretions. The most significant of all hepatitis viruses for humans is HBV. HBV is responsible for 80 percent of hepatocellular carcinoma (HCC) in the world. Annually, 250,000 people die of HCC (100,000 in China alone), and an estimated 300 million people are infected with HBV (HBV carriers). Seventy-five percent of these carriers live in Asia. Hepatocellular cancer is one of the leading cancers in Asia.

HBV has strong implications for Asian/Pacific Americans because it is responsible for a majority of cases of HCC and for a significant portion of chronic liver diseases such as chronic hepatitis and cirrhosis among Asians (Beasley, 1988). HBV is distributed worldwide and perpetuated among humans through a large reservoir of chronic carriers. More than 200 million people around the world, 5 percent of the entire world population, are chronically infected with HBV (i.e., are HBV carriers) (Zuckerman, 1983). However, the distribution of HBV carriers is skewed; 75 percent of these 200 million carriers live in Asia.

Chronic infection with HBV may lead to the development of chronic hepatitis (chronic persistent and chronic active), postnecrotic cirrhosis, and hepatocellular cancer. There is a striking epidemiological correlation between the incidence of HCC and the prevalence of chronic HBV carrier state. Globally, HBV is probably responsible for 75 percent–95 percent of HCC (Beasley, 1988). HCC is rare in the United States and Western Europe, but it is one of the leading cancers in the world and perhaps the most common (Beasley, 1988). HCC is the most prevalent malignant neoplasm in much of Asia, especially China, Taiwan, and Korea and is one of the leading causes of death in these countries (Beasley et al., 1981; Beasley, 1988; Li & Shiang, 1980).

Ninety percent of infected individuals develop antibodies against HBV and become protected from infection by HBV, The other 5 percent to 10 percent of infected persons remain chronically infected with the virus and chronic carriers and become the source of infection of other individuals who do not have immunity against HBV.

If HBV transmission occurs during the perinatal period, up to 90 percent of infected infants will remain chronic carriers of HBV (Rizzetto et al., 1982). Forty to fifty percent of the chronic carriers in Korea and Taiwan are infected during childhood, approximately half by their mothers at birth (Beasley et al., 1982). Many new infants infected neonatally who become chronic HBV carriers may develop chronic hepatitis B, cirrhosis, and hepatocellular cancer later in life.

In the United States alone, there are more than 200,000 cases of new HBV infection annually; of these, 12,000 to 20,000 become chronic HBV carriers each year (Advisory Committee on Immunization Practices, 1985). Furthermore, with the large wave of immigration from Asia, the newly arriving Asians have brought with them their high HBV carrier rate (5% to 20% compared with 0.2% in the United States) and the increased risk of chronic liver disease and HCC.

When adults are exposed to HBV, they respond in one of three patterns: *acute symptomatic hepatitis* (30–40%), *self-limited and subclinical hepatitis B infection* (50%), or *development of the chronic carrier state* (5%-10%). If a child is infected at birth, nearly 90 percent of these individuals will develop the chronic carrier state (Hoofnagle, 1981). For those who are infected during childhood, the chronic carrier state affects from 29 percent to 40 percent (Stevens et al., 1975).

Chronic infection with HBV may lead to the development of chronic hepatitis (chronic persistent and chronic active), cirrhosis (both active and silent), and HCC. Of chronic carriers, 40 percent of men and 15 percent to 20 percent of the women will die of long-term HBV infection, such as chronic active hepatitis, cirrhosis, and HCC. Some fortunate chronic carriers remain free of serious liver disease.

Acute symptomatic hepatitis patients have jaundice, malaise, fever, nausea, and abdominal pain. Self-limited and subclinical hepatitis B infections do not become clinically apparent hepatitis but cause transient subclinical infections. Patients in the chronic carrier state can live for months or years, or for life.

As of 1990, there were more than 6.5 million Asian Americans; by the year 2,000, they are expected to total 9.9 million, representing 4 percent of the U.S. population. According to the 1989 U.S. Census, the proportions of foreign-born (immigrant) Asian Americans in the six largest groups were 28 percent Japanese, 63 percent Chinese, 66 percent Filipinos, 70 percent Asian Indians, 82 percent Koreans, and 91 percent Vietnamese. Studies have shown that foreign-born Asian Americans have higher chronic carrier rates than those born in the United States (London, 1990). Although Asian Americans represent less than 3 percent of the total U.S. population at present, they contribute to a significant number of carrier pools in the United States. Chronic HBV carrier rates have been estimated from 5 percent to 15 percent in the Asian/Pacific American population (Franks et al., 1989; London, 1990).

Perinatal transmission is the most common mode of HBV transmission, and the remainder of carriers are infected during earlier childhood, and a lesser number during the teenage years (Franks et al., 1989). An estimated 54 percent of all HBV-carrier infants born in the United States were born to Asian/Pacific women, the majority of whom were foreign-born. Because many foreign-born Asian/Pacific women receive late or no prenatal care, they are more likely to transmit the virus to their babies. Therefore, prevention of perinatal transmission is of the utmost importance in the Asian/Pacific American population. To carry out proper screening and immunization and to reduce the risk of HBV transmission to children, childbearing Asian/Pacific American women, particularly immigrant and refugee women, will need to be identified for outreach as a high-risk target group and encouraged to seek early screening, prenatal care, and immunization.

Treatment. The time interval between HBV infection and the development of serious liver disease and hepatocellular cancer is usually more than 40 years. During the interim, HBV carriers may remain "healthy," asymptomatic, with or without underlying progressive chronic liver disease, or may develop symptomatic liver diseases such as chronic active hepatitis and/or cirrhosis.

There is no effective treatment for healthy carriers at the present time, except regular follow-ups for the early detection of HCC in adult carriers. If detected early, hepatocellular cancer can be treated by surgical resection with great success. If detected late, HCC is inoperable and the survival rate is extremely low.

Prevention. There are two ways to approach HBV: (a) through primary prevention, that is, through immunization, whether of all uninfected individuals or of all infants born to HBV-carrier mothers; and (b) secondary prevention, through follow-ups every six months with HBV-carriers for early detection of HCC. The ultimate goal is to eliminate HBV infection by immunization of all susceptible individuals. HBV vaccines such as Recombivax-B and Engerix B are available in the United States.

A Brief Look at Other Types of Hepatitis

There at least four other types of viral hepatitis. Each is caused by a different virus.

Hepatitis A What was formerly called *infectious hepatitis* is common in children in developing countries but seen more frequently in adults in the Western world. It accounts for about 40 percent of all reported cases of hepatitis. It is often transferred in unsanitary conditions and can be caught from unclean foodhandlers, fecal matter, and water. There is a new hepatitis A vaccine available.

Hepatitis C The most commonly acquired hepatitis transmitted by a blood transfusion.

Hepatitis D This type of hepatitis is found mainly in IV-drug users who are carriers of the hepatitis B virus, which must be present for the hepatitis D virus to spread.

Hepatitis E This form of hepatitis resembles hepatitis A but is caused by a virus commonly found in the Indian Ocean area.

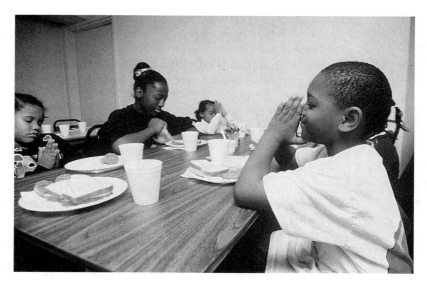

Photo by Robert Harbison.

The healing system is the way the body mobilizes all its resources to combat disease.
The belief system is often the activator of the healing system.

—Norman Cousins

Tuberculosis: The World's Deadliest Infectious Disease

Pan American Health Organization, an office of the World Health Organization (1996), reported that tuberculosis (TB) is the world's deadliest infection, killing 3 million people (including 300,000 children) each year. TB currently kills more adults each year than AIDS, malaria, and tropical diseases combined, and causes 26 percent of avoidable deaths in the developing world.

Approximately one-third of the world's population is infected by the tuberculosis bacterium (*Mycobacterium tuberculosis*). Someone in the world is newly infected with TB literally with every tick of the clock, one person per second. Left untreated, one person with active TB will infect 10 to 15 people in a year's time. In the next decade, it is estimated that 300 million more people will become infected, that 90 million people will develop the disease, and 30 million people will die from it.

The infectious bacteria that causes TB lodges in the lungs and can eventually spread to the rest of the body. The TB bacilli invades the respiratory system, causing a severe inflammatory response that can cause the buildup of fibrosis and calcified materials that engulf the bacilli. These encasements are called *tubercles*. The TB is arrested at this point, not cured, and can be reactivated when immunity becomes depressed. This period of arrest is known as *primary tuberculosis*.

Secondary tuberculosis is due to reactivation of bacilli that were encased in tubercles during primary TB. This reactivation leads to extensive lesions and cavitation in the upper portion of the lungs. Over time the infected person may develop the following symptoms: persistent coughing, weight loss, fever, night sweats, and spitting up blood (Purtilo, 1978). Persons whose immune systems have been weakened or compromised by debilitating disorders such as AIDS, diabetes mellitus, malnutrition, or alcoholism are more vulnerable to TB. TB is becoming the leading cause of death among HIV-positive people (WHO, 1996).

Only persons who are actually sick with TB can infect others. It is spread through the air and by casual contact. When infectious people sneeze, cough, talk, or expectorate, the TB bacilli in their lungs are propelled in the air where they can remain suspended for hours and be inhaled by others (WHO, 1996). However, only 5–10 percent of people who are infected with TB actually become sick or infectious themselves, because the immune system "walls off" the TB organisms (WHO, 1996).

In the United States, TB was one of the leading causes of death in the early 1900s, but as researchers began to understand the infectious process of tuberculosis, it was brought under reasonable control. Through improved sanitation, isolation of the infected person, and treatment with drugs, the incidence of TB was steadily decreasing until the mid 1980s, when the downward trend abruptly reversed.

Two major factors have contributed to the rise of TB in the United States. First, the accelerated spread of human immunodeficiency virus (HIV), the causative agent for AIDS, increases the possibility of TB infecting the patient because of his or her compromised immune system. TB and HIV form a deadly combination, each having a synergistic effect on the other. As more TB cases become infectious, more people will carry and spread TB to healthy populations.

The second factor is the number of new immigrants and refugees entering the United States. The largest number of foreign-born people with TB originated from Mexico, the Philippines, Haiti, India, the People's Republic of China, and Vietnam. In 1993, about one-fourth of reported tuberculosis cases were in people who were born outside of the United States. During 1986–1994, the number of TB cases reported annually among foreign-born persons in the United States increased 55 percent (from 4925 to 7627) (CDC, no date). In 1995, TB cases reported among people born outside of the United States and its territories accounted for 35.7 percent of the total reported cases, compared with 31.3 percent in 1994. Each consecutive year from 1993, the percent of foreign-born people with tuberculosis in the United States has increased. Table 9.3 presents the number and percentage of tuberculosis cases diagnosed among individuals from Mexico, the Philippines, and Vietnam residing in Hawaii and Los Angeles for the year 1993.

In 1994, 24,361 cases of TB were reported in the United States. Of these cases, only 26.7 percent were in non-Hispanic whites. Non-Hispanic blacks, some 12 percent of the population, accounted for 34.2 percent of the TB cases. Hispanics, 9.5 percent of the population, accounted for 20.8 percent of the TB cases (American Lung Association, 1996).

Diagnosis and Treatment.   There is a distinct difference between being infected with TB and active TB disease. If infected but not active, the TB bacteria is in the person's body, a skin test will be positive, the chest X-ray will be normal, and the person is not contagious. When a person has active TB, the bacteria is in the body, the skin test is positive, the chest X-ray is abnormal, the sputum is usually positive, and the symptoms associated with TB are usually present. This person is contagious. A recently developed sputum test can

TABLE 9.3   Number and Percentage of Tuberculosis Cases among Foreign-Born Persons Who Had Resided in Hawaii and Los Angeles County, 1993

Area of Origin	Hawaii (n = 261)		Los Angeles (n = 261)	
	No.	(%)	No.	(%)
Asia				
Philippines	211	(80.8)	71	(27.2)
Vietnam	16	(6.1)	36	(13.8)
Other Asian	27	(10.3)	48	(18.4)
Mexico and Central America				
Mexico	1	(0.4)	79	(30.3)
Central America	0		9	(3.4)
Other	6	(2.3)	18	(6.9)

Source: CDC WONDER Home Page (no date). Tuberculosis article http://wonder.cdc.gov/WONDER/static/^SYSTEM=PREGUID^LEVEL=topics.htm

tell if a person has active tuberculosis within four to five hours. The most commonly used skin test to check for tuberculosis is the Purified Protein Derivative. This test confirms that a person has been infected with the bacilli but it does not confirm if he or she has "active" tuberculosis. The most cost-effective way to stop the spread of tuberculosis in communities with high incidence is by curing it.

The best curative method for TB is known as Directly Observed Treatment, Short Course (DOTS), in which health workers ensure that TB patients take their full course of anti-TB drugs by watching them swallow each and every dose. By guaranteeing that treatment regimens are completed, DOTS prevents further spread of infection and the development of drug-resistant TB (WHO, 1996).

Intestinal Parasitic Infestations

Intestinal parasitic infestations are very common in immigrants and refugees entering the United States, in particular, in refugees from Indochina. Barrett-Conner (1989) reported a prevalence rate of intestinal parasitic infestations as high as 80 percent in screened refugees.

The distribution and frequency of parasites varies among different ethnic groups and countries. The most commonly identified parasites are nematodes, cestodes, protozoa, and trematodes.

Nematodes

Over 30 roundworms are human parasites. A common intestinal parasite, *Ascaris,* is about 10 inches in length and spends its adult life in the human intestine, where it survives by ingesting partly digested food. Ascariasis affects roughly 1 billion people throughout the world, but is most prevalent in tropical countries. *Ascaris* eggs leave the human body with the feces. In many parts of the world, human waste is used as fertilizer. People become infected most commonly when it is transferred from hand to mouth. It can also be transferred when individuals ingest the *Ascaris* eggs on unwashed vegetables or fruit, or from hands dirty with contaminated soil.

During their migration through the human digestive tract, the *Ascaris* larvae can damage the lungs and other tissues. When they settle in the small intestine, they may cause abdominal pain, allergic reactions, or malnutrition. Sometimes a tangled mass of these worms blocks the intestine (Solomon et al., 1996).

Other roundworms include the hookworm, *Ancylostoma duodenale,* and *Necator americanus,* which affects close to one quarter of the world's population. Trichina worms are acquired when humans eat poorly cooked, infected pork or bear. *Pinworms* are found in children. Mild manifestations of pinworm may result in discomfort, irritation of the anal region, and injury to the intestinal wall.

Another common symptom of both roundworm and tapeworm is gastroenteritis ("Montezuma's revenge"). Signs and symptoms of acute gastroenteritis are: (a) nausea, (b) vomiting, and (c) water diarrhea (Purtilo, 1978).

Cestodes (tapeworm)

There are more than 1000 different species of the Cestoda. Cestoda live as parasites in the intestines of every kind of vertebrates, including humans. Tapeworms are long, flat, ribbonlike animals strikingly specialized for their parasitic mode of life. Humans become infected when they eat poorly cooked meat or fish containing the tapeworm larvae. The three tapeworms found in humans are the pork tapeworm, found in poorly cooked, infected pork; the fish tapeworm, found in raw, or poorly cooked, infected fish; and the beef tapeworm, which can be passed on by someone eating rare infected steak.

Tapeworm can cause severe chronic gastroenteritis in addition to malnutrition and anemia. Blood is lost from the parasitized mucosa, and absorption of food is often impaired.

Protozoa

Amebiasis is a very common disease common in the tropics, especially in Southeast Asia, where more than 40 percent of the population may be infected (Martinez-Palomo & Marines-Baez, 1983). Intestinal ulcerations, dysentery, and hepatic abscess can result from this disease. Malaria is transmitted to humans by *Anopheles* mosquitoes that carry the protozoa that causes the disease. Around the world, some 270 million people each year develop malaria, but it is only a minor problem in the United States. *Amebic dysentery* is a common symptom of malaria. The protozoan parasite ulcerates the mucosa of the colon and causes acute inflammation. Diarrhea characterized by extensive mucus production and hemorrhage results (Purtilo, 1978).

Giardia or giardiasis is the most common protozoan disease found in the United States. Its prevalency rate is approximately 2 out of 10,000 people in the United States, making it the most prevalent enteric parasite and the leading infectious agent identified in waterborne outbreaks of diarrhea (Applied Medical Informatics, 1996). This protozoan is found in human and animal feces. Day care centers and campers and hikers who drink contaminated water are at high risk. Once ingested, these parasites stick to the intestinal walls and absorb nutrients from their host. Symptoms include nausea, lack of appetite, gas, diarrhea, fatigue, abdominal cramps, and bloating. Dehydration from diarrhea can be life-threatening in small children and the elderly.

Trematodes (flukes)

Blood flukes are widespread in tropical areas of the world. Liver flukes are common in Asia, particularly where human feces are used to fertilize crops. Liver flukes may infect some 25 percent of the Hong Kong population and a small portion of Chinese immigrants and Southeast Asian refugees in the United States. The snail that thrives in ponds, rice paddies, and the marshy areas that form when dams are built acts as the intermediate host for the fluke. Free-swimming larvae leave the snail and burrow in through the skin of people who work in the water environment, entering the bloodstream of the host and inhabiting the intestinal veins. Eggs are passed in to intestines and are excreted through human feces. The eggs eventually find their way to water where they hatch; the larvae are eventually consumed by the snail to complete the cycle.

Diagnosis and Treatment of Parasitic Infestations.   Most parasitic infestations can be diagnosed through the inspection of the patient's feces and treated with designated medications for the specific parasite.

Preventing Communicable Diseases: Childhood Immunizations

There are now nine contagious diseases for which there are effective childhood vaccines. However, three in 10 infants and toddlers are going without adequate immunizations, leaving them at risk for life-threatening or disabling illnesses. In 1990, for example, almost 28,000 cases of measles were reported in the United States, and 89 children died (ARC of the United States, n.d., 1994).

The U.S. Preventive Services Task Force National Headquarters recommends that children should be vaccinated against the following diseases: Diptheria, tetanus, and pertussis (DTP); haemophilus influenza type b conjugate vaccine (HIB); live measles, mumps, and rubella viruses in a combined vaccine (MMR); oral polio virus vaccine (OPV); and tetanus diptheria toxoid (TD).

Arc (1994) reported that:

1. Three thousand to 28,000 cases of measles have been reported yearly in the United States. Measles can cause encephalitis, which can lead to convulsions, hearing loss, mental retardation, and possible death.
2. In recent years, 4,500 to 13,000 cases of mumps have been reported in the United States, and occasional outbreaks still occur. Mumps can cause meningitis.

TABLE 9.4   Recommended Immunization Schedule for Children

Recommended Age	Immunization(s)
2 months	DTP, OPV
4 months	DTP, OPV
6 months	DTP
15 months	DTP, OPV, MMR
18 months	HIB
4–6 years	DTP, OPV
14–16 years	TD, every 10 years thereafter

3. Prior to the HIB vaccine, one in every 200 children contracted HIB disease within the first five years of life. One in 20 children dies of the illness and 25 to 35 percent suffer permanent brain damage, including mental retardation.
4. Hepatitis B can cause hepatitis and often leads to cirrhosis or cancer.

The U.S. Preventive Services Task Force (n.d.) recommends the immunization schedule in Table 9.4 for children.

The total number of cases of vaccine preventable diseases for 1992–1993 are given in Table 9.5.

Among the unvaccinated adolescents in the United States, 40 percent of inner-city populations are not properly immunized (Reagan and Brookins-Fisher, 1997). Table 9.6 displays the percent of children immunized in 1994.

TABLE 9.5   Vaccine Preventable Diseases: Annual Cases, 1992–1993

	Total Cases	
Disease	1992	1993
Congenital rubella syndrome	9	7
Diptheria	3	0
Haemophilius influenza	1,412	1,264
Hepatitis B	16,126	12,396
Measles	2,231	281
Mumps	2,485	1,640
Pertussis	2,485	6,335
Poliomyelitis, paralytic	—	—
Rubella	157	195
Tetanus	44	43

Source: Adapted from CDC (Feb. 4, 1994). MMWR, Vol. 43, no. 4, p. 58.

TABLE 9.6   Percent of Children Immunized, 19 to 35 Months (1994)

Vaccination	White	Black	Other
DTP (3 doses)	89.4%	82.6%	84.5%
Polio	79.8%	73.4%	80.8%
Haemophilus influenza B	57.0%	44.8%	56.9%
Measles	86.9%	76.9%	72.5%
Hepatitis B	16.3%	16.0%	16.6%
Combined series	75.7%	69.2%	68.0%

Source: Adapted from CDC: MMVR, Oct. 7, 1994, Vol 43, No. 39, p. 708.

Many of the children who do not get immunized are from families that do not have health insurance. This population often includes minorities, in particular, Hispanic Americans and African Americans. Many public health programs are targeting children who do not have medical insurance. For those who do not have insurance coverage and cannot afford to pay for immunizations, public health clinics provide them at no cost. Clinics that receive vaccines from the government are forbidden by law from denying vaccinations for those who cannot pay.

REFERENCES

Advisory Committee on Immunization Practices. Recommendations for protection against viral hepatitis. *Morbidity and Mortality Weekly Report* 34 (1985), 313–315.

American Academy of Pediatrics. *School health: A guide for health professionals.* Evanston, IL: Author, 1977.

American Lung Association. *Tuberculosis in diverse communities,* a pamphlet on the internet, 1996. http:/www. lungusa.org/noframes/learn/health/heaaboutast.html

Applied Medical Informatics *Giardiasis,* 1996. http:// www.familyinternet.com/peds/scr/000288sc.htm

ARC of the United States. *Questions and answers on immunizations.* Arlington, TX: Arc National Headquarters, 1994. hppt://TheArc.org/faqs/vaccineq.html

Barrett-Connor, E. Latent and chronic infections imported from Southeast Asia. *Journal of the American Medical Association* 239 (1989), 1901–1906.

Beasley, R. P. Hepatitis B virus: The major etiology of hepatocellular carcinoma. *Cancer* 61 (1988), 1942–1956.

Beasley, R., Hwang, L., Lin, C., Leu, M., Stevens, C., Szmuness, E., and Chen, K. Incidence of hepatitis B virus infections in preschool children in Taiwan. *Journal of Infant Development* 146 (1982), 198–204.

Beasley, R. P., Lin, C., Hwang, L. Y., and Chien, C. Hepatocellular carcinoma and hepatitis B virus. A prospective study of 22,707 men in Taiwan. *Lancet* 2 (1981), 1129–1132.

Cantor, E., Kimmel, P., and Bosch, J. Effect of race on expression of acquired immunodeficiency syndrome-associated nephropathy. *Archives of Internal Medicine,* 151 (1991), 125–128.

Centers for Disease Control and Prevention (CDC). *HIV/ AIDS surveillance report.* Atlanta, GA: CDC, 1990.

Centers for Disease Control and Prevention (CDC). *HIV/ AIDS surveillance report.* Atlanta, GA: CDC, 1994.

Centers for Disease Control and Prevention. *Morbidity and Mortality Weekly Report: Tuberculosis Morbidity—US, 1995. Newsline* 45, 18 (1996).

Centers for Disease Control and Prevention. Mortality attributable to HIV infection/AIDS-United States, 1981–1990. *Morbidity and Mortality Weekly Report,* 40 (1991), 41–44.

Centers for Disease Control. Recommendations for the Prevention and Management of Chlamydia trachomatis infections. *Morbidity and Mortality Weekly Report 42,* No. RR-12, (August 6 1993), 1–39.

Centers for Disease Control and Prevention. The second 100,000 cases of acquired immuno-deficiency syndrome-United States, June 1982-December 1991. *Morbidity and Mortality Weekly Report* 41 (1992), 218–229.

Centers for Disease Control. Sexually transmitted disease surveillance. In *The Women's Health Data Book,* Washington, DC: Jacobs Institute of Women's Health (2nd ed.), p. 38, 1995.

Centers for Disease Control and Prevention. *Tuberculosis.* CDC WONDER/PC e-mail, n.d. http://wonder.cdc.gov/ WONDER / static / ^ SYSTEM = PREGUID ^ LEVEL= topics.htm

Centers for Disease Control and Prevention (CDC). *U.S. AIDS cases reported through December 1992, HIV/ AIDS Surveillance.* Report, Year-End Edition, Jan, 1993.

Chu, S., Peterman, T., Doll, L., Buehler, J., and Curran, J. AIDS in bisexual men in the United States: Epidemiology of transmission to women. *American Journal of Public Health* 82 (1992), 220–224.

Franks, A., Berg, C., Kane, M., Browne, B., Sikes, R., Elsea, W., and Burton, A. Hepatitis B virus infection among children born in the United States to Southeast Asian refugees. *New England Journal of Medicine* 321 (1989), 1301–1305.

Greaves, W. The black community. In H. L. Dalton and S. Burris (Eds.), *AIDS and the law: A guide for the public* (pp. 281–289). New Haven: Yale United Press, 1987.

Hann, R. "Parasitic Infections." In N. Zane, D. Takeuchi, and K. Young. *Confronting Critical Health Issues of Asian and Pacific Islander Americans.* Thousand Oaks, CA: Sage, 1994.

Hoofnagle, J. Serologic markers of hepatitis B virus infection." *Annual Review of Medicine* 32 (1981), 1–11.

Kelley, P., and Holman, S. The new faces of AIDS. *American Journal of Nursing* 93 (March, 1993), 26–35.

Li, F., and Shiang, E. Cancer mortality in China. *Journal of the National Cancer Institute* 65 (1980), 217–221.

London, W. Prevention of hepatitis B and hepatocellular carcinoma in Asian residents in the United States. *Asian Journal of Clinical Science Monograms: Hepatitis B Virus Infections* 11 (1990), 49–57.

Margolis, H., Alter, M., and Hadler, S. "Hepatitis B: Evolving epidemiology and implications for Control." *Seminars in Liver Disease,* 2, 84–86, 1991.

Martinez-Palomo, A., and Martines-Baez, M. Selective primary health care: Strategies for control of disease in the developing world: X. Amebiasis. *Review of Infectious Disease,* 5, 1093, 1983.

Mays, V. M. "AIDS prevention in black populations: Methods of a safer kind." In V. M. Mays, G. W.

Albee, J. Jones, and S. F. Schneider (Eds.), *Primary prevention of AIDS: Psychological approaches* (pp. 264–278). Newbury Park: Sage, 1989.

Med Help International. *Cervical Dysplasia,* no date. Http://medhlp.netusa.net/general/womens/displas.txt

Midland Family Physicans. *HPV and Cervical Dysplasia: Patient Information.* LSUMC Family Medicine Patient Education Home Page, 1996. http://lib_sh. lsumc.edu/fammed/pted/hpymid.html

National Center for Health Statistics. *Health United States, 1989.* DHHS Pub. No. 1232. Hyattsville, MD: Public Health Services, 1990.

National Commission on AIDS. *Special report: The challenge of HIV/AIDS in communities of color.* San Francisco: National Commission on AIDS (pp. 3–6, 27–30), 1993.

Novic, L., Glebatis, D., Stricof, R., McCubbin, P., Lessner, L., and Berns, D. "Newborn seroprevalence study: Methods and results." *American Journal of Public Health,* 81(Suppl.), 15–21, 1991.

Pan American Health Organization. *Tuberculosis: A threat to each of us.* Washington, DC: Pan American Health Organization, 1996. Http://www.paho.org/english/ DPI/rlmar22a.htm.

Purtilo, D. *A survey of human diseases.* Menlo Park, CA: Addison-Wesley, 1978.

Ramalingaswami, V. and Purcell, R. "Waterborne non-A., non-B hepatitis." *Lancet,* 2, 571–573, 1988.

Reagan, P., and Brookins-Fisher, J. *Community health in the 21st century.* Boston: Allyn and Bacon, 1997.

Rizzetto, M., Bonino, R., Sakuma, K., Takahara, T., Okuda, F., and Mayumi, M. "Prognosis of hepatitis B surface antigen carriers in relation to routine liver function states: A retrospective study." *Gastroenterology,* 83, 114–117, 1982.

Rolfs, R. T., and Nakashima, A. K. "Epidemiology of primary and secondary syphilis in the United States, 1981 through 1989." *JAMA* 264:1432–7, 1990.

Rural Center for the Study and Promotion of HIV/STD Prevention. *HIV Infection and Women.* Bloomington, IN: Indiana University, n.d. http://monticello.avenue.gen.vor.us/Health/Svc Providers/ASG/edwo0695 htm

Smith, P., Mild, J., and Truman, B. HIV infection among women entering the New York State correctional system. *American Journal of Public Health,* 8, 35–39, 1991.

Solomon, E., Berg, L., Martin, D., and Villee, C. *Biology.* Fort Worth, TX: Saunders College Publishing, 1996.

Stevens, C., Beasley, R., Tsui, J., and Lee, W. "Vertical transmission of hepatitis B antigen in Taiwan." *New England Journal of Medicine,* 292, 771–774, 1975.

Stricof, R., Kennedy, J., Nattell, T., Weisfuse, I., and Novick, L. "HIV-seroprevalence in a facility for runaway and homeless adolescents." *American Journal of Public Health,* 81(Suppl.), 50–53, 1991.

Syphalis rate at all-time U.S. low, Atlanta (AP). (1998, June) San Luis Obispo County Telegram-Tribune, page C-10.

Toomey, K., Oberschelp, A., and Greenspan, J. "Sexually transmitted diseases and Native Americans: Trends in reported gonorrhea and syphillis morbidity, 1984–1988." *Public Health Reports,* 104(6), 1989.

U.S. Department of Health and Human Services, Public Health Service. Division of STD Prevention. *Sexually transmitted disease surveillance, 1994.* Atlanta, GA: Centers for Disease Control and Prevention. September 1995.

U.S. Preventive Services Task Force. *Recommended immunization schedule for children.* http://www.phcs.com/healthy/immunize.html (no date)

Wilkinson, W. "Asian/Pacific Islander women and HIV: The risk is real." *Focus,* 3, 1, 3, 1992.

World Health Organization (WHO). "Statistics: AIDS toll hits 339, 250 with influx from expanded definition." *AIDS Weekly,* pp. 2–4, November 8, 1993,

Zuckerman, A. "World Health Organization Report of a W.H.O. scientific group." *Lancet,* 1, 463–465, 1983.

CHAPTER

10 Sex-Specific Issues and Concerns

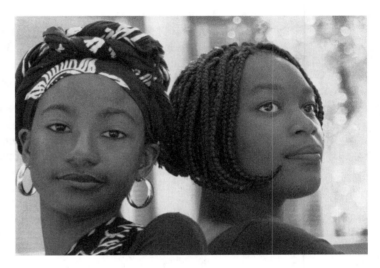

Presume not that I am the thing that I was.

—Shakespeare

Photo by Evarardo Martinez-Inzunzo.

It is important for every person to gain knowledge and understanding of his or her body and how it is related to his or her health and well-being. It is important to research the health of both men and women. This chapter explores many of the sex-specific health issues and concerns that affect both men and women. The reason for this focus is that the individual research on both men and women's sex-specific health problems is still in its early stages and, therefore, limited. Much of the past research focused on health problems without distinguishing the medical differences between men and women. Research is just beginning to concentrate on the differences between men and women by recognizing their different responses to interventions such as medications, diet, and surgery. The sex-specific medical movement parallels the limited research on minority U.S. health concerns and issues.

The last decade of the 20th century has given rise to a new focus in medicine, sex-specific medicine. In 1990, the National Institutes of Health (NIH) declared that no grant applications for studies would be accepted unless both men and women were adequately represented. In 1991, the NIH established the Office for Research on Women's Health.

One of the most intriguing long-range studies is the Women's Health Initiative (WHI), initiated in 1991. This 15-year study focuses on over 160,000 postmenopausal women between the ages of 50 and 79 years. The study is divided into four major parts:

1. The lifestyles of 100,000 women will be "observed" through periodic physical examinations and annual surveys that will focus on heart disease, cancer, osteoporosis, and other health issues.
2. A number of women will be involved in a randomized hormone replacement therapy (HRT) trial to determine the benefits and risks of this therapy.
3. The effects of a low-fat, high-fiber, and high-fruit-and-vegetable diet on women will be studied to determine its relationship to breast and colon cancer rates.
4. The effects of calcium and vitamin D supplements on women will be evaluated to determine their relationship to osteoporosis and colon cancer risks.

Because of the WHI, other projects, such as the Study of Women's Health across the Nation (SWAN) for younger women between the ages of 40 and 55 was inaugurated in 1995. The focus of the study is to help determine the connections between women's hormonal and menstrual changes and the onset of such common chronic diseases as arthritis, hypertension, diabetes, heart disease, and osteoporosis. This study is also unique because it deliberately includes African Americans, Hispanic Americans, and Asian Americans. Corporations have also teamed with different universities to study gender-based medicine. It will be a few years before some of the questions concerning gender-based medicine will be answered, but the impetus towards recognizing health similarities and differences between the sexes has begun.

The remainder of this chapter is divided into the following areas: (1) sex-specific health problems for women, and (2) sex-specific problems for men.

Sex-Specific Health Problems for Women

This section of the chapter is divided into the following five areas: the monthly cycle, vaginal infections and irritations, the uterus, cervical dysplasia and cancer, infant and maternal mortality, other women's health issues, fertility control, and contraceptive use.

The Monthly Cycle

Menstrual Cramps (dysmenorrhea).   Menstruation is a regular event in a woman's life. It usually begins (menarche) at about ages 12–13 and continues until a woman is about 50 years old (menopause). Menstruation, sometimes referred to as the "period," is the monthly bleeding that occurs as part of a woman's reproductive cycle. Some women have mild to severe cramps associated with menstruation. *Dysmenorrhea* is the medical term for painful menstrual cramps. Menstrual cramping is not premenstrual syndrome (PMS), but can be a symptom of PMS (PMS is discussed in the next section of this chapter). More than half of menstruating women have cramps associated with their periods. The amount of discomfort varies from woman to woman. Some women hardly even know they are. their menstrual period while others become incapacitated. Symptoms can include cran. like spasms, lower back and leg pain, dizziness or nausea, general achiness, vomiting, and constipation or diarrhea. Some women describe cramps as a dull ache or sense of pressure in the lower abdomen. Many women have cramps severe enough to keep them home from school and work.

The uterus is a muscle. Like all muscles, it contracts and relaxes. During menstruation, the uterus contracts more strongly than at other times of the month. The contractions produce the cramps. Just as the uterus contracts to open the cervix (neck of the uterus) and push out a baby, it contracts to expel menstrual blood.

There are two types of dysmenorrhea, *primary* and *secondary*. Primary dysmenorrhea occurs in women who have higher levels of prostaglandins and this is thought to be what causes more intense muscle spasms. The contractions are caused by prostaglandin hormones, natural substances made by cells in the wall of the uterus and other parts of the body. Prostaglandins made in the uterus make the muscle of the uterus contact. When the contractions are too strong and frequent, the blood supply of the uterus is cut off temporarily. This deprives the muscle of oxygen, causing pain. Secondary dysmenorrhea may be caused by underlying problems such as, endometriosis, tumors, and fallopian tube infection.

Menstrual Bleeding and Toxic Shock Syndrome.   The amount of bleeding varies from woman to woman, but if you're bleeding excessively—soaking one or more tampons or pads an hour—you should see a doctor. If a woman is expelling blood clots during her period, she is not in danger (Rarick, 1997). Women who use tampons should be aware of toxic shock syndrome, or TSS, a rare but serious, and sometimes fatal, disease associated with tampon use. Because TSS mostly affects 15-to-19-year-olds, it's especially important for teenagers to know the following signs (Rarick, 1997):

Sudden fever over 102 degrees Fahrenheit
Vomiting
Diarrhea
Dizziness, fainting, or near fainting when standing up
A rash that looks like a sunburn

Treatment of Primary Dysmenorrhea.   The first important step in treatment is to see a gynecologist to rule out any underlying disease or anatomical abnormality as the cause of dysmenorrhea. If cramps are mild and unobtrusive in a woman's life, she may not need any treatment. However, if primary dysmenorrhea interferes with work, school, or sleep, medications may be recommended. Menstrual cramps can be treated with prescription anti-prostaglandin medications that prevent the formation of the prostaglandins that cause menstrual cramps. Analgesic and anti-inflammatory drugs such as aspirin and ibuprofen can be used to relieve pain by reducing the production of prostaglandins. Oral contraceptives often relieve or reduce the pain of primary dysmenorrhea. Birth control pills reduce menstrual cramping by preventing the lining of the uterus from building up so much, so there's less bleeding. This results in less prostaglandin production and blood vessel narrowing, because there's less lining to separate, and fewer contractions, because there's less tissue to push out (Rarick, 1997).

Premenstrual Syndrome (PMS). Premenstrual syndrome is not menstrual cramps, and many articles do not always distinguish between the two. Some women with PMS have completely pain-free menstrual periods. Many women with severe cramps have no premenstrual distress. Menstrual cramps are caused by excess prostaglandin hormones that result in uterine contractions and cramping. Researchers have not been able to identify a specific cause for PMS. PMS appears to be multifactoral and must be approached holistically.

Premenstrual syndrome involves a group of symptoms, both physical and emotional. PMS refers to the time of the month that the symptoms appear, prior to the onset of menstruation. It also improves shortly after the onset of menstrual bleeding. PMS occurs in 30 percent to 40 percent of all women 19 to 45 years of age. The highest risk group in women are between the ages of 25 to 35 (Health Education Associates, 1990). Some 50 million women suffer from PMS in the United States.

Symptoms. The symptoms of PMS range in severity from compulsive behavior, a craving for sweets and/or salty foods, headache, depression, irritability, to fatigue and insomnia. Some people have described a common sign of PMS as a Ms. Jekyll to Ms. Hyde personality change. Many women become very frustrated from not being able to control their emotions and reactions to the situations occurring during that period. PMS can negatively affect family and work relationships. In addition, PMS may also have a significant impact on a woman's daily life because symptoms may lead to absence from school or work. For some patients, PMS is so severe that it causes suicidal and homicidal feelings that may be acted on.

One hundred and fifty to more than two hundred symptoms have been reported to be attributed to PMS. Patients normally report 30 to 40 multisymptom complaints during any single cycle (Premenstrual Syndrome, 1997). Listed below are some commonly reported symptoms of PMS sufferers (Health Education Associates, 1990; Premenstrual Syndrome, 1997):

diarrhea/constipation	anxiety
headache	pimples/acne
fainting	chest pain
weight gain/loss	depression
loneliness	insomnia
body aches	craving sweets
irritability	panic attacks
edema	forgetfulness
uncontrollable crying	feelings of paranoia
abdominal bloating	rapid heart rate
dizziness	clumsiness
sensations of prickly skin	extreme resentment
breast swelling/tenderness	mood swings
fatigue	shortness of breath
joint pain	change in vision
loss of emotional control	abdominal bloating
emotional outbursts	

Causes of PMS.   The cause of PMS is still not clearly understood. Health Education Associates (1990) reported two possible theories: (1) PMS appears to be due to an imbalance of the two female hormones, estrogen and progesterone, and (2) it may be due to a nutritional deficiency, a deficiency of the mineral magnesium and vitamin B_6.

Northrup (1994) summarized a series of nutritional factors that contribute to PMS. She reported that women with PMS tend to have the following nutritional and physiological characteristics: (1) High consumption of dairy products, caffeine, refined sugars, and animal fat, (2) low consumption of whole grains, vegetables, vitamins C and E and the minerals selenium and magnesium, and (3) high blood levels of estrogen, excessive body weight, and inadequate exposure to natural sunlight (p. 136–137).

Diagnosis and Treatment.   Diagnosis is difficult because PMS has so many symptoms and no clear cause. Women should chart their symptoms for three months and fill out a PMS evaluation questionnaire. When seeking a professional, a woman should look for a specialist in PMS, preferably one who treats PMS with nutrition therapy.

Vitamin B_6 and oral contraceptives are the most commonly used medications. At the same time, nutritional recommendations of increasing vitamin and mineral intake, a low-fat, high complex carbohydrate diet, and the elimination of caffeine, salt, alcohol, refined sugar, and refined flour products should be followed. In addition, a woman should exercise more and practice relaxation techniques to help reduce the symptoms of PMS. For women who suffer seasonal affective disorder (SAD), exposure to full spectrum light for two hours each evening and morning from either natural light or a full spectrum lighting source is recommended. In summary, the treatment of premenstrual syndrome starts with a better understanding of the symptoms and possible causes, enabling a woman to better plan her life and activities when PMS occurs.

Menopause.   Menopause is the point along the aging process that is marked by the cessation of menses or the monthly menstrual cycle. At this point, the ovaries cease the production of mature ova (eggs). Estrogen output slows down, although the ovaries do continue some estrogen production. The average age of menopause is about 52, with a range of 45 to 55 (Northrup, 1994). There is a strong tendency for a woman's menopause to occur at about the same time her mother's did. The years surrounding menopause are known as the *climacteric*. The climacteric is a process and not an "event" (Northrup, 1994). It takes place over six to ten years. Menopause usually does not start with a complete cessation of menses. It is often sporadic in the beginning: periods may stop for several months and then return. Periods may also vary in intensity and flow from light to heavy. Most women tend to have lighter periods that gradually become further apart until they cease altogether. However, some women simply stop having periods and have no symptoms. Others experience a variety of symptoms, from hot flashes, sweats, insomnia, tingling of the hands and feet, to fatigue and vaginal dryness.

Our culture has given the word *menopause* many meanings. The negative stereotype suggests that menopausal women are upset, capricious, impulsive, irrational, and depressed (Rosen and Rosen, 1981). It has also been suggested that our culture mistakenly views menopause as a time of decreased physical vigor, and a period when "femininity" declines. Finally, the menopausal woman is mistakenly thought to have lost her capacity and desire for sexual activity.

It is important to note that menopause and the "change of life" are often thought to be synonymous terms. They are not. The word *menopause* refers to the cessation of menses, while the change of life represents the sum total of all normal hormonal readjustments, from a gradual decline in estrogen production to the body's adaptation when it reaches a new and different state of hormonal balance (Lanson, 1977).

Hot flashes are vasomotor flushes and are experienced by 80 to 90 percent of American women during the menopausal years (Northrup, 1994). Hormones influence the vasomotor system, so as hormone levels fluctuate during menopause, the diameter of blood vessels may change. Hot flashes are related to the lower estrogen levels that occur during the climacteric. Rapid dilation of the vessels may cause the woman to experience a rush of heat. Hot flashes can occur several times a day and during sleep. They were once thought to be imaginary, but actual skin temperature changes do take place. Hot flashes are characterized by a feeling of sweating, usually involving the head and neck to a great degree. In one moment a woman may feel cool and comfortable and in the next hot and uncomfortable. During sleep, she may wake up sweating with the sheets soaked, and within a few minutes need blankets because she is too cold.

Some menopausal women complain of vaginal dryness and thinning, which cause irritation (Northrup, 1994). These changes result from a decrease in circulating hormones. The vaginal mucosa becomes thinner. Both the length and width of the vagina decreases, and these changes contribute to diminished expansive ability of the inner vagina during sexual arousal (Crooks & Baur, 1980). Crooks and Baur also reported that the vagina may also have diminished lubrication during the sexual response, which can lead to uncomfortable and painful intercourse and cause irritation and increased susceptibility of infection. Artificial lubricants may provide a satisfactory solution.

Treatment.   Treatment for menopause falls into three basic categories: estrogen replacement, natural progesterone, and nutritional treatment. Estrogen replacement therapy (ERT) can be very helpful to some women by controlling hot flashes and vaginal dryness. Current research suggests that a menopausal woman may wish to evaluate the potential benefits and risks of ERT against symptoms of hormone deficiency (Crooks & Baur, 1980).

Natural progesterone, provided as a skin cream or capsule, has been used by many women to alleviate the symptoms of hot flashes and headache. Nutritional treatment involves eliminating sugar, caffeine, and alcohol and following a high complex carbohydrate, low-fat diet. Many women have also been helped by the use of various herbal preparations, in particular, Chinese herbal remedies. Finally, many women who exercise regularly, practice meditation or relaxation techniques, and/or use acupuncture have an easier time going through menopause.

Vaginal Infections and Irritations

Vaginitis.   *Vaginitis* is a general term that indicates an inflammation (*itis*) of the vagina characterized by discharge, irritation, and/or itching. There are a variety of different organisms that can cause vaginitis, so the cause of vaginitis cannot always be adequately determined solely on the basis of symptoms or a physical examination. Laboratory tests may be required for correct diagnosis.

Just about every woman is susceptible to a vaginal infection at some point in her life. Common organisms that produce infection under the right circumstances are gardnerella, trichomonas, and yeast. The vagina normally contains many different microorganisms. Yeast and gardnerella, for example, normally lie in the vagina. These organisms are usually in balance within the vagina and cause no problem. Only when the environment or flora within the vagina are disrupted will an infection occur.

Monilia (yeast infection, vuvlovaginal candidiasis (VVC)).   The yeast infection is the most prevalent and perhaps the most stubborn to treat. It has been estimated that approximately 75 percent of all women will experience at least one episode of monilia during their life time (U.S. Department of Health and Human Services, 1992). Monilia is caused by an overabundance or overgrowth of yeast cells (primarily *Candida albicans*) that are normal vaginal inhabitants and part of the natural *flora* of the vagina of most women. The yeast cells are also found in the mouth and intestines of both sexes. All of these areas are potential sources of vaginal infection or reinfection. However, certain conditions must exist before growth and propagation occur, otherwise the yeast (monilia) remains unobtrusive.

Symptoms.   The most frequent symptoms of monilia are itching, burning, and irritation of the vagina. For many women, the itching is almost intolerable, The itching, of course, is followed by scratching, and an itch–scratch cycle begins. As this cycle continues, the labial structures surrounding the opening of the vagina become inflamed and swollen. Lesions in the skin from excessive scratching can invite secondary infections and cause a burning sensation when urine comes into contact with the raw and irritated tissues during urination. Pain in the labial area during intercourse is also common when a woman has monilia.

An abnormal vaginal discharge produced by this infection may also be seen but the amount will vary from woman to woman. In some cases it will be minimal or not present at all and for others it may be profuse. The discharge is typically described as a cottage cheese, curdlike substance that is whitish in color mixed with a watery discharge that may be seen at the vaginal opening (Lanson, 1980). Male partners of women with monilia usually do not experience any symptoms of the infection. On occasion, a male may feel a transient rash and burning sensation of the penis after intercourse. These symptoms disappear over a short period of time.

Causes of Fungal Flare-Ups.   Many things, including oral contraceptives, increased blood sugar levels, pregnancy, antibiotics, and various unknown factors, are related to monilia (Northrup, 1994). Birth control pills and pregnancy raise estrogen levels in a woman. Estrogen, in turn, causes glycogen to be deposited within the vaginal cells. Higher estrogen levels will affect the balance of the internal environment or flora of the vagina by increasing vaginal cellular glycogen. The fungus grows, multiples, and thrives in a glycogen-rich environment. On occasion, a persistent vaginal infection may even be aggravated by an excessive intake of sweets. During pregnancy, vaginal yeast infections are common but usually disappear after delivery.

The use of antibiotics has also been closely correlated with monilia. One theory is that the antibiotics suppress the normal protective vaginal bacteria that normally exert an antifungal effect, although the exact mechanism by which antibiotics cause monilia is not completely understood (Lanson, 1980). Other factors that may increase the incidence of monilia include the use of douches, perfumed feminine hygiene sprays, tight, poorly venti-lated clothing and underwear, and not drying carefully enough in the vaginal area after bathing. Almost anything that can disrupt the normal balance of the environment or flora within the vagina has the potential of causing monilia.

Diagnosis and Treatment.   Diagnosis should be done through microscopic examination of vaginal secretions for evidence of yeast forms. Treatment varies from antifungal vaginal creams and suppositories to oral antifungal drugs (U.S. Department of Health and Human Services, 1992). Condoms, switching to low-dose estrogen oral contraceptives, wearing cotton rather than nylon underwear to allow proper ventilation, and drying carefully in the vaginal area after bathing are some preventive measures to help reduce the possibility of infection or reinfection.

Gardnerella Vaginalis (bacterial vaginosis, haemophilus vaginalis, corynebacte-rium vaginale, nonspecific vaginitis).   Bacterial vaginosis (BV) is a common cause of vaginitis symptoms among women of childbearing age (U.S. Department of Health and Human Services, 1992). BV is due to a change in the balance among different types of bac-teria in the vagina. Instead of the normal predominance of lactobacillus bacteria, increased numbers of bacterial organisms such as *Gardnerella vaginalis* begin to upset the balance of the vaginal flora. When present in large numbers, gardnerella causes annoying symptoms of an abnormal vaginal discharge that is slightly grayish or yellowish in color, with a fishy odor, and especially noticeable after intercourse (University of Toronto Sexual Education & Peer Counseling Office, 1996). These symptoms may also be accompanied by painful urination, irritation, and itching of the female genital area. However, nearly half the women with clinical signs of BV report no symptoms. It is especially rare in males. If symptoms do appear in the male, they appear as a mild itching or burning with urination or unusual discharge from the penis.

Gardnerella can be spread by genital contact with an infected person. Use of an intrauterine device may also increase the risk of acquiring bacterial vaginosis. Some common causes include (Northrup, 1994; University of Toronto, 1996):

Repeated intercourse over a short period of time. The repeated deposit of the alkaline fluid from the male prostate gland can disrupt the pH balance of the vagina.

Prolonged dampness (sweating) in the vulvar area. Exercising in restrictive and non-absorbent clothing can lead to infection.

Chemical irritants (bubble bath, vaginal deodorants, chemicals in pools and spas) and antibiotics can also disrupt the balance of the vaginal flora.

Diagnosis and Treatment.   A sample of vaginal fluid can be examined under a micro-scope to detect the presence of the organisms associated with BV. Treatment may be nec-essary if the symptoms are unpleasant or bothersome. Some women choose not to be treated if they are asymptomatic or have few symptoms. The long-term effects of this infection are presently unknown. If treatment is requested, antibiotics are available. A homeopathic remedy that includes douching with vinegar (1 tsp.) and warm water (1 qt.) in conjunction with insertion of yogurt (lactobacillus acidophilus) capsules in the vagina for five to seven nights is an alternative to antibiotics (Northrup, 1994). The yogurt capsules can be purchased at any health food store.

Trichomonas Vaginalis (trichomoniasis, "trich," or "TV"). *Trichomonas vaginalis* is a common sexually transmitted infection that affects 2 to 3 million Americans a year (Donnelly, n. d.). TV is a one-celled microscopic protozoan (parasite) that can produce a copious, watery, malodorous, yellowish or greenish-white discharge in women (UCLA Student Health Services, n. d.). The associated itching, soreness, and inflammation of the vaginal opening and vulva make this infection very annoying and uncomfortable. Males with trichomoniasis usually do not experience symptoms. However, when symptoms do appear, they include a puslike or watery penile drip, pain on urination, and a tingly feeling inside the penis.

The protozoan *Trichomonas vaginalis* is not a normal inhabitant of the vagina or any other area in the human body nor is it acquired by either fecal contamination of the vagina or by oral–genital sex. Condoms may help prevent the spread of this infection. Trichomoniasis, like many other sexually transmitted infections, often occurs without symptoms. Because many victims are asymptomatic, the majority of TV vaginal infections are acquired through contact of sexual organs with an unknowing infected partner. When symptoms occur, they usually appear within 4 to 20 days after being infected, although symptoms can appear years after infection.

Trichomoniasis is almost always spread sexually. However, because this protozoan can survive several hours on moist objects, it can be spread by coming in contact with infected objects such as linen, towels, and toilet seats (Bod Squad, 1995). A person can also be reinfected an infinite number of times. Treatment of a case of trichonomas does not ensure immunity against future exposures. If left untreated, trichomoniasis can cause inflammation of the cervix, urethra, and the bladder. Recent studies have linked trichomoniasis to an increase risk of transmission of HIV and may cause delivery of low birthweight or premature infants (U.S. Department of Health and Human Services, 1992). Additional research is needed to explore these relationships fully.

Diagnosis and Treatment. Trichomoniasis is usually diagnosed in women by examining their vaginal fluid under a microscope. Evidence of the protozoan in vaginal or penile fluid can also be obtained from a culture growth in the laboratory. Although symptoms of trichomoniasis in men may disappear within a few weeks without treatment, they may still be infectious even without the symptoms. Therefore it is preferable to treat both partners to eliminate the parasite. Flagyl, an oral antibiotic, is often used to treat TV. This medication has side effects of nausea, vomiting, and headaches. In addition, mixing alcohol with this antibiotic can cause severe nausea and vomiting (Donnelly, n. d.).

The Uterus

Endometriosis. Endometriosis is a puzzling disease characterized by the appearance of endometrial tissue on the outside of the uterine cavity and, on rare occasions, outside of the pelvic area entirely. This tissue is histologically identical to the same tissue that is found on the inside lining of the uterus shed during the monthly menstrual cycle, thus its name comes from the word *endometrium* (Lanson, 1980). This increasingly common condition occurs when abnormal endometrial growth appears on the external surface of the ovaries, behind the uterus (cul-de-sac), fallopian tubes, ligaments that support the uterus, the area between the vagina and rectum, outer surface of the uterus, and lining of the pelvic cavity (Endometriosis Association, 1992).

The most common site of endometriosis is the ovaries. Ovarian endometriosis probably starts as a surface lesion but eventually becomes invasive and grows into the ovarian tissue. Over time, the endometrial cysts become filled with a chocolate-colored liquid. These are commonly called *chocolate cysts,* or *endometrium A* (Lanson, 1980).

Endometriosis also leads to scarring or the formation of adhesions on pelvic structures. The endometrial lesions will irritate and inflame tissue, which eventually leads to scarring. These adhesions are most commonly found in the immobile pelvic structures.

Symptoms of Endometriosis.   Unlike the lining of the uterus, endometrial tissue outside the uterus has no way of leaving the body. The result is pelvic pain, abnormal menstrual cycles, internal bleeding, inflammation of surrounding areas, formation of scar tissue, the degeneration of the blood and tissue shed from the growths, and infertility.

The symptoms of endometriosis vary from one patient to another. The magnitude of the symptoms may not correlate with the extent of the disease. For example, a patient with severe disease may have very little pain. Nor is the amount of pain necessarily related to the extent or size of growths. Tiny growths (called *petechiae*) are known to cause great discomfort in most patients (Endometriosis Association, 1992). The most common symptom is pelvic pain before and during periods (usually worse than "normal" menstrual cramps) and during and after sexual intercourse. Other symptoms are abnormal bleeding, spotting prior to periods, low back pain during periods, diarrhea or constipation and other intestinal upset with periods, painful bowel movements with periods, and infertility. The symptoms, of course, will vary from woman to woman.

How Common Is Endometriosis?   Endometriosis is one of the most common gynecological diseases. With the recent use of laparoscopy, diagnosis of endometriosis in women in their mid to late twenties is very common. Endometriosis occurs in millions of women in the United States and has been estimated to affect about 5 percent of women who are in their reproductive years. However, in women with severe menstrual cramps, the incidence of endometriosis may be as high as 25 to 35 percent (Babahnia, 1990; Perloe, 1996). The women who are most susceptible to endometriosis are:

Women who are in their reproductive years; the disease is normally not seen in women before age 15 or after menopause,

Women who have a sister or mother who has already had endometriosis; there is a familial tendency with endometriosis, but, having a sister with endometriosis does not guarantee that you will have it too;

Women who are Caucasian; the prevalence of endometriosis in white American women is twice that of African American women, but this may be due to the fact that African American women in the past were not getting appropriate medical care; women of color should not believe that they are not at risk for this disease;

Women who begin their menstrual cycle at a significantly younger age;

Women who have a regular cycle as opposed to women who have irregular menstrual cycles;

Women who have severe menstrual cramps and women who have prolonged menstrual flows; these two symptoms, of course, may be caused by the endometriosis and are not precursors for the condition.

Some Common Myths about Endometriosis

Intercourse during the menstrual cycle increases the risk of endometriosis: There are no studies to bear this out. This has not been proven.

There is a relationship between endometriosis and the use of tampons: There has been no scientific evidence to indicate that the use of tampons or douching increases the risk of endometriosis.

"Career" women have a higher risk of developing endometriosis: There is no evidence to bear this out. This myth developed because women with careers are more likely to seek medical diagnosis and care.

Etiology of Endometriosis. There are a number of theories as to how endometriosis is developed, but the most commonly mentioned theory is the retrograde menstruation theory. Many researchers believe the theory of retrograde menstruation is the main cause for the initiation of endometriosis. This theory posits that, during menstruation, some of the menstrual tissue backs up through the fallopian tubes, implants in the abdomen, and grows (Sampson, 1984). Since retrograde menstruation probably occurs in every menstruating woman at some point, this doesn't explain why some women get the disease and others do not. Other theories suggest the spread of endometrial cells through lymphatic channels or blood vessels may be a congenital condition present at birth.

Diagnosis. Endometriosis of the pelvic cavity can be diagnosed only by laparoscopy, a minor surgical procedure done under anesthesia in which a laparoscope (a thin tube with a light in it) is inserted into the abdomen to explore the abdominal and pelvic areas (Babahnia, 1990). Once endometriosis is identified, the physician and patient can discuss long-range treatment based on the extent and location of the endometriosis.

Treatment. Treatment for endometriosis has varied over the years but no sure cure has yet been discovered. Treatments range from hormone therapy, minor surgery through the use of lasers, cautery, or small surgical instruments, to radical surgery involving hysterectomy and removal of all growths and the ovaries (Tureck, 1997; Northrup, 1994). Because each patient is different and each condition is unique to that individual, no one single approach is acceptable for all women. Menopause also generally ends the activity of mild or moderate endometriosis.

Fibroid Tumors. Fibroid tumors (*uterine fibroids, myomas, leiomyomas*) are benign (noncancerous) growths of the uterus. They grow in various locations on and within the uterine wall itself or in the uterine cavity. They are found in about 30 percent of women over the age of 30 (Bradley, 1996). They are usually detected during a routine pelvic examination, and the vast majority of cases will rarely produce symptoms if the tumors are small. In fact, many women are unaware that they have them until they are discovered during a routine pelvic examination. Whether a fibroid is symptomatic has to do with its size and location within the uterus. The size of a single fibroid may be smaller than a pea or larger than a melon. Sometimes they are single or multiple fibroids that vary in size.

The fibroids develop from cells in the wall and are composed of muscle cells, not fibrous tissue. No one knows what causes the growth of fibroids but evidence suggests that their growth is tied to estrogen. These benign tumors appear to need estrogen for maintenance, as they are extremely rare before puberty or after menopause, and they sometimes grow rapidly in pregnancy (Lanson, 1980). Also, when a woman takes certain birth control pills, which increases estrogen levels, the normally slow growth rate of the fibroid often accelerates.

The size of fibroids is gauged by comparing them to the size of the uterus containing a fetus of that size. Thus, a woman will be told that she has a 14-week-size fibroid (e.g., a large grapefruit), if her uterus is as big as it would be if she were 14 weeks pregnant (Lanson, 1980). Fibroids are hard, white, gristly tissue with a spiral-like pattern. In some instances, a fibroid tumor can outgrow the size of the uterus.

Fibroids can also degenerate in size. If a rapidly growing or large fibroid outgrows its blood supply, the center of the fibroid cannot get enough oxygen from the blood, and the tissue dies. The fibroid will slowly degenerate and sometimes disappear completely. This process is usually accompanied by a few weeks of pain, but it is not a life-threatening situation.

Symptoms.   Most women do not have symptoms from their fibroids. Fibroids that cause no symptoms should be observed and the patient followed conservatively. However, when a fibroid is symptomatic, the physician and patient must work closely together to determine the best option for care.

Bleeding.   Fibroids that grow into the uterine lining itself often cause heavy or irregular bleeding, resulting in anemia and fatigue. As the fibroids expand, they can stretch the endometrium, causing heavy menstrual bleeding and severe pain as the uterus tries to expel the mass (Bradley, 1997).

Pelvic pressure.   Sometimes the fibroid causes symptoms by pushing into adjacent organs, such as the bladder or rectum. As this slow process evolves, the patient may become aware of a "heaviness" or "pressure" in the lower back or abdomen. It may also result in the need for urinary frequency or having to void in frequent small amounts. Pressure on the rectum will contribute to constipation or a sensation of not having a completely emptied bowel. Large fibroids can also cause discomfort with intercourse and increased menstrual pain.

Some Common Facts about Fibroid Tumors (Perloe, 1996; Lanson. 1980; Bradley, 1997)

No one knows what causes fibroid tumors.

Fibroid tumors are the most common type of abnormal pelvic growth in women and account for about one-third of all gynecological hospital admissions. They are the number one reason for hysterectomies in the United States (Hutchins, 1990).

Every year over 650,000 American women undergo hysterectomies of which 40 percent are related to fibroid tumors.

Fibroid tumors are 3 to 9 times more common in African American women than Caucasians.

Fibroid tumors are almost never cancerous.

Fibroids can run in families, but a family predisposition is not an inevitable "sentence" that one will get the disease.

Fibroids can interfere with pregnancy depending on their size and location. Fibroids can result in miscarriage or even infertility. However, many women with fibroids have normal labor and delivery without any problems. Whether or not fibroids should be removed before attempting pregnancy should be a decision between a women and her doctor after all the options have been discussed.

Fibroids do grow sometimes, but not always. Sometimes they go away completely on their own.

Fibroids can change size during ovulation and just before the menstrual period begins. They can also grow during times of stress.

Treatment.   Do fibroids need to be removed? For the vast majority of patients, the answer is definitely no. However, when symptoms create problems for the patient, then a number of treatment options are available to both the patient and physician. Listed below are some recommendations for treatment.

Observation or "watch and wait."   If the fibroid uterus is "silent," and no symptoms are present, conservative observation is appropriate. The patient should have a pelvic exam every six months to a year, depending on her situation.

Hormone therapy.   The use of hormones is considered temporary therapy because, once stopped, the fibroid uterus will return to its pretreatment status within six months. Hormone therapy provides a temporary relief period in which the patient and doctor can make decisions about the future.

Hysteroscopic submucous resection.   A small telescopelike instrument is introduced through the cervix, which allows certain tumors found in the inner lining of the uterus to be shaved down to a smaller size. This procedure is appropriate for those women who want to maintain their fertility. This procedure is limited to certain tumors, determined by their location.

Myomectomy.   This is the process of surgically removing the individual fibroids. This can be accomplished using a minimally invasive technique called *laparoscopy*. The disadvantages are that postoperative adhesions may develop, the procedure is very lengthy, there is a high recurrence rate of fibroids, and it is difficult to be sure that all tumors are removed, especially those within the uterine wall.

Hysterectomy.   A hysterectomy should be considered only after a patient has had a history of both fibroid tumors and medical consultations. Only when situations such as prolonged and excessive bleeding, extremely large protrusions, consistency in unpredictable bleeding, and excessive pressure on the bladder occur should hysterectomy be considered. A woman must be both physically and emotionally prepared for a hysterectomy because it will have long-term effects on her physical and emotional health as well as her body image.

Cervical Dysplasia and Cervical Cancer

For many young women, cancer is an abstraction. But a precancerous condition called *dysplasia of the cervix,* detectable by a Pap test, is increasing among young women in their late teens and early twenties. Dysplasia is easily treatable and rarely recurs if caught early. But left untreated, approximately 30 percent of moderate to severe cases eventually develop into cervical cancer later in life. In 1995, an estimated 103,600 new cases of uterine cancer were diagnosed in the United States. Thirty percent of the 10,700 uterine cancer deaths in 1995 affected the cervix.

Dysplasia is a condition in which the cells of the cervix change in either shape or size. It is a premalignant or precancerous change to the cells of the cervix. The medical term for dysplasia is *cervical intra-epithelial neoplasia* (CIN). CIN-I is a mild cell abnormality that will, in some cases, regress without treatment. About 60 to 70 percent of mild dysplasia cells resolve on their own. CIN-I is by far the most common abnormality and is not considered a true premalignant disease by many physicians. CIN-I generally represents a tissue response to the human papilloma virus (HPV), commonly called the wart virus (Midland Family Physicians, 1996), a sexually transmitted virus responsible for most of the nearly 16,000 new cases of cervical cancer diagnosed in the United States. Several of the HPV's many different strains cause genital warts or lesions that have been linked to both dysplasia and cancer. For more information about HPV see Chapter 9's section on sexually transmitted infections.

CIN-II is a moderate abnormality, and CIN-III is a severe and premalignant lesion or a carcinoma confined to the site of origin (carcinoma in situ). Moderate and severe dysplasia are treated when they are discovered, because of their higher rates of turning into cancer. CIN-III is virtually 100 percent curable (Med Help International, n. d.). If CIN-III is not treated, cancer develops and spreads deeper into the cervix. This process may take anywhere from 6 months to 10 years. Even with early cancer or precancer, 90 percent are cured with relatively simple local treatment (GenneX, 1996). For women with HIV, who may be at greatly increased risk of developing cancer, this test should be done once every six months (ARIC, 1996). Table 10.1 reports the incidence of uterine cancer cases and deaths by race.

The incidence of cervical cancer is on the rise for Hispanic American women, in particular, among Puerto Rican women. On the other hand, many Hispanic Americans have lower than average rates of other varieties of cancer.

Risk Factors.   Having sex before age 18 or having more than three sexual partners in a lifetime increases a woman's likelihood of contracting HPV and cervical cancer. Smoking has also been linked to increased risk for cervical cancer (Midland Family Physicians, 1996).

Diagnosis.   The Pap smear is a simple test that involves collecting a small number of cervical cells and examining them for dysplasia or cancer. Although the Pap smear occasion-

TABLE 10.1   Uterine Cancer Cases and Deaths by Race

Number of cases of uterine/cervical cancer:	48,600
Number of deaths from uterine/cervical cancer:	10,700
Number of deaths from uterine/cervical cancer by race	
African American	1,904
Native American	42
Japanese and Chinese American	27
Hispanic American	292

Source: "Cancer Facts and Figures, 1995"

ally produces false negatives, it is still the best screening test available. The Pap smear is very effective for detecting dysplasia and early-stage cancer, but is not as effective for detecting cancers of the uterine lining. Early signs of uterine cancer include bleeding outside the normal menstrual period or after menopause or persistent unusual vaginal discharge (American Cancer Society, 1995).

Treatment.   When the diagnosis is dysplasia, the most common treatment is cryosurgery or the freezing of the abnormal cells. This procedure only takes about 10 minutes. There may be some watery discharge for a few days after the procedure. Laser surgery is often used in more advanced cases. Once treated, dysplasia usually does not occur. Only 5 to 10 percent of women will need additional treatment. Although medication can control symptoms, there is no cure for HPV. Cryosurgery and laser surgery do not kill off all of the virus. Some usually remain after treatment.

Infant and Maternal Mortality

Infant Mortality.   In 1990 the six leading causes of infant death were, in order, congenital anomalies, sudden infant death syndrome, disorders relating to short gestation, unspecified low birth weight, respiratory distress syndrome, and newborns affected by maternal complications of pregnancy. Except for congenital anomalies, the risk for each of these was substantially higher for black infants than for white infants, with the largest discrepancy in disorders relating to short gestation and unspecified low birth weight (National Center for Health Statistics, 1990). Black infant mortality from this cause was 3.4 times that of white infants.

Low birth weight infants—those weighing less than 2,500 grams (5 pounds, 8 ounces)—are at greater risk not only for dying during the first year of life but also for developing long-term health and neurological disabilities. Of all infants who die, about 60 percent are of low birth weight. African Americans have a greater proportion of very low birth weight babies than do whites.

Ectopic pregnancies are related to pelvic inflammatory disease and sexually transmitted diseases, both of which occur more often among poor women. Ectopic pregnancies are the leading cause of death of the mother during the first three months of pregnancy and the leading cause of death among African American women of childbearing age (McBarnette, 1988).

The issue of infant mortality in African American communities needs to be more clearly linked to women's health, nutritional status, and the high rates of both intended and unintended pregnancies among young unmarried African American women. In African American communities, more than 500,000 infants are born each year to women under 20 years of age (Carol et al., 1988). Teenage pregnancy, which is associated with high infant mortality and other serious lifestyle problems, has become a national concern. Appropriate nutrition and low usage of alcohol and cigarettes are some key preventative measures that can improve the birth status of black infants.

It is known that economic factors play a role in the excess of black infant mortality rates, but not all things can be attributed to poverty. For example, if education is used as an index, the black infant mortality rate exceeds the white rate at each level of education. In fact, blacks with some college education have higher infant mortality than whites with no more than an eighth-grade education.

Health care professionals (Institute of Medicine, 1985) have concluded that prenatal care is effective in increasing birth weight and reducing infant mortality, yet over 20 percent of white women and nearly twice as a many black women get no prenatal care during the first trimester (National Center for Health Statistics, 1990). Teenagers have even lower rates of prenatal care, some 52 percent of all women under 18 have no care during the first trimester and black teenagers have a slightly higher rate of no care, 56.7 percent (National Center for Health Statistics, 1990).

Maternal Mortality.   Maternal mortality—death from complications of pregnancy—disproportionately affects blacks. Maternal deaths result from a number of causes, including preexisting health problems aggravated by the pregnancy, pregnancy-related conditions such as pre-eclampsia, and complications of labor and delivery. For blacks the main causes of maternal mortality are ectopic pregnancy, eclampsia, toxemia, and pre-eclampsia, in that order (Hughes et al., 1988). Even though there has been a decline in maternal mortality, black women are three to four times more likely to die from complications of childbirth than white women. Black women are seven more times more likely to die as a result of preventable problems, such as anemia, and five to nine times more likely to die from anesthetic-related causes during uncomplicated deliveries (Hughes et al., 1988).

Maternal morbidity among women having cesarean sections is 12 times higher than for those having vaginal childbirth. Embolism, hypertensive disease, and obstetrical hemorrhage lead the list of causes of death in pregnancies not ending in live births. McBarnette (1988) reported that black women in the United States were three times more likely to die in childbirth (because of living conditions and inadequate access to prenatal care).

The birth rate for American Indians is almost twice the national rate. The Indian birthrate for 1987 through 1989 was 28.8 births per 1,000 population, compared with 15.9 births for the United States, all races (U.S. Indian Health Service, 1993). Native American women also have extremely high infant and maternal deaths for many of the same reasons that African American women do. Native American women are also at risk for developing gestational diabetes, glucose intolerance during pregnancy. Gestational diabetes can cause significant health risks for both the woman and the fetus and thus creates increased risk for infant mortality and morbidity.

Mexican American women have high birth rates, which would indicate the need for greater access to prenatal and postnatal care for Mexican American women and children. The birth weight pattern of Mexican Americans resembles that of upper-income, non-Hispanic whites, rather than that of comparable lower income African Americans. Distinctive cultural factors, such as less frequent smoking and lower alcohol intake by Hispanic women, probably contribute to this counterintuitive finding. Given the lower education, lower income, and limited access to health care of Latinas, one would expect that Latina birth outcomes would be substantially more negative than African Americans or Anglos. In fact just the opposite has been consistently observed.

Other Women's Health Issues

Fibrocystic Breast Disease (mammary dysplasia, chronic cystic mastitis).   Fibrocystic breast disease, also known as mammary dysplasia and chronic cystic mastitis, is the most common disease of the female breast, affecting up to one-third of women between the ages of 30 and 50 (Saint Francis Hospital, n. d.). Many physicians, in fact, believe it is a normal variant of the breast. Many physicians do not like to call it a disease and prefer the term *fibrocystic breast "condition"* or *"change"* (American House Call Network, 1996). The breasts have a fibrous or cystic feeling. For some women, the first symptom will be finding one or more cysts or nodules in the breast. This fibrocystic condition may affect one or both breasts. The nodules or cysts are nonmalignant but are often tender and painful (Lanson, 1980). Most women with chronic fibrocystic breast changes are not at higher risk for developing breast cancer (Saint Francis Hospital, n. d.). However, if the breast conditions contain abnormal breast cells, the probability of cancer is much higher.

The cause of fibrocystic tissue is not completely understood but is believed to be a result of estrogen changes during the menstrual cycle. The hormonal relationship is based on the fact that it is most common in women 30 to 50 years old, rare in postmenopausal women, and the incidence is lower in women taking oral contraceptives. In addition, the pain is usually worse prior to the menstrual period when estrogen levels are dropping. Many clinicians also believe there is a link to dietary fat, smoking, and caffeine intake (Rx Med, n. d.). Excessive intake of these substances is associated with a higher incidence and greater extent of fibrocystic breast disease.

Signs and Symptoms.   Fibrocystic breast disease is associated with the appearance of a dense, irregular,3 only and bumpy "cobblestone" consistency in the breast tissue (Lanson, 1980). The cysts can be either solitary or multiple and are usually found in the outer quadrants of the breast. The breasts become swollen, tender, and painful during premenstrual periods. The symptoms may range from mild to severe and typically reach their peak just before the menstrual period and improve immediately after the menstrual period.

Diagnosis and Prevention.   Diagnostic tests include the mammogram, ultrasonograph, and surgical diagnostic procedures such as biopsy or cyst aspiration (Rx Med, n. d.; Saint Francis Hospital, n. d.). Regular breast self-examination is also important in monitoring the size of the cysts. Performing a breast self-examination at the same time each month, and using the same technique, will give a woman the same feel of the breast from month to month, help her become familiar with the feel and location of the cysts, and give her a reference or guide for each monthly exam. Any changes should be reported to the physician immediately. She should also reduce dietary fat, excessive caffeine, and avoid cigarettes.

Fibrocystic breast disease is presently incurable, but it does not jeopardize health. Some cysts can be aspirated in the doctor's office, causing the lump to disappear. In severe cases, doctors may utilize drug therapy.

Pelvic Inflammatory Disease (PID).   Pelvic inflammatory disease (PID) is a general term used to refer to infection of the uterus, fallopian tubes, or ovaries. PID can be acute (short-term) or chronic (long-term) and may have symptoms ranging from asymptomatic (no symptoms) to very severe. PID can lead to infertility, tubal pregnancy, chronic pelvic pain, and even death (Health Trek, 1996).

The incidence of acute PID has risen to an estimated one million diagnosed cases per year in the United States (Centers for Disease Control Wonder, n. d.). This, of course, does not include the millions of cases that are believed to go undiscovered. About 1 in 7 women are treated for PID at some point in their lives. Of the one million who contract PID each year in the United States, about 250,000 are hospitalized, many require surgery because of severe infection, and more than 150 women will die from this infection (Pelvic Inflammatory Disease, n. d.).

Causes of PID.   PID usually affects sexually active women during their childbearing years. It occurs when disease-causing microorganisms move toward the reproductive organs from the vagina and the cervix. Many cases of PID are thought to develop from sexually transmitted diseases, in particular, gonorrhea (*Neisseria gonorrhea*) and chlamydia (*Chlamydia trachomatis*). These infectious organisms attach themselves to sperm during intercourse, enabling travel into the uterus and fallopian tubes. *Mycoplasma hominis* and other such bacteria can also cause PID. The organisms may also gain easier access during menstruation.

Symptoms.   Not all women who develop PID will experience the same physical symptoms. Possible symptoms include the following:

> No symptoms;
> Lower abdominal pain;
> Elevated temperature (fever);
> Vaginal discharge that may include bleeding;
> Vaginal discharge with an unpleasant odor;
> Chills;
> Nausea and/or vomiting;
> Difficult or painful urination;
> Painful or difficult sexual intercourse;
> Spotting or pain between menstrual periods;
> Unusually long or painful periods.

> (University of Illinois at Urbana-Champaign Health Resource Center, 1996; Health Trek, 1996)

Who Is At-Risk of Developing PID.   While any woman can develop PID, certain women share characteristics of higher risk. These risk factors include:

Women under 25 years old;

Women who have had or have more than one sexual partner;

Women who use an intrauterine device (IUD) for contraception (especially during the first few months after insertion);

A woman whose partner has more than one sexual partner;

Women who have a previous history of a sexually transmitted disease;

Women who have a previous history of PID;

A woman who has a sexual partner with gonorrhea or nongonococcal urethritis (NGU is an inflammation of the urethra, generally caused by chlamydia).

(University of Illinois at Urbana-Champaign Health Resource Center, 1996; Planned Parenthood League of Massachusetts, n. d.)

Reducing the Risk of PID.   Women can reduce their risk of PID by:

Limiting the number of sexual partners;

Having the male partner use a condom to help protect against sexually transmitted disease (the use of a spermicide and diaphragm may also protect against the spread of sexually transmitted infectious diseases);

Having regular pelvic examinations;

Being aware of the symptoms of PID.

Diagnosis and Treatment.   PID is diagnosed through an oral or written assessment and a physical examination that includes a number of lab tests. The medical practitioner will usually obtain a written or oral history of the patient and the problems that she is experiencing. The next step is a physical examination, which will include a pelvic examination, at which time the fallopian tubes and ovaries are also checked for tenderness and pain. Special laboratory tests, such as the pap test, gonorrhea and chlamydia cultures, urine analysis (for bacteria, blood and white cells), and a blood test for elevated white cell count (indicates infection) may be included. Under special circumstances diagnosis may require laparoscopy or ultrasound.

Treatment for PID includes antibiotics, bed rest, and abstinence from sexual intercourse until the follow-up examination and laboratory test results are completed. Antibiotics alone are usually enough to get rid of the infection. PID can be caused by more than one type of organism, and no one antibiotic kills all of the organisms thought to cause PID. For this reason, two or more antibiotics are usually prescribed. The two most common antibiotics are ampicillin and tetracycline (Health Trek, n. d.)

All recent sexual partners should also be examined by the doctor and treated if they have gonorrhea and/or chlamydia infection. A woman should not have sex again until her sexual partners have been treated.

Osteoporosis.   Osteoporosis, sometimes called "brittle bone disease," is a condition in which bones become weakened due to calcium loss. Because bone loss in later life appears to be a natural process, osteoporosis is experienced with the aging process. Osteoporosis is a common condition affecting 20 million Americans (Women's Health, 1997). Both men and women can develop osteoporosis, but excessive calcium loss is seen more often in elderly women. The reason is that osteoporosis is gender-, genetic-, and hormonally related. Women have less bone mass or density than men and the reduction of the sex hormone estrogen after menopause effects new bone development. There is also a strong tendency for osteoporosis to occur in individuals who have a family history of it. Other risk factors associated with osteoporosis are: (1) women who reach menopause before the age of 50, (2) white American ancestry, (3) thin, small-boned women, and (4) cigarette smokers (Women's Health, 1997).

Although osteoporosis is usually associated with the elderly, young male and female athletes whose caloric intake is inadequate, teenagers on junk food diets, and young women suffering from eating disorders can develop osteoporosis (Tortora and Grabowski, 1993). As bone strength decreases from the loss of calcium, bones become more susceptible to breaking, and osteoporosis is responsible for 1.3 million fractures of the spine, hip, and forearm each year.

Treatment.   Because bone loss in later life appears to be a natural process, the best strategy to minimize the effects of osteoporosis is to build maximally dense bones during the years of growth (Aveoli, 1984). The following three strategies are used to help build maximum bone density: (a) eating a calcium rich diet, (b) weight-bearing exercises, and (c) hormone replacement therapy after menopause. Getting enough dietary calcium is essential to preventing bone loss. The daily recommended amount for women is 1000–1500 mg of calcium (Women's Health, 1997). This is equivalent to three 8-ounce glasses of milk per day. The Women's Health organization has made some of the following dietary recommendations to help boost calcium intake.

> Drink skim or lowfat milk, which contains calcium;
> Use milk to replace part of the water in cooked cereals and soups;
> Use plain yogurt to replace mayonnaise in salad dressings and other recipes;
> Use farmers cheese, cottage cheese, or ricotta cheese as a spread on toast;
> Choose milk instead of coffee, tea, or a soft drink with meals;
> Sprinkle Parmesan cheese on vegetables, salads, soups, and popcorn,
> Choose foods with high calcium content.

Because calcium-rich diets often have a higher fat content, lowfat dieters need to be conscious of their fat intake. Before taking calcium supplements, individuals should first check with their health practitioner.

Regular impact or weight-bearing exercises, such as walking, jogging, or aerobics, stimulates bone formation and may strengthen bones and increase bone mass. Exercises such as swimming will increase fitness but do not stress (impact) the bones and have minimal effect on the increase of bone density. Hormonal replacement therapy is an effective way to prevent osteoporosis for some women.

Bladder Infections (cystitis, urinary tract infections (UTIs)).   Cystitis, an infection of the urinary bladder, is a problem that seems to occur with annoying regularity for many women. Women get bladder infections much more frequently than men. When bladder infections occur, the patient feels an urgent and frequent need to urinate, often with little result (Ryan, 1996). Many will also have symptoms of pain in the pelvic area as well as pain and a burning sensation during urination. Depending on the infection, the urine appears to be more concentrated, looks darker in color, and becomes malodorous. If not treated, the infection may spread to other organs such as the kidney, prostate, or urinary pathways. Cystitis is not a sexually transmitted disease, nor is it contagious.

Cystitis is caused by bacteria that get into the urinary tract and work their way back to the bladder to cause the infection. The bacteria can come from a variety of sources— vaginal secretions, fecal matter, or even the bloodstream. The reason that women are more susceptible to this problem is their anatomy. The urethra or urinary tract of a woman is rel- atively short, slightly over one and a half inches in length (Lanson, 1980). Furthermore, the presence of bacteria around the vulvar mucosa and the closeness of the urethral opening to the vagina enhance the potential for bacterial invasion of the bladder. If any bacteria are able to invade the urinary opening, they do not have to travel very far to reach the bladder. In contrast, the male urinary tract is much longer, with the average length from the tip of the penis to the bladder measuring about seven to eight inches (Lanson, 1980). If bacteria invade the male urethra, the body will usually respond with painful urination and the indi- vidual often seeks help before the bacteria has time to reach the bladder.

Because invading bacteria normally take a day or so to establish themselves, acute cystitis usually strikes about 30 to 36 hours after invasion. Bladder infections are quite serious and they require treatment.

Factors That Promote Cystitis:

Sexual intercourse is the most common way of introducing bacteria into the urethra. The upper wall of the female vagina is also the floor of the urethra and bladder that sits above it. The pumping action of the penis during the conventional missionary position (man-on-top) irritates these structures above the vaginal wall and pushes bacteria from the outside vulvar area into the woman's urethra and bladder. Any foreplay involving massaging of the vaginal area will also massage the urethra and push the bacteria upward through the urethra and into the bladder.

Some irritants, such as bubble bath, strong soaps, and feminine hygiene products, can irritate the urinary opening, making it easier for bacteria to invade.

Although controversial, some physicians recommend that, after urinating, women should wipe from front to back. This will wipe the bacteria that are normally present away from the bladder. Many physicians feel that the "wiping" precaution is an "old wives tale" and does not decrease the possibility of infection (Northrup, 1994). Other questionable beliefs about the cause of UTIs are wearing tight jeans, douching, oral contraception, tampons, urination before intercourse, excessive washing of the genital area, and the direction of wipe after a bowel movement. Recent research (University of Wisconsin, 1996) suggests that the above activities do not promote UTIs.

Using a diaphragm as a contraceptive device may lead to infections. It is recommended that if a woman is having repeated urinary tract infections, she should choose another method of contraception.

Chemotherapy may also contribute to bladder infections by changing the lining of the bladder and the vagina, which allows bacteria to adhere much more easily.

Preventing Bladder Infections.   There are a number of ways to help prevent this irritating and often painful condition (Ryan, 1996; Health Centre Online, 1996).

Drink plenty of fluids, which flushes bacteria out before they can get established. Drink the recommended eight glasses of water a day. If you are prone to frequent infections, 10 to 15 glasses of water may be necessary.

Urinate immediately after sexual intercourse. It may be beneficial to drink two glasses of water before sexual activity.

Abstain from intercourse while you are having symptoms.

Antibacterial medications from a physician are available. Most medications will improve the situation within one to two days.

Fertility Control

The ideal birth control method should be safe, effective, easily obtainable, unobtrusive, reversible, and inexpensive. Unfortunately, this ideal birth control method has not been developed. Although a wide variety of birth control methods are available, each has its own shortcoming. No contraceptive method other than abstinence is 100 percent effective. Each contraceptive method has a theoretical effectiveness rate if all aspects of its use are absolutely perfect. However, people make mistakes, diminishing the effectiveness of the method. This is called the "user" rate. It is a more realistic measurement of effectiveness in the real world.

Unfortunately, except for condoms and surgical sterilization (vasectomy), all birth control methods currently available must be used by women. With the options available, women must consider their medical history, personal preference, and lifestyle to determine what is right for them. Among the compromises a woman must consider are the method's effectiveness, ease of use, cost, and potential side effects and risks. Another consideration involves the possibility of acquiring AIDS and/or other sexually transmitted infections. Consequently, choosing the right birth control method requires the individual to make some degree of compromise in his or her choice.

Contraception is a specific term for any procedure that is used to prevent the fertilization of an ovum. *Birth control,* a term often used interchangeably, refers to all available contraceptive measures, as well as sterilization, the use of the intrauterine device, and abortion procedures. This section will focus only on birth control methods.

Over-the-Counter Methods

Over-the-counter methods are the least expensive of contraceptive methods but are also the least effective. There are two types of contraceptive methods that can be purchased at the drugstore: spermicides (jellies, creams, foams, films, and suppositories) and barrier methods, which include condoms (for both males and females) and contraceptive sponges.

Spermicides have special applicators that place the chemicals in the vagina close to the cervix before sexual intercourse in order to kill sperm. In addition to killing sperm, the active ingredient in most spermicides, nonoxynol-9, helps reduce (not eliminate) the chances of acquiring the AIDS virus and other sexually transmitted disease during intercourse. When used in conjunction with other barrier methods, such as the condom, diaphragm, or cervical cap, their effectiveness is greatly increased. Aside from minor skin irritations in some women with sensitive skin, spermicides have no side effects. Spermicides must be applied 5 to 30 minutes prior to intercourse and their estimated effectiveness for use rate is 75 percent–85 percent.

Contraceptive sponges are round and concave on one side. That side fits against the women's cervix. The other side has a string attached to it so the woman can pull the sponge out. The sponge can be left in place for 24 hours and be placed in position hours in advance before having intercourse. It must be moistened before inserting it. Another advantage is that a woman may have intercourse as many times as she desires in that time. It does not have to be replaced after each sexual act. However, it must be left in place for six hours after intercourse. The use effectiveness rate is 75 percent–85 percent.

The male *condom* ("rubber") is a latex sheath shaped to cover the erect penis and retain semen on ejaculation and keep it from entering the woman's vagina. The familiar condom is a safe and effective contraceptive device. The condom also provides a measure of protection against sexually transmitted diseases. For maximum effectiveness, the condom should be placed on the erect penis before genital contact. Early application is particularly important in the prevention of sexually transmitted diseases. After ejaculation, be certain that the condom does not become dislodged from the penis. If semen should escape the from the condom, a spermicide agent should be immediately placed into the vagina. If a lubricant is used during intercourse, it must be a water-soluble lubricant and not a petroleum-based product, such as petroleum jelly, mineral oil, baby oil, vegetable oil, shortening, and certain hand lotions. Petroleum based lubricants can damage a condom. The use effectiveness rate is 80 percent–90 percent.

The *female condom* is similar to the condom in terms of protecting against sexually transmitted diseases and pregnancy. The female condom consists of a prelubricated sheet of polyurethane with two flexible rings at each end and is inserted like a tampon. The smaller inner ring is pushed to the back of the vagina and covers the cervix, and the polyurethane sheath lines the inner contours of the vagina. The larger ring extends outside the vagina and covers the labia. The condom is inserted before any penis–vagina contact occurs and carefully removed after ejaculation. It must be replaced with another condom after each act of intercourse. The polyurethane is stronger and more resistant to oils than is the latex sheath used for condoms. The use effectiveness rate is 74 percent–79 percent.

Prescription Contraceptives

Prescription contraceptives, hormonal contraception, and barrier methods are the most reliable methods and must be acquired from a doctor. Hormonal methods include oral, injected, and implanted contraceptives. Barrier methods include the diaphragm and cervical cap.

The *pill* (oral contraceptive) is one of the most popular and reliable forms of contraception in the United States. Although earlier versions of the pill raised questions of safety, it is now considered reasonably safe for nonsmoking women up to about the age of 45. Any woman considering the pill should have a thorough examination and discussion with her physician before making a final decision. Breakthrough bleeding (spotting between periods) and nausea are common side effects. The use effectiveness rate is 97 percent–98 percent.

Depo-Provera is the injectable progestin that circumvents some of the side effects of the oral birth control pills because it is not metabolized in the liver. As a result, lower doses of hormone can be used. The hormone is injected in the woman's buttock every three months. Some women experience irregular menstrual spotting in early months of use. The use effectiveness rate is 99+ percent.

Hormone implants (*Norplant*) are the six matchstick-sized silicone rubber capsules, each containing synthetic progesterone, that are implanted by a doctor into the fleshy underside of a woman's upper arm. The hormone is gradually released into the woman's system and is effective for the next five years, during which time she is unable to conceive. Irregular bleeding, nausea, breast tenderness, and weight gain are some of the side effects. The use effectiveness rate is 99+ percent.

The Diaphragm and Cervical Cap.

The *diaphragm* is a rubber dome that fits inside the vagina and covers the cervix, and should always be used in conjunction with a spermicidal cream or jelly. Because each woman is different, a doctor must fit each woman for a diaphragm. The major role of the diaphragm is essentially to hold the spermicide in place, which provides the major share of the contraceptive effect. The diaphragm with spermicide is placed in the vagina prior to intercourse but must be left in place six to eight hours after intercourse. This amount of time gives the spermicide enough time to kill all the sperm. The use effectiveness rate is 80 percent–90 percent.

The *cervical cap* works much like a diaphragm, but it is much smaller and shaped like a thimble. Whereas the diaphragm covers the cervix and part of the vaginal wall around it, the smaller cervical cap fits directly onto the cervix and is held on by suction. The cervical cap must also be used in conjunction with a spermicide. Like the diaphragm, the cervical cap should be left in place at least six to nine hours after intercourse. The use effectiveness rate is 82 percent.

The Intrauterine Device (IUD).

The *intrauterine device* is a small object inserted by a clinician into the uterus to prevent pregnancy. They come in various shapes and sizes, with some containing chemicals such as copper or progesterone. No one knows exactly how they work, but any foreign object in the uterus seems to prevent pregnancy. Using an IUD appears to increase the risk of pelvic inflammatory disease and impaired fertility, particularly in women who have not yet had children. Therefore, it is an unlikely choice for college women because they probably would not want to hurt their chances for having children later. For this reason most clinicians will not insert an IUD in a woman who has not yet completed her family. The use effectiveness rate is 95 percent–98 percent.

Sterilization.   Sterilization can be performed on both men and women and is considered a permanent procedure that is more than 99 percent effective in preventing pregnancy. Although it is sometimes possible to reverse a sterilization procedure with microscopical techniques, anyone choosing to be sterilized should not count on reversal as a realistic option.

    Vasectomy, the male form of sterilization, is a minor surgical procedure in which the spermatic tubes (the sperm-carrying tubes called the *vas deferens*) are tied so that the sperm is prevented from being ejaculated in man's semen. The clinician makes a small incision on each side of the scrotum, isolates the vas deferens on each side, and cuts and ties them off. Small sutures are used to close the incisions on the scrotum surface. The male's ejaculate becomes sperm-free. Sperm constitutes less than 10 percent of the male's total ejaculate. The patient is asked to use alternate means of birth control for six to eight weeks after the procedure, or until he receives a negative semen analysis. It is simpler and safer to do a vasectomy procedure than tubal ligation. The use effectiveness rate is 99+ percent.

    Tubal ligation is the most common sterilization procedure for women. This procedure involves cutting or banding the fallopian tubes so that the sperm cannot reach any egg that is released by the ovary. A small incision is made near the navel and a special lighted tube, called a *laparoscope,* is inserted to locate the fallopian tubes. A special instrument is threaded through the laparoscope to cut and tie each tube. This surgery is usually considered minor and generally an outpatient procedure. As soon as the surgery is complete, a woman can regard herself as infertile and does not have to use any other form of birth control. The use effectiveness rate is 99+ percent.

Natural Family-Planning Methods

Withdrawal and *periodic abstinence* are the two natural family-planning methods practiced most frequently. Periodic abstinence is based on being aware of ovulation and fertility and avoiding sexual intercourse during the female's fertile period. The four basic periodic abstinence approaches are: (1) the calendar method, (2) the basal body temperature (BBT) method, (3) the cervical mucus method, and (4) the symptothermal method (a combination of the cervical mucus and basal body temperature methods). Many women combine one or more of these four approaches with barrier methods of birth control during the time of the month when they are fertile. The use effectiveness rate for the different methods is 75 percent–85 percent.

    Withdrawal, also known as *coitus interruptus,* is a practice in which the erect penis is removed from the vagina just prior to ejaculation of semen. The effectiveness of this method requires good timing, enormous self-control on the part of the male, and good luck because of its poor effectiveness rate in actual practice. Because men generally prefer deep penetration at the moment of ejaculation and women generally prefer consistent thrusting, withdrawal tends to inhibit complete sexual enjoyment. The use effectiveness rate is 75 percent–85 percent.

Abortion

No matter how many precautions are taken, mistakes happen or contraceptive methods fail and pregnancy occurs. When an unwanted pregnancy occurs, a decision must be made whether to terminate or carry the fetus to full term. To have an abortion is a personal decision and is based on a woman's personal beliefs, values, and resources after careful consideration of all alternatives. *Abortion* is the medical term for terminating a pregnancy, therefore, it is included in the discussion of birth control. However, it must be restated that abortion is not a contraceptive method. More than 1.6 million abortions are performed in

---

BOX **10.1**

How safe are the options?

Birth control method	Risk of death in any given year
Oral Contraceptives	
Nonsmoker	1 in 63,000
Smoker	1 in 16,000
Barrier methods	
Condoms, diaphragm, or cervical cap	0
Intrauterine devices	1 in 100,000
Sterilization	
Tubal ligation (via laparoscopy)	1 in 67,000
Hysterectomy	1 in 1,600
Vasectomy	1 in 300,000
Natural birth control methods	
Withdrawal, abstinence, fertility observation	0
Abortion	
Illegal	1 in 3,000
Legal	
Before 9 weeks	1 in 500,000
Between 9 and 12 weeks	1 in 67,000
Between 13 and 16 weeks	1 in 23,000
After 16 weeks	1 in 8,700
Pregnancy and childbirth	1 in 14,300

Source: K. Carlson, S. Eisenstat, and T. Ziporyn (1996). The Harvard Guide to Women's Health. Cambridge MA: Harvard University Press, p. 80.

the United States every year, representing almost a fourth of all pregnancies (Lacayo, 1992).

The type of abortion procedure used is determined by how many weeks pregnant the woman is. Abortions are safer and easier early in a pregnancy. Vacuum curettage (or aspiration) is the preferred method for abortions up to the 12th week of pregnancy. A special pump sucks the contents of the pregnancy off the uterine wall. Dilation and curettage (D & C) is a procedure that is used when the pregnancy moves into the second trimester. This process utilizes a special instrument to scrape embryonic tissue off the uterus wall. Dilatation and evacuation (D & E) is a procedure used between the 13th and 15th weeks of pregnancy. This process removes the fetus with special surgical instruments.

Contraceptive Use in Minority Populations

Although much has been written about different birth control methods, very little research has focused on usage rates by ethnicity. Consequently, the following data are limited. In 1987, 92 percent of sexually active women were using some form of contraception, including sterilization, and 8 percent were not. The highest percentage of unprotected women were black. In all, 66 percent of women between the ages of 15–44 were using some type of contraceptive method (Muller, 1990). An issue that potentially effects all women of reproductive age is easy access to healthy reproductive care, which disproportionately impacts certain groups of women such as low-income, black, and teenage clients who may have unmet needs for contraception, prenatal, or maternity services, and pregnant women needing programs addressing drug abuse, HIV infection, and other conditions (Muller, 1990).

The need for family planning services among sexually active women wishing to avoid pregnancy depends on the method of contraception selected. The pill, the leading method among young and never-married women, requires visits, whereas sterilization, the leading method among older women, does not. Black women tend to use methods requiring more visits and are less likely to use sterilization (Muller, 1990). For black women, 56.5 percent of all family planning visits were to clinics, versus 31.3 percent for whites, and blacks were less likely to use private sources (Mosher, 1990).

Health care services must be sensitive to the needs of their patients. The Native American Women's Health Education Center (1993) reported in 1991 that the Indian Health Service (IHS), a division of the U.S. Public Health Service, began providing Norplant to Native Americans living on reservations without adequate contraceptive counseling. Among the unsafe side effects associated with Norplant are acute liver disease, unexplained vaginal bleeding, breast cancer, and blood clots. Norplant is contraindicated for patients who smoke and suffer from diabetes, high blood pressure, or gall bladder disease. Unfortunately, Native people suffer from the highest rates of diabetes, alcoholism, and related diseases in the United States, such as cirrhosis of the liver, obesity, and gall bladder disease. They also have high rates of hypertension and cancer and many are smokers. For the average Native American woman living on a reservation, Norplant is a poor contraceptive choice.

In the national study *Women and HIV Prevention: Unintended Effects,* Davis et al. (1996) reported that, among cultures in which the accepted view is that men, by virtue of nothing other than their sex, are dominant, this perception detracts power from women in general and in their sexual relationships in particular. In these cultures, the subject of sex is not easily open for discussion by most women. This lack of control in their sexual relationships precludes any opportunity for women to negotiate condom use as a means to control their fertility and to prevent disease (Mays & Cochran, 1988). Many Latino, Asian, and African American men resist the use of condoms.

Latinas are less likely to use family-planning services than non-Latino white women and African American women (Garcia et al., 1985/1996). The use of family-planning services is an important determinant of use of birth control methods. Giachello (1996) summarized the results of the 1988 National Family Growth Survey (NFGS) and the 1982–84 HHANES data. The NFGS showed that the pill is the contraceptive method most often reported by Latinas between ages 15 and 44 (33&). This percentage is slightly higher than those reported for non-Latino whites (30%) but lower than those reported by African American women of the same age group (38%). The HHANES found that 15.7 percent of Mexican American women, 9.7 percent of Puerto Rican, and 8.2 percent of Cuban American women reported current use of oral contraceptives.

The 1988 National Family Growth Survey also found that condom use was reported by 14 percent of the Latino population. The percentage use is similar to whites (15%), but higher than that for African Americans (10%). Those most likely to use condoms for the total 1988 sample were teenagers, never-married women, and those who intended to have children in the future. The intrauterine device (IUD) and the diaphragm were the contraceptives least used by Latinas (5% and 2% respectively).

Male-Specific Health Problems and Concerns

This section of the chapter is divided into three areas: urinary tract infection in men, prostate problems, and testicular cancer.

Urinary Tract Infection in Men

Urinary Tract Infection (UTI) is an overgrowth of bacteria in the urinary tract or urethra, bladder, and kidneys. The most common form of UTI in young men is caused from sexually transmitted infections such as gonorrhea and chlamydia. Nonsexually transmitted UTIs seldom occur before age 50. Urinary tract infection is more common in women than men because of the length of the urethra. In women, the length is relatively short, whereas the male urethra is much longer, making it more difficult for the bacteria to ascend the urinary tract. UTIs include various disorders:

■ *urethritis or the inflammation of the urethra (urinary tract).* The most common cause for this condition is gonorrhea. Nongonoccocal urethritis (NGC) is caused by two separate organisms, chlamydia and T-strain mycoplasma. NGC is quite common in males and most often produces symptoms (discharge and mild burning during urination) while leaving most women asymptomatic. Occasionally, NGC may result from trichomonas infection, allergic reactions to vaginal secretions, or irritation by soaps, vaginal contraceptives, and deodorant sprays.

- Prostatitis or inflammation of the prostate gland. Prostatitis causes intense pain, urinary complications, sexual dysfunction, infertility, and a significant reduction in the quality of life. Almost no research has taken place to find diagnostic techniques or a cure. No research has been shown that it does not lead to prostate cancer or BPH (benign prostatic hyperplasia). Prostatitis is a non-fatal but often disabling disease affecting young men between the ages of 25 and 50. This inflammation is often overlooked, avoided, dismissed, or ignored by the medical profession. Besides gonorrhea, prostatitis may also be caused by the reflux of bacteria strains that are usually normal flora in the reproductive area. Sufferers are offered, at best, a life-long course of antibiotics, and at worst, a state of constant agony and neglect (Prostatitis Foundation, 1996).
- Cystitis or the infection of the bladder occurs more frequently in women and commonly occurs following initial intercourse or during pregnancy. It does, however, also affect men. The symptoms of acute cystitis are a burning sensation on urination (dysuria) and increased frequency of urination, and hematuria (blood in the urine) can result. The major danger of cystitis is that the infection can ascend to the kidneys and cause pyelonephritis (inflammation of the kidneys).
- Pyelonephritis, or infection of the kidney, results in patients experiencing pain in the flanks, chills, fever, and weakness, with a possible reduction in renal function. The kidney swells and develops multiple small abscesses on its external surfaces. If repeated episodes of acute pyelonephritis occur, chronic pyelonephritis can develop and renal tubules are destroyed. Severe damage to the kidney can occur leading to uremia (excess urea and waste accumulation), which can cause convulsions and coma.

The symptoms (Healthy Devil Online, 1994) of urinary tract infection include:

- pain and discomfort (burning, itching) when urinating;
- frequent and urgent need to urinate (especially at night);
- urethral discharge; a clear fluid or small amount of pus from the penis, more common with sexually transmitted diseases;
- abdominal pain;
- fever;
- blood in the urine;
- back pain; low back pain can be associated with prostatitis and high back pain with pyelonephritis.

Diagnosis of UTI requires an examination of the urinary tract, prostate, and rectal area. A urine test and an examination of the urethral discharge is usually requested. UTI is treated with antibiotics such as sulfonamide or amoxicillin. The symptoms usually go away within 24 hours after treatment begins. The patient is also requested to drink plenty of fluids and to empty the bladder completely when urinating.

Prostate Problems

Benign Prostatic Hyperplasia (prostate hypertrophy).   The prostate gland normally increases in size as a man moves into his 50s. This enlargement can squeeze the urethra and interfere with the normal flow of urination. In some cases, excess urine can build up in the bladder because of the pinched urethra and urine can back up causing damage or failure in the kidney. Symptoms before this occurs include a weakened urine stream, frequent urination, and a feeling of urgency.

BPH is not the first sign of prostate cancer and BPH does not mean a Turp operation, a new one-hour outpatient treatment now available.

Prostate Cancer.   Prostate cancer is the third most common form of cancer in males, and approximately 1 out of 11 men will develop the disease. Although it is the second leading cause of cancer deaths in males, killing an estimated 40,400 men in 1995, of those who develop prostate cancer, most will have very serious problems with it. African American males have the highest rate of prostate cancer, at 180.6 per 100,000 (National Cancer Institute, 1996). The average man who develops prostate cancer is well over 60, although cases have occasionally developed in young men in their twenties.

The chance that a man over 60 years will develop a microscopic focus of "latent" prostate cancer tissue is nearly 42 percent (that is, 42 of 100 older men will get such a microscopic focus). However, the chance that the same man will get clinically significant prostate cancer is only 9.5 percent. Finally, of the same 100 men, only about three will actually die of prostate cancer (CoMed Communications Internet Health Forum, 1996). Because prostate cancer tends to stay localized and progress slowly, many elderly men with prostate cancer will die of other causes before dying of prostate cancer. Table 10.2 shows prostate cancer cases and deaths by race in 1995.

Symptoms of Prostate Cancer.   Prostate cancer is not like benign prostate hyperplasia. It normally begins to grow in the outer area of the prostate gland and therefore does not announce its presence by showing the same symptoms of BPH. The following symptoms

TABLE 10.2   Prostate Cancer Cases and Deaths by Race (1995)

Prostate cancer cases	244,000
Prostate cancer deaths	40,000
Prostate cancer deaths by race	
African American	5,299
Native American	71
Chinese Americans	32
Japanese Americans	47
Hispanic American	833

Source: "Cancer Facts and Figures, 1995"

have been identified by the National Cancer Institute as possible indicators of prostate cancer:

> Frequent urination (especially at night);
> Inability to urinate;
> Trouble starting to urinate or trouble holding back urination;
> Pain during ejaculation;
> A weak or interrupted urine flow;
> Pain or a burning feeling during urination;
> Blood in the semen or in the urine;
> Frequent pain or stiffness in the lower back, hips, or upper thighs
>
> (CCIHF, 1995).

Because all of these symptoms may be related to other problems, a man should visit a trained physician who will be able to diagnose whether the symptoms are prostate cancer.

Risk Factors for Prostate Cancer.   No one really knows exactly what causes some men to get prostate cancer while others do not. Some of the factors that appear to be related to the development of prostate cancer include:

1. Genetics: If you have a brother or father or uncle that has had prostate cancer, you are greater risk of getting it. However, this does not mean that you will absolutely get prostate cancer.
2. Race: Prostate cancer is much more common in some races than in others. For example, Japanese men living in Japan have an extremely low incidence of prostate cancer. By comparison, African American men are at very high risk for this disease. The incidence is 30 percent higher among African American men than it is among white Americans. Why? Nobody has an answer. Even more intriguing is the fact that Japanese American men who were born in America have a risk of prostate cancer similar to any other average American man living in the same area, and Japanese men who move to America increase their of risk of developing prostate cancer (CCIHF, 1996).
3. Age: As a man grows older, his risk of prostate cancer increases. The longer he lives, the possibility of prostate cancer goes up proportionally. As previously stated, the average man who develops prostate cancer is well over 60, although cases have occasionally developed in young men in their twenties.

Diagnosis of Prostate Cancer.   The initial diagnostic procedures for prostate cancer are the digital rectal examination (DRE) and a prostate specific antigen (PSA) test (CCIHF, 1997). If the physician feels any suspicious growth on the prostate gland or an elevated PSA level is discovered, the urologist will usually recommend a prostate biopsy. This requires that a piece of tissue be removed from the prostate and tested to determine a positive or negative diagnosis of prostate cancer.

Recommendations of the American Urological Association (1997) include:

All males of 50 years or more should have an annual prostate examination comprising a digital rectal examination and a PSA test.

All males of 40 years or more with a family history of prostate cancer should have an annual prostate examination comprising a digital rectal examination and a PSA test.

Treatment for Prostate Cancer.   There is a great deal of controversy within the medical profession about appropriate treatment for prostate cancer. The options range from radical prostatectomy (removal of prostate gland), to radiation, to "wait and see." Prostate cancer has a high incidence rate in older men (40 percent) but only 2–3 percent die from it. Stated differently, prostate cancer has a relatively high incidence but low rate of fatalities. Asian Americans have the same 40 percent prostate cancer incidence rate but fewer than 1 percent die from it (National Prostate Cancer Coalition, 1997). Should radical surgery or radiation therapy be done on all patients diagnosed with prostate cancer or is the risk of these procedures worse than the disease? Because prostate cancer appears so late in life and grows slowly, many men who have it will die of other causes before they die of prostate cancer. A patient must educate himself and discuss all the options with his physician before making a decision about treatment.

Testicular Cancer

Testicular cancer is the most common tumor found in young men between the ages of 20 to 35 years of age. Fortunately, it is one of the least common forms of cancer. Two risk factors associated with testicular cancer are a family history of testicular cancer and undescended testicles during childhood.

Symptoms of cancer of the testicles include a small painless lump on the side of a testicle, a swollen testicle, or a dragging sensation in the groin or scrotum. If left untreated, testicular cancer can metastasize to other organs and/or the lymph nodes.

To detect testicular cancer, the American Cancer Society (1990) recommends a process of self-examination.

1. The best time to perform the examination is after a warm bath or shower, when the scrotal skin is most relaxed. (*Scrotal* refers to the scrotum, the pouch in which the testicles normally lie.)
2. Roll each testicle gently between the thumb and fingers of both hands. A normal testicle is smooth, egg-shaped, and somewhat firm to the touch. At the rear of each testicle is a tube called the *epididymis,* which carries sperm away from the testicle; this is a normal part of your body.
3. If a man finds any hard lumps or nodules, or if there is any change in the shape, size, or texture of the testicles, consult a physician promptly. These signs may not indicate a malignancy, but only a physician can make a diagnosis.

Repeat this examination every month. It is important that men know what their own testicles feel like normally so that they can recognize any changes.

REFERENCES

American Cancer Society. *Cancer facts & figures—1994.* Atlanta, GA: American Cancer Society, 1995.

American Cancer Society. *For men only: Testicular cancer and how to do TSE (a self-exam).* Atlanta, GA: American Cancer Society, 1990.

American House Call Network. *Health information: Fibrocystic breast disease.* http://www.housecall.com./databases/ami/convert/000912html nd estrogen use." *New England Journal of Medicine, 300* (1996), 9–13, 1979.

American Urological Society. Fundamentals of prostate cancer: Detection and treatment." In CCIHF-CoMed Communications Internet Health Forum (1997). *Detection and diagnosis of prostate cancer.* http://www.comed.com:80/Prostate/index.html

ARIC. AIDS Research Information Center (1996) *ARIC's AIDS medical glossary on-line: Cervical dysplasia, www.critpath.org/aric/gloss/cervical-dysplasia.htm*

Aveoli, L. Calcium and osteoporosis. *Annual Review of Nutrition* 4(1984), 471–491.

Babahnia, A. *Endometriosis: The 90's outlook.* FBS Home Journal Library Index: Atlanta Reproductive Health Center, 1990. http://www.bioscience.org/bioscience/books/endomet/end01.33.htm

Bod Squad. *What is trichomonas?* Washington, DC: National Women's Health Resource Center, 1995. http://www.women.com/wwi...qabod/951129.qa.bod.html

Bradley, J. *Uterine fibroids: What every women should know.* MedSeek Publishing Services, 1996. http:/medseek.com/glennbradley/fibroids.html

Carlson, K., Eisenstat, S., and Ziporyn, T. *The Harvard guide to women's health.* Cambridge MA: Harvard University Press, 1996, p. 80.

Carol, F., Kalmuss, K., and Lopez, I. Barriers to prenatal care: An examination of use of prenatal care among low-income women in New York City. New York: Community Service Society of New York, 1988.

CCIHF-CoMed Communications Internet Health Forum (1996). *The causes of prostate cancer.* http://www.comed.com:80/Prostate/index.html

CCIHF-CoMed Communications Internet Health Forum (1997). *Detection and diagnosis of prostate cancer.* http://www.comed.com:80/Prostate/index.html

CCIHF-CoMed Communications Internet Health Forum (1995). *The symptoms of prostate cancer.* http://www.comed.com:80/Prostate/index.html

Centers for Disease Control Wonder (no date). *PID: An introduction.* CDE Prevention Guidelines. wwwonder.cdc.gov/wonder/prevguid/p0000133/body0002htm

Crooks, R. and Baur, K. *Our sexuality.* Menlo Park, CA: Benjamin/Cummings, 1980.

Davis, D., Brown, P., Alegria, M., Bayne-Smith, M., and Smith, V. (1993-December). Women and HIV/AIDS prevention efforts: Unintended effects. Final report of national research project funded by the Centers for Disease Control and Prevention, Grant #U50/CCU304522–04. In M. Bayne-Smith (Ed.), *Race, gender, and health.* Thousand Oaks, CA: Sage, 1996, p. 30–31.

Donnelly, M. (no date). *Trichomonas (trich).* The Trichomonas Information Page. http://linux.coe.missour...pecinfs/trichomonas.html

Endometriosis Association. *Endometriosis: What is it?* Educational Support Research, 1992. http://www.ivf. com/endoassn.html

GeeneX (1996) *Cervical cancer.* Healthcare Technologies. www.healthwire.com/women/ask/cervihnc.htlm

Giachello, A. Latino Women. In M. Bayne-Smith (Ed.), *Race, gender, and health.* Thousand Oaks, CA: Sage, 1996 (p. 121–171.).

Health Centre Online. *Preventing bladder infections,* 1996. http://cii2.cochran.com/pharmasave/healthnotes/2/3/bladder.html

Health Education Associates. *Premenstrual syndrome (PMS).* Maui, HI: Health Education Associates, 1990. http://planet-hawaii.com/Wellnet/PMS/pmsla-html

Health Trek. *Pelvic inflammatory disease,* n. d. http://www.healthtrek.com/lpelvic.htm

Healthy Devil Online. Urinary tract infection in men. Duke University, 1994. http://h-devil-www.mc.duke.edu/h-devil/men/uti.htm

Hughes, D., Johnson, K., Rosenbaum, S., Butler, E., and Simons, J. *The health of America's children: Maternal and child health data book.* Washington, DC: Children's Defense Fund, 1988.

Hutchins, F. "Uterine fibroids: Current concepts in management." *Female Patient* 15, p. 29, October, 1990.

Institute of Medicine. *Preventing low birth weight.* Washington, DC: National Academy Press, 1985.

Lacayo, R. "Abortion: The future is already here, *Time,* 4 May 1992, 28.

Lanson, L. *From woman to woman.* New York: Alfred A. Knopf, 1977.

Mays, V. and Cochran, S. (1988). Issues in the perception of AIDS risk and risk education activities by black and Hispanic/Latino women. *American Psychologist, 432,* 949–957. In M. Bayne-Smith (Ed.), *Race, gender, and health.* Thousand Oaks, CA: Sage, 1996, p. 31.

McBarnette, L. "Women and poverty: Effects on reproductive." In C. Perales and L. Young (Eds.), *Women, health, and poverty* (pp. 55–81). New York: Haw-thorne, 1988.

Midland Family Physicians (1996). *HPV and cervical dysplasia: Patient information.* LSUMC Family Medicine Patient Education Home Page. http://lib-sh.lsumc.edc/fammed/pted/hpymid.html

Mosher, W. Use of family planning services in the United States: 1982 and 1988. Advanced Data No. 184. Hyattsville, MD: National Center for Health Statistics, April 11, 1990. In C. Muller, (Ed.), *Health care and gender.* New York: Russell Sage Foundation, 1990, p. 175.

Muller, C. (Ed.)., *Health care and gender.* New York: Russell Sage Foundation, 1990.

National Cancer Institute. *Prostate Cancer.* Bethesda, MD: National Cancer Institute, 1996. Http://www. nci.nih,gov/htm

National Center for Health Statistics. *Health, United States, 1990.* Hyattsville, MD: Public Health Services, 1990.

National Institutes of Health (NIH) Office. *Extramural Research (OER) Grants: Grants Policy,* 1998. http:// www.nih.gov/grants/policy/policy.htm

National Prostate Cancer Coalition (1997). *Fundamentals of prostate cancer: Detection and treatment.* http:// rattler.cameron.edu/ww/

Native American Women's Health Education Resources Center, Native American women uncover Norplant abuses," *Ms.* (Sept.–Oct., 1993) Vol. IV, p.69.

No author (1997). *Description of Premenstrual Syndrome.* http://www. bairpms.com/descrip.html

Northrup, C. *Women's bodies, women's wisdom: Creating physical and emotional health and healing.* New York: Bantam Books, 1994.

Pelvic Inflammatory Disease (PID). (no date). http:/www. medica/arts.com/MA-Pages/pid.html

Perloe, M. (1996). *Endometriosis.* Atlanta, GA: Atlanta Reproductive Health Centre WWW. http://www. ivf.com/endomp.html

Planned Parenthood League of Massachusetts. (no date). *Pelvic inflammatory disease,* a pamphlet published by the Planned Parenthood League of Massachusetts. http://www.pplm.org/pid.html

Premenstrual syndrome. (1997). http://www.cgocable.ca: 80/jvi/sante/health/e53.htm

Prostatitis Foundation. *Prostatitis.* Smithshire, IL: author, 1996. Http://prostate.org/aboutpf.html

Rarick, L. (1997). In M. Segal (ed.), *On the teen scene: A balanced look at the menstrual cycle.* For your

health: Health care articles. MedAcess Corporation, 1997.

Rosen, R. and Rosen, L. *Human sexuality.* New York: Alfred A. Knopf, 1981.

Rx Med (no date). *Fibrocystic breast disease.* http:// www.ixmed.com/illnesses/fibrocystic_breast-disease. html

Ryan, S. (1996). *Bladder and 'yeast' infections: Prevention and cure.* The Physician and Sportsmedicine, 24. 7, July 96. http://www.physsportsmed.com/ issues/jul-96pa.htm

Saint Francis Hospital (no date). *Fibrocystic breast condition,* a pamphlet by Saint Francis Hospital in Tulsa, Oklahoma http://www. saintfrancis.com.fibrocys. html

Sampson, H. "Peritoneal endometriosis due to the menstrual dissemination of endometrial tissue into the peritoneal cavity." *American Journal of Obstetrics and Gynocology,* 1984.

Tortora, G., and Grabowski, S. *Principles of anatomy and physiology,* 7th. ed. New York: Harper-Collins, 1993.

Tureck, R. *Treatment of endometriosis.* PA: University of Pennsylvania Health System, 1997.

UCLA Student Health Service (no date). *Trichomonas.* http://www.saonet.ucla.e...Ithed/HANDOUTS/trich. html

U.S. Department of Health and Human Services (USDHHS). *Vaginal infections and vaginitis.* Bethesda, MD: Office of Communications National Institute of Allergy and Infectious Diseases, National Institutes of Health, 1992.

U.S. Indian Health Service. *Trends in Indian health.* Washington, DC: USDHHS, 1993.

University of Illinois (UIUC) Health Resource Center (1996). *Pelvic inflammatory disease,* a pamphlet by the University of Illinois Board of Regents. http:// www.uiuc.edu/deptments/mckinley.info/womenhlt/ pid.html

University of Toronto Sexual Education & Peer Counseling Centre (1996). *Gardnerella vaginalis.* hhp:// www.campuslife.ut...ervices/sec/gardvag.html

University of Wisconsin Health Service. *Bladder infections of cystitis,* a pamphlet of the University Health Center: The Board of Regents of the University of Wisconsin System, 1996.

Women's Health (1997). *Osteoporosis.* hhp://www.stay-healthy.com/wh-o.htm

INDEX